ADVANCED TOPICS IN NEUROLOGICAL DISORDERS

Edited by **Ken-Shiung Chen**

Advanced Topics in Neurological Disorders
Edited by Ken-Shiung Chen

Published by InTech
Janeza Trdine 9, 51000 Rijeka, Croatia

Publishing Process Manager Martina Durovic

Technical Editor Teodora Smiljanic

Cover Designer InTech Design Team

Additional hard copies can be obtained from orders@intechopen.com

Advanced Topics in Neurological Disorders, Edited by Ken-Shiung Chen
p. cm.
978-953-51-0303-5

For EU product safety concerns:
IN TECH d.o.o., Prolaz Marije Krucifikse Kozulić 3, 51000 Rijeka, Croatia,
info@intechopen.com or visit our website at intechopen.com.

Meet the editor

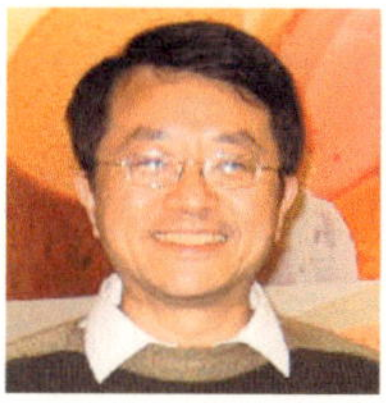

Dr Ken-Shiung Chen received both his M.A. and Ph.D. degrees from the University of Texas, Austin, USA and held the position of an Assistant Professor at the Baylor College of Medicine, Houston, USA. Currently, he is an Associate Professor at the School of Biological Sciences, Nanyang Technological University, Singapore. Dr Chen's research interests are focused on the elucidation of the molecular mechanism of chromosomal deletion/duplication syndrome as well as on epigenetic regulation in genomic imprinting. The human genome project and the concomitant race to map and sequence the mice genomes have created the basis for interspecies comparisons. Together with the recent advancement in mouse mutagenesis, conditional knockout and chromosomal engineering techniques have given us the ability to define gene function and to model human disease in a mammalian system.

Contents

Preface

The study of our brain and associated neurological disorders represent one of the most fascinating frontiers in the biomedical sciences. Recent research studies using multidisciplinary approaches not only provide a molecular understanding of disease mechanisms but also suggest novel tools for therapeutic interventions. *Advanced Topics in Neurological Disorders* presents reports on a wide range of areas in the field of neurological disorders, including bioengineering, stem cell transplantation, gene therapy, proteomic analysis, and alternative treatments to neuropsychiatry illnesses.

Chapter 1 presents a review of the history of the bionic eye and provides an update on the current state and future prospects of the field. Chapter 2 describes an accurate method for the simultaneous evaluation of the eye, head and shoulder positions in neurological practice. Possible applications and perspectives for clinical practice are also described in the chapter. Chapter 3 provides a review for the clinical application of using mesenchymal stem cells to treat brain injury. Ongoing clinical trials, issues of delivery timing, route and donor source, dosage and mechanisms of action underlying beneficial effects are discussed. Chapter 4 provides a review for the use of foamy virus vector as a carrier to deliver therapeutic genes for neurological disorders and other diseases. Chapter 5 presents a review of existing methods to extract the morphology of intracranial pressure (ICP). A novel probabilistic framework to track the ICP morphology in real time is introduced and a successful study for the real-time prediction of ICP hypertension is described. Chapter 6 introduces methods for protein analysis and profiling techniques in clinical practice, and further discusses the application of new methods for cerebrospinal fluid analysis as a primary biological media for the study of neurological diseases. Chapter 7 describes the use of a proteomic approach to study the Angelman syndrome (AS) mouse model. The results indicate that proteins involved in neuronal cell differentiation, learning processes, energy production, actin disassembly and neuronal signal transduction are affected in AS. Chapter 8 discusses the molecular basis, metabolites, biomarkers, triggers and polymorphisms associated with migraines. This chapter further discusses the pharmacotherapy for migraines and the effects of herbal medicine in migraine treatments. Chapter 9 argues that substance dependence should be considered a brain disease associated with cellular and neurocircuitry dysfunction. This review compares the relationship between anatomical and functional changes in the prefrontal cortex, executive abilities, and substance dependence by describing this relationship across multiple classes of drugs and polysubstance dependence.

I would like to sincerely thank all the authors who contributed to this book. In preparing this book, we have included information from a wide range of fields involved in neurological research that not only provides researchers, clinicians and graduate students with insight on the most recent advances in neurological research but also highlights the importance of applying multidisciplinary approaches to the study of neurological disorders.

Ken-Shiung Chen Ph.D.
Associate Professor
Nanyang Technological University, School of Biological Sciences,
Singapore

Part 1

Bioengineering in Neurological Disorders

1

Image Analysis for Automatically-Driven Bionic Eye

F. Robert-Inacio[1,2], E. Kussener[1,2], G. Oudinet[2] and G. Durandau[2]
[1]*Institut Materiaux Microelectronique et Nanosciences de Provence, (IM2NP, UMR 6242)*
[2]*Institut Superieur de l'Electronique et du Numerique (ISEN-Toulon)*
France

1. Introduction

In many fields such as health or robotics industry, reproducing the human visual system (HVS) behavior is a widely sought aim. Actually a system able to reproduce even partially the HVS could be very helpful, on the one hand, for people with vision diseases, and, on the other hand, for autonomous robots.

Historically, the earliest reports of artificially induced phosphenes were associated with direct cortical stimulation Tong (2003). Since then devices have been developed that target ùany different sites along the visual pathway Troyk (2003).These devices can be categorized according to the site of action along the visual pathway into cortical, sub-cortical, optic nerve ane retinal prostheses. Although the earliest reports involved cortical stimulation, with the advancements in surgical techniques and bioengineering, the retinal prosthesis or artificial retina has become the most advanced visual prosthesis Wyatt (2011).

In this chapter, both applications will be presented after the theoretical context, the state of the art and motivations. Furthermore, a full system will be described including a servo-motorized camera (acquisition), specific image processing software and artificial intelligence software for exploration of complex scenes. This chapter also deals with image analysis and interpretation.

1.1 Human visual sytem

The human visual system is made of different parts: eyes, nerves and brain. In a coarse way, eyes achieve image acquisition, nerves data transmission and brain data processing (Fig. 1).

The eye (Fig. 2) acquires images through the pupil and visual information is processed by retina photoreceptors. There exist two kinds of photoreceptors: rods and cones. Rods are dedicated to light intensity acquisition. They are efficient in scotopic and mesopic conditions. Cones are specifically sensitive to colors and require a minimal light level (photopic and mesopic conditions). There are three different types of cones sensitive for different wavelengths.

Fig. 3a shows the photoreceptors responses and Fig. 3b their distribution accross the retina from the foveal area (at the center of gaze) to the peripheral area. At the top of Fig. 3b, small parts of retina are presented with cones in green and rods in pink. This outlines that the repartition of cones and rods varies on the retina surface according to the distance to the

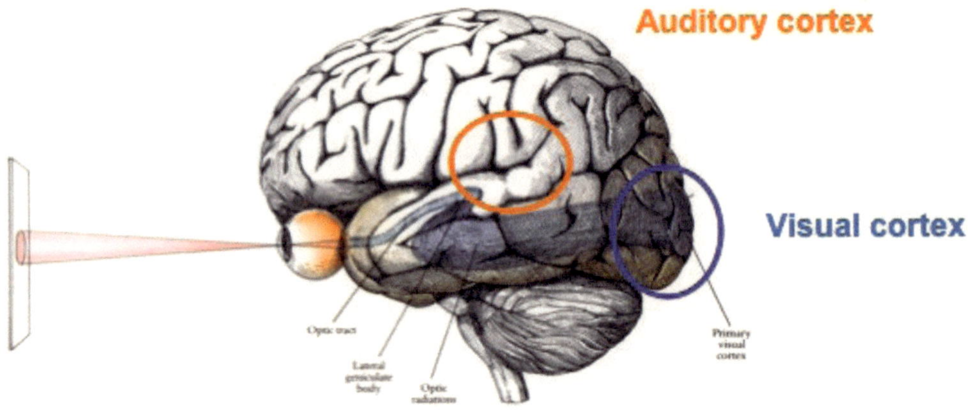

Fig. 1. Human visual system

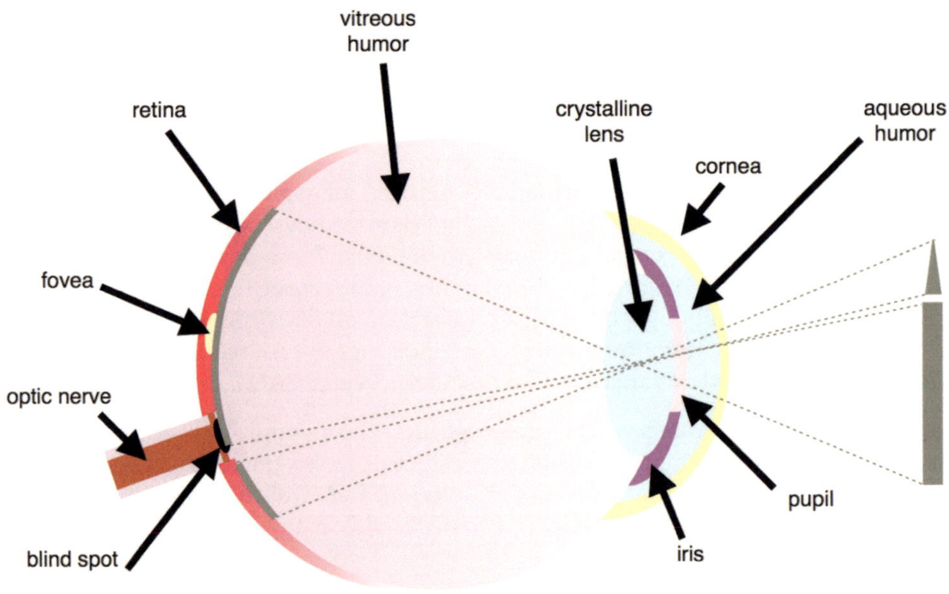

Fig. 2. Human eye

center of gaze. Most of the cones are located in the fovea (retina center) and rods are essentially present in periphery. Then light energy data are turned into electrochemical energy data to be carried to the visual cortex through the optic nerves. The two optic nerves converge at a point called optic chiasm (Fig. 4), where fibers of the nasal side cross to the other brain side, whereas fibers of the temporal side do not. Then the optic nerves become the optic tracts. The optic tracts reach the lateral geniculate nucleus (LGN). Here begins the processing of visual data with back and forth between the LGN and the visual cortex.

1.2 Why a bionic eye?

Blindness affects over 40 millions people around the world. In the medical field, providing a prosthesis to blind or quasi-blind people is an ambitious task that requires a huge sum of

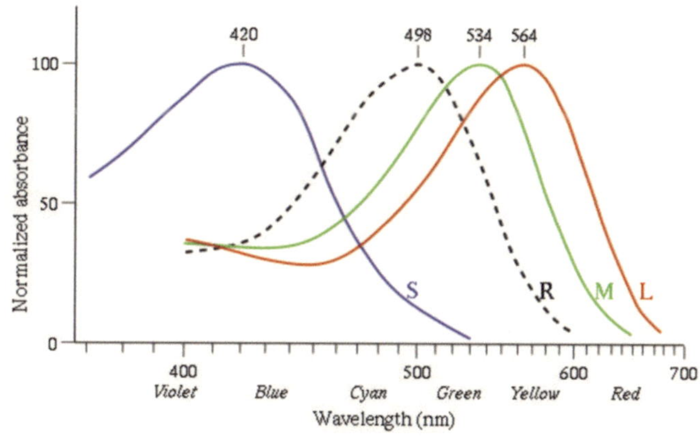

(a) Rods (R) and cones (L, M, S) responses

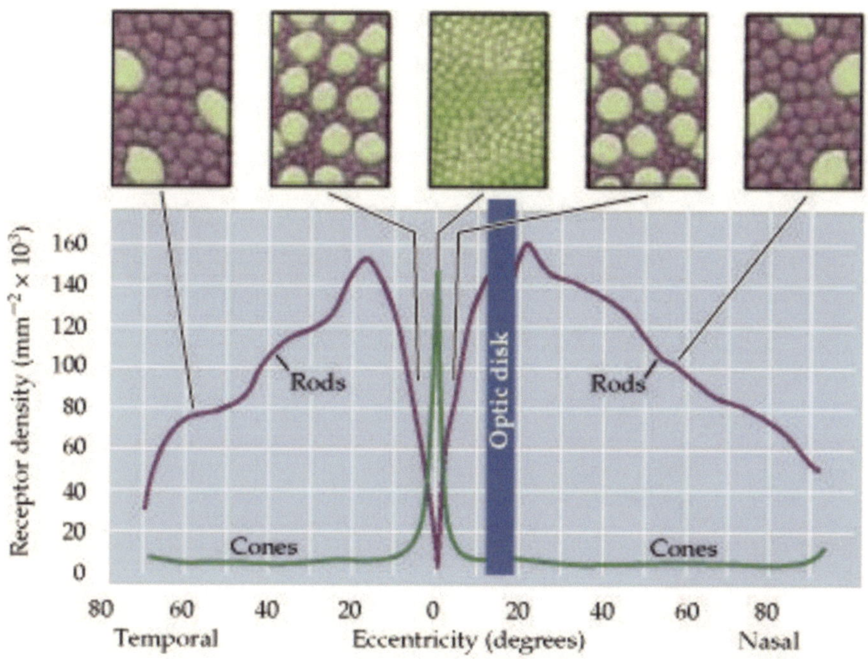

(b) Rods and cones distribution accross the retina (from http://improveeyesighttoday.com/improveeyesight-centralization.htm)

Fig. 3. Rods and cones features

knowledge in different fields such as microelectronics, computer vision and image processing and analysis, but also in the medical field: ophtalmology and neurosciences. Cognitive studies determining the human behavior when facing a new scene are lead in parallel in order to validate methods by comparing them to a human observer's abilities. Several solutions are offered to plug an electronic device to the visual system (Fig. 4). First of all, retina implants can

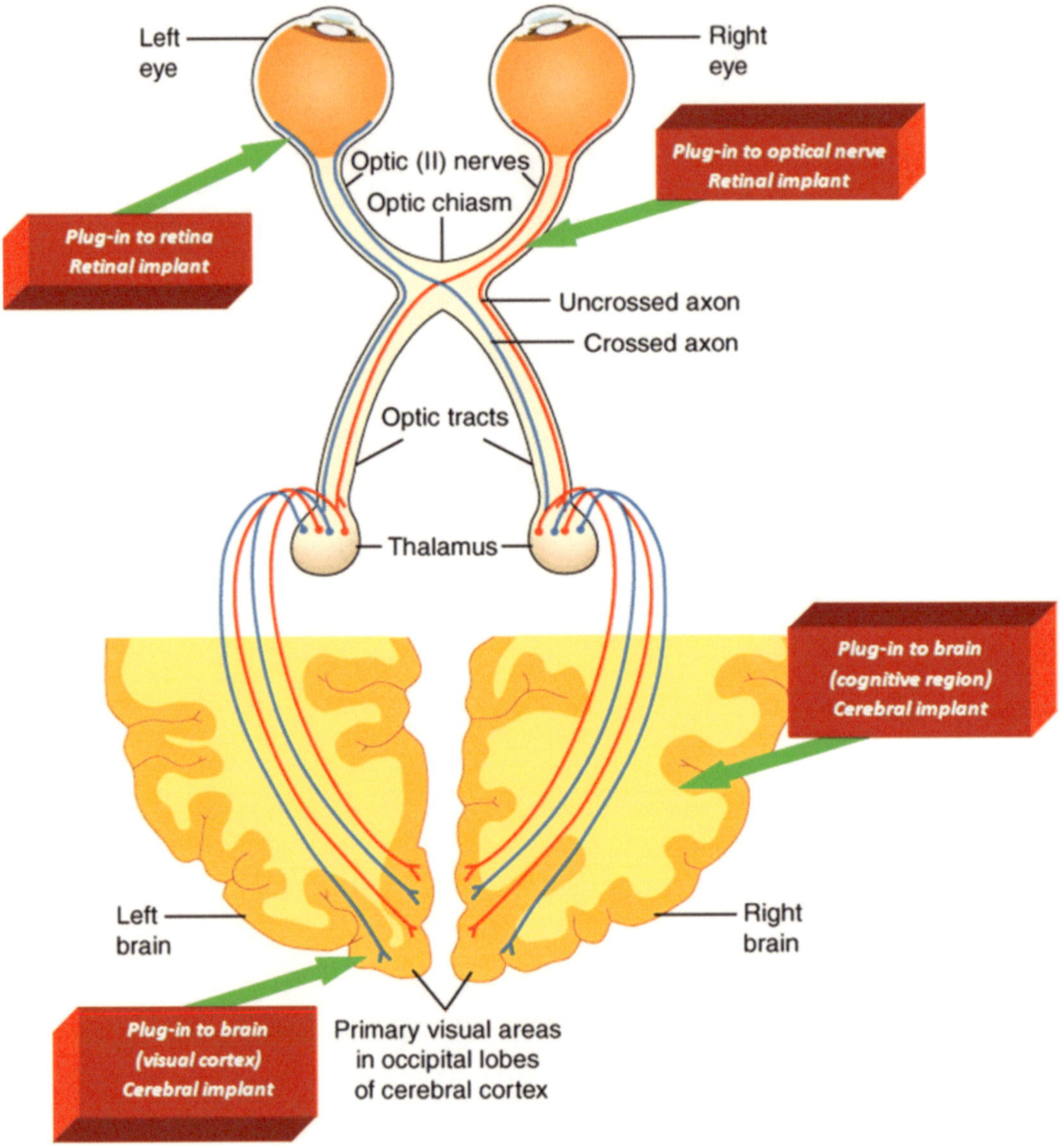

Fig. 4. Human visual system and solutions for electronic device plugins

be plugged either to the retina or to the optic nerve. Such a solution requires image processing in order to integrate data and make them understandable by the brain. No image analysis is necessary as data will be processed by the visual cortex itself. But the patient must be free of pathology at least at the optic nerve, so that data transmission to the brain can be achieved. In another way, retina implants can directly stimulate the retina photoreceptors. That means that the retina too must be in working order. Secondly, when either the retina or the optic nerve is damaged, only cerebral implants can be considered, as they directly stimulate neurons. In this context, image analysis is required in order to mimick at least the LGN behavior.

1.3 Why now?

The development of biological implantable devices incorporating microelectronic circuitry requires advanced fabrication techniques which are now possible. The importance of device stability stems from the fact that the microelectronics have to function properly within the relatively harsh environment of the human body. This represents a major challenge in developing implantable devices with long-term system performance while reducing their overall size.

Biomedical systems are one example of ultra low power electronics is paramount for multiple reasons [Sarpeshkar (2010)]. For example, these systems are implanted within the body and need to be small, light-weighted with minimal dissipation in the tissue that surrounds them. In order to obtain implantable device, some constraints have to be taken into account such as:

- The size of the device
- The type of the technology (flexible or not) in order to be accepted by the human body
- The circuit consumption in order to optimize the battery life
- The performance circuit

The low power hand reminds us that the power consumption of a system is always defined by five considerations as shown on Fig.5:

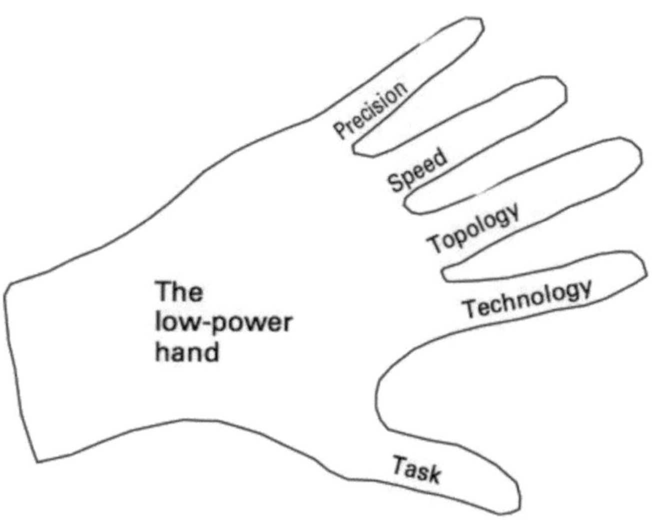

Fig. 5. Low power Hand for low power applications

2. State of the art: Overview

Supplying visual information to blind people is a goal that can be reached in several ways by more or less efficient means. Classically blind people can use a white cane, a guide-dog or more sophisticated means. The white cane is perceived as a symbol that warns other people and make them more careful to blind people. It is also very useful in obstacle detection. A guide-dog is also of a great help, as it interprets at a dog level the context scene. The dog is trained to guide the person in an outdoor environment. It can inform the blind person and advise of danger through its reactions. In the very last decades, electronics has come to reinforce the environment perception. On the one hand, several non-invasive systems have been set up such as GPS for visually impaired [Hub (2006)] that can assist blind people with orientation and navigation, talking equipment that provides an audio description in a basic way for thermometers, clocks or calcultors or in a more accurate way for audio-description that gives a narration of visual aspects of television movies or theater plays, electronic white canes [Faria (2010)], etc. On the other hand, biomedical devices can be implanted in an invasive way, that requires surgery and clinical trials. As presented in Fig. 4, such devices can be plugged at different spots along the visual data processing path. In a general way the principle is the same for retinal and cerebral implants. Two subsystems are linked, achieving data acquisition and processing for the first one and electrostimulation for the second one. A camera (or two for stereovision) is used to acquire visual data. These data are processed by the acquisition processing box in order to obtain data that are transmitted to the image processing box via a wired or wireless connection (Fig. 6). Then impulses stimulate cells where the implant is connected.

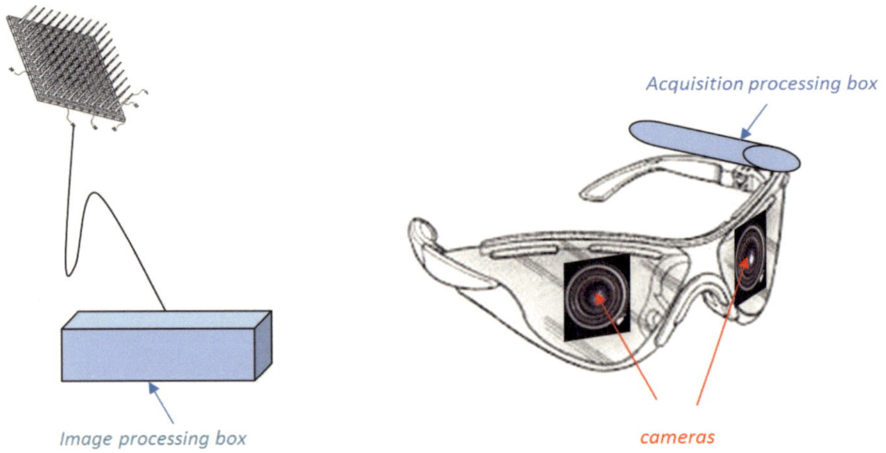

Fig. 6. General principle of an implant

2.1 Retina implant

For retinal implants, there exist two different ways to connect the electronic device: directly to the retina (epiretinal implant) or behind the retina (subretinal implant). Several research teams work on this subject worldwide. The target diseases mainly are:

- retinitis pigmentosa, which is the leading cause of inherited blindness in the world,
- age-related macular degeneration, which is the leading cause of blindness in the industrialized world.

2.1.1 Epiretinal implants

The development of an epiretinal prosthesis (Argus Retinal Prosthesis) has been initiated in the early 1990s at the Doheny Eye Institute and the University of California (USA)[Horsager (2010)Parikh (2010)]. This prosthesis was implanted in patients at John Hopkins University in order to demonstrate proof of principle. The company Second Sight[1] was then created in the late 1990s to develop this prosthesis. The first generation (Argus I) has 16 electrodes and was implanted in 6 patients between 2002 and 2004. The second generation (Argus II) has 60 electrodes and clinical trials have been planned since 2007. Argus III is still in process and will have 240 electrodes.

VisionCare Ophtalmic Technologies and the CentralSight Treatment Program [Chun (2005)Lane (2004)Lane (2006)] has created an implantable miniature telescope in order to provide central vision to people having degenerated macula diseases. This telescope is implanted inside the eye behind the iris and projects magnified images on healthy areas of the central retina.

2.1.2 Subretinal implants

At University of Louvain, a subretinal implant (MIVIP: Microsystem-based Visual Prosthesis) made of a single electrode has been developped [Archambeau (2004)]. The optic nerve is directly stimulated by this electrode from electric signals received from an external camera.

In the late 1980s, Dr. Joseph Rizzo and Professor John Wyatt performed a number of proof-of-concept epiretinal stimulation trials on blind volunteers before developing a subretinal stimulator. They co-founded the Boston Retinal Implant Project (BRIP). The collaboration was initiated between the Massachusetts Eye and Ear Infirmary, Harvard Medical School and the Massachusetts Institute of Technology. The mission of the Boston Retinal Implant Project is to develop novel engineering solutions to restore vision and improve the quality-of-life for patients who are blind from degenerative disease of the retina, for which there is currently no cure. Early results are actually a reference for this solution. The core strategy of the Boston Retinal Implant Project [2] is to create novel engineering solutions to treat blinding diseases that elude other forms of treatment. The specific goal of this study is to develop an implantable microelectronic prosthesis to restore vision to patients with certain forms of retinal blindness. The proposed solution provides a special opportunity for visual rehabilitation with a prosthesis, which can deliver direct electrical stimulation to those cells that carry visual information.

The Artificial Silicon Retina (ASR)[3] is a microchip containing 3500 photodiodes, developed by Alan and Vincent Chow. Each photodiode detects light and transforms it into electrical impulses stimulating retinal ganglion cells (Fig. 8).

In France, at the Institut de la Vision, the team of Pr Picaud has developed a subretinal implant [Djilas (2011)]. They have also set up clinical trials.

As well, in Germany [Zrenner (2008)], a subretinal prosthesis has been developed. A microphotodiode array (MPDA) acquires incident light information and send it to the chip located behind the retina. The chip transforms data into electrical signal stimulating the retinal ganglion cells.

In Japan [Yagi (2005)], a subretinal implant has been designed at Yagi Laboratory[4]. Experiments are mainly directed to obtain new biohybrid micro-electrode arrays.

[1] 2-sight.eu/
[2] http://www.bostonretinalimplant.org
[3] http://optobionics.com/asrdevice.shtml
[4] http://www.io.mei.titech.ac.jp/research/retina/

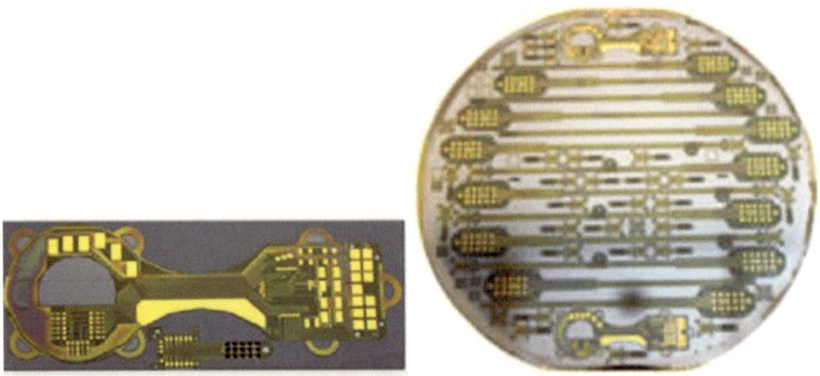

(a) Silicon wafer wit flexible polyalide iridium oxide electrode array (b) Close up of a flx circuit to which IC will be attached

Fig. 7. BRIP Solution

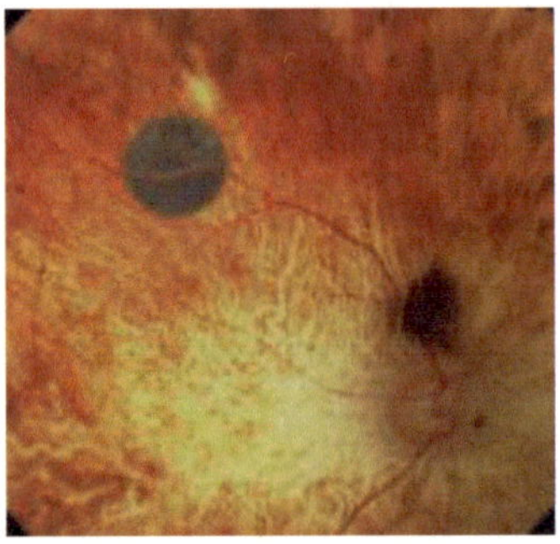

Fig. 8. ASR device implanted in the retina

At Stanford University, a visual prosthesis[5] (Fig. 9) has been developed [Loudin (2007)]. It includes an optoelectronic system composed of a subretinal photodiode array and an infrared image projection system. A video camera acquires visual data that are processed and displayed on video goggles as IR images. Photodiodes in the subretinal implant are activated when the IR image arrives on retina through natural eye optics. Electric pulses stimulate the retina cells.

In Australia, the Bionic Vision system[6] consists of a camera, attached to a pair of glasses, which transmits high-frequency radio signals to a microchip implanted in the retina. Electrical impulses stimulate retinal cells connected to the optic nerve. Such an implant improves the perception of light.

2.2 Cortex implant

William H. Dobelle initiated a project to develop a cortical implant [Dobelle (2000)], in order to return partially the vision to volunteer blind people [Ings (2007)]. His experiments began in the early 1970s with cortical stimulation on 37 sighted volunteers. Then four blind volunteers

[5] http://www.stanford.edu/ palanker/lab/retinalpros.html
[6] http://bionicvision.org.au/eye

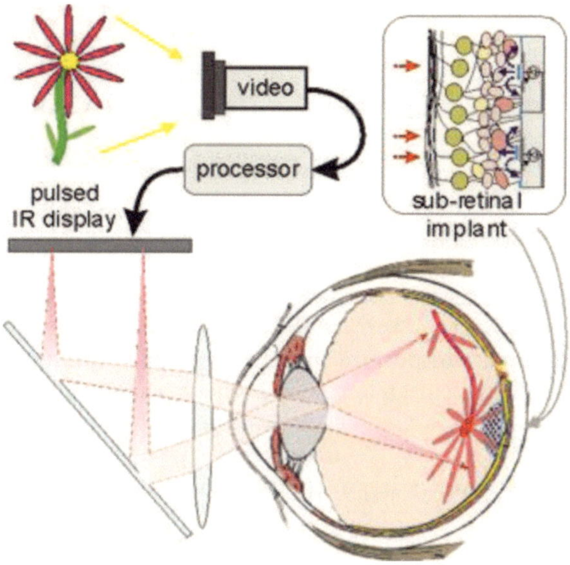

Fig. 9. Stanford University visual prosthesis

were implanted with permanent electrode arrays. The first volunteers were operated at the University of Western Ontario, Canada. A 292 × 512 CCD camera is connected to a sub-notebook computer in a belt pack. A second microcontroller is also included in the belt pack and it is dedicated to brain stimulation. The stimulus generator is connected to the electrodes implanted on the visual cortex through a percutaneous pedestral. With this system a vision-impaired person is able to count his fingers and recognize basic symbols.

In Canada, the research team of Pr Sawan [Sawan (2008)] at Polystim Neurotechnologies Laboratory[7] has begun clinical trials for an electrode array providing images of 256 pixels (Fig. 10). Such images are not very accurate but they allow the patient to guess shapes. Furthermore clinical trials have proved that it was possible to directly stimulate neurons in the primary visual cortex.

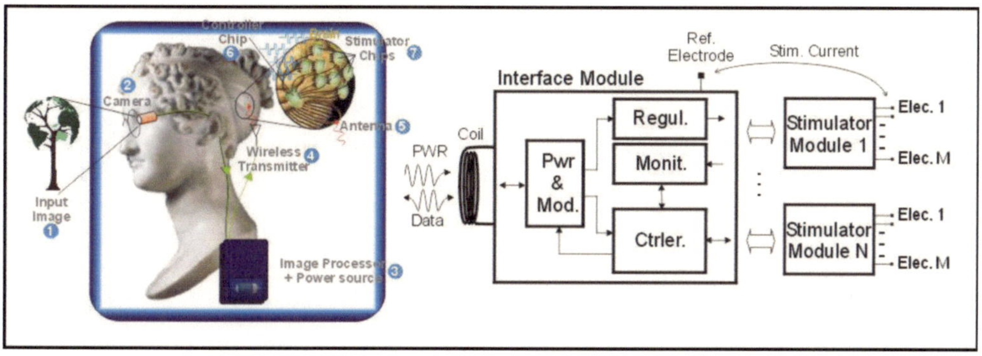

Fig. 10. Principle of Polystim Laboratory visual prosthesis

[7] http://www.polystim.ca

3. Bionic eye

Such a system has to mimick several abilities of the human visual system in order to make visual information available for blind people. The system is made of a camera acquiring images, an electronical device processing data and a mechanical system that drives the camera. Outputs can be provided on cerebral implants, in other words, electrodes matrices plugged to the primary visual cortex. When discovering a new scene the human eye processes by saccades and the gaze is successively focused at different points of interest. The sequence of focusing points enables to scan the scene in an optimized way according to the interest degree. The interest degree is a very complex criterion to estimate because it depends on the context and on the nature of elements included in the scene. Geometrical features of objects as well as color or structure are important in the interest estimation (Fig. 11). For example, a tree (b) is of a great interest in a urban landscape whereas a bench (a) is a salient information in a contryside scene. In the first case, the lack of geometrical particularities and the color difference make the tree interesting. In the second case the structure and the geometrical features of the bench make it interesting in comparison to trees or meadows.

Several steps are carried out successively or in parallel to process data and drive the camera. First of all a detection of points of interest is achieved on a regular image, in other words, on an image usually provided by a camera. One of the points best-scoring with the detector is chosen as the first focusing point. Then the image is re- sampled in a radial way in order to obtain a foveated image. The resulting image is blurred according to the distance to the focusing point [Larson (2009)]. Then a detection of points of interest is achieved on the foveated image in order to determine the second focusing point. These two steps are repeated as many times as necessary to discover the whole scene (Fig. 12). This gives the computed sequence of points of interest. In parallel a human observer faces the primary image while an eye- tracker follows his eye movements in order to determine the observer sequence of points of interest, when exploring the scene by saccades [Hernandez (2008)]. Afterwards the two sequences will have to be compared in order to quantify and qualify the computer vision process, in terms of position and order.

4. Circuit and system approach

4.1 Principle and objective

The proposed solution is based on Pr. Sawan research [Coulombe (2007)Sawan (2008)]. The implementation is a visual prosthesis implanted into the human cortex. In the first case, the principle of this application consists in stimulating the visual cortex by implanting a silicium micro-chip on a network of electrodes made of biocompatible materials [Kim (2010)Piedade (2005)] and in which each electrode injects a stimulating electrical current in order to provoke a series of luminous points to appear (an array of pixels) in the field of vision of the sightless person [Piedade (2005)]. This system is composed of two distinct parts:

- The implant lodged in the visual cortex wirelessly receives dedicated data and associated energy from the external controller. This electro-stimulator generates the electrical stimuli and oversees the changing microelectrode/biological tissue interface,
- The battery-operated outer control includes a micro-camera which captures the image as well as a processor and a command generator. They process the imaging data in order to:
  1. select and translate the captured images,

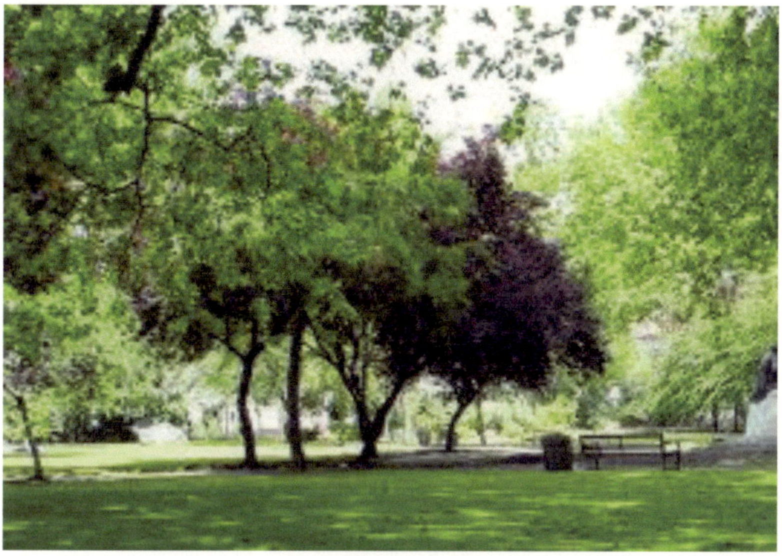

(a) Bench in a park

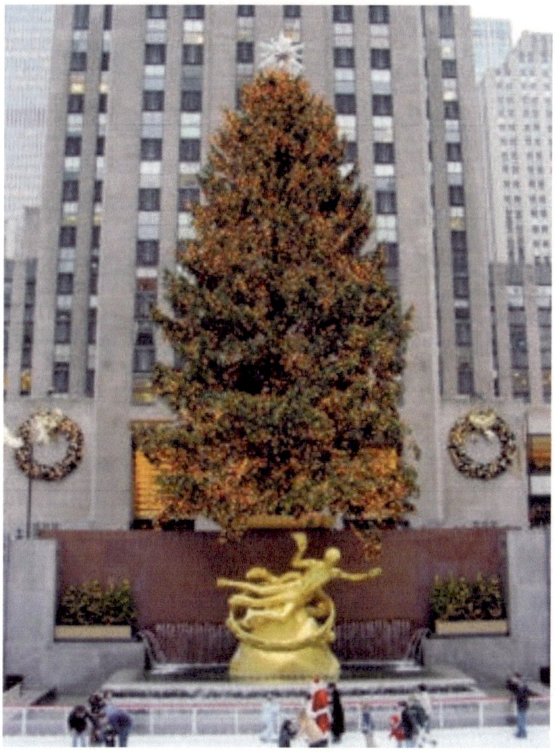

(b) Tree in a town

Fig. 11. Image context and points of interest

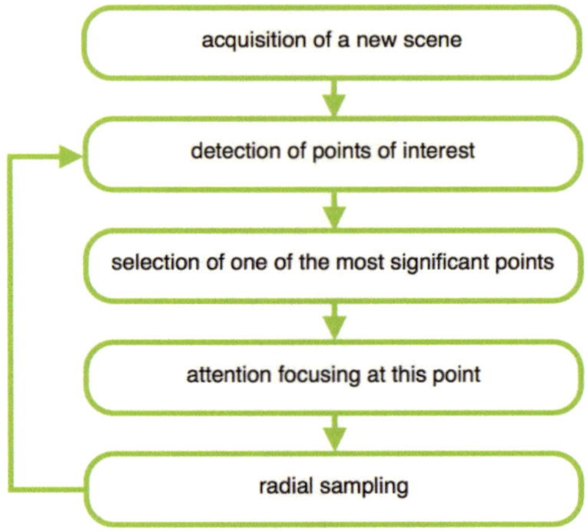

Fig. 12. Scene exploration process

2. generate and manage the electrical stimulation process
3. oversee the implant.

The topology is based on the schematic of Fig. 13.

An analog signal captured by the camera provides information to the DSP (Digital Signal Processor) component. The image is transmitted by using the FPGA which realizes the first Image Pre-processing. A DAM (Direct Access Memory) is placed at the input of the DSP card in order to transfer the preprocessing image to the SDRAM. The DSP realizes then the image processing in order to reproduce the eye behavior and a part of the cortex operation. The LCD screen is added in order to achieve debug of the image processing. In the final version, this last one will be removed. The FPGA drives two motors in two axes directions (horizontal, vertical) in order to reproduce the eye movements. We will know focus on the different components of

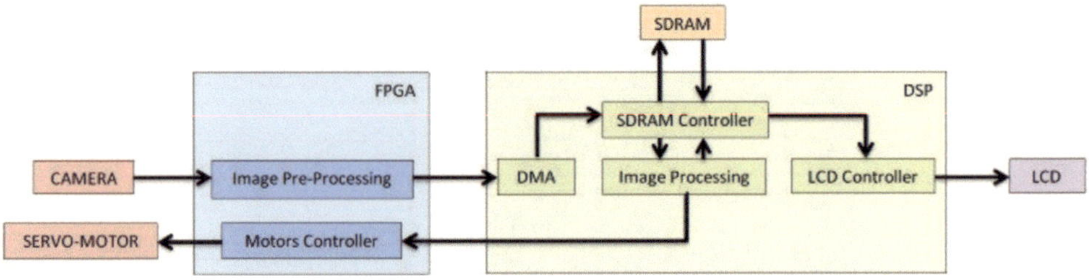

Fig. 13. Schematic principle of bionic eye

this bionic eye topology.

4.2 Camera component

With the development of the mobile phone, the CMOS camera became more compact, lower powered, with higher resolution and quicker frame rate. As for biomedical systems, the constraints tend to be the same, this solution retained our attention. Indeed, for example, Omnivision has created a 14 megapixel CMOS camera with a frame rate of 60 fps for a 1080p frame and a package of 9 mm $\times$ 7 mm. In this project, we have retained a choice of a 1.3 megapixel camera at a frame rate of 15 fps for mainly two reasons: the package who is easy to implement and the large number of different outputs thanks to the internal registers of the camera. The registers allow us to output a lot of standard resolutions (SXVGA, VGA, QVGA etcÉ), the output formats (RGB or YUV) and the frame rate (15 fps or 7.5 fps). These registers are initialized by the I2C controller of the DSP. This allows a dynamic configuration of the camera by the DSP. The camera outputs are 8 bits parallel data that allow a datastream up to 0, 3 Gb/s with 3 control signals (horizontal, vertical and pixel clocks). For the prototype we output at a VGA resolution in RGB 565 at 15 fps.

In order to reproduce of the eye movement, two analog servo motors have been used (horizontal and vertical) mounted on a steel frame and controlled by the FPGA.

4.3 FPGA (Field-Programmable Gate Array) component

The FPGA realizes two processes in parallel. The first one consists in controlling the servo motor. The FPGA transforms an angle in pulse width with a refresh rate of 50 Hz (Fig. 13). The angle is incremented or decremented by two pulse updates during the signal of a new frame (Fig. 15). For 15 fps a pulse is 2 degrees for a use at the maximal speed of the servo motor (0.15s @ 60ą).

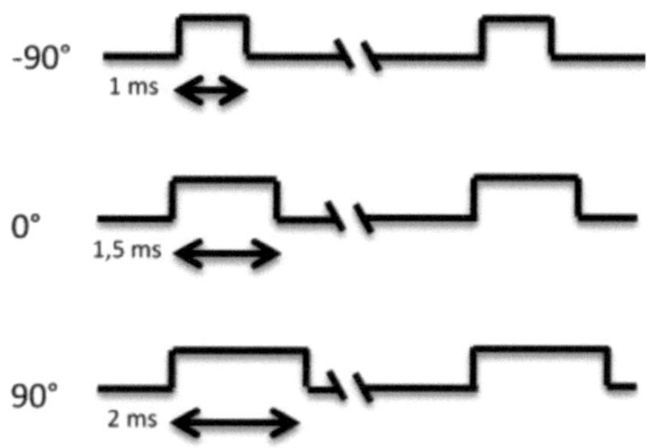

Fig. 14. Time affectation of the pulse width

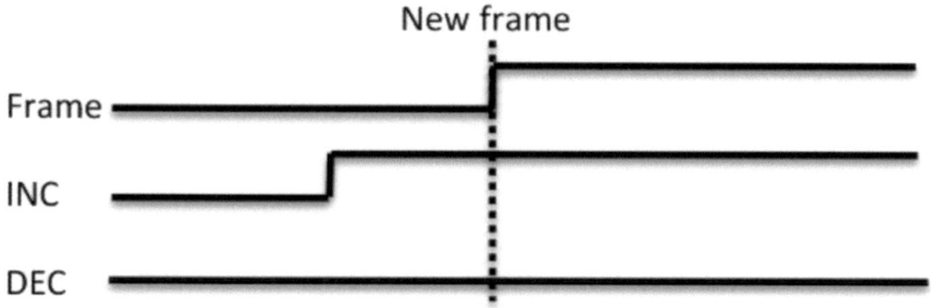

Fig. 15. New frame: increment/decrement signal

The second process is the image preprocessing. This process consists of the transformation of 16 bits by pixel image with 2 clocks by pixel into 24 bits by pixel image with one clock by pixel. For this, we divide the pixel clock by two and we interpolate the pixel color with 5 or 6 bits to a pixel color with 8 bits.

4.4 DSP (Digital Signal Processor) component

For a full embedded product, we need a core that can run a heavy load due to the image processing in real-time. This is why we focus our attention on a DSP solution and precisely on the DSP with an integrated ARM core by Texas Instrument, in fact the OpenCV library[8] is not optimized for DSP core (the mainline development of openCV effort targets the x86 architecture) but it has been successfully ported to the ARM platforms[9]. Nevertheless, several algorithms require floating-point computation and the DSP is the most suitable core for this thanks to the native floating point unit (Fig. 16).

Function Name	ARM9™ (ms)	ARM Cortex-A8 (ms)	C674x DSP (ms)
cvCornerEigenValsandVecs	4746	2655	402
cvGoodFeaturestoTrack	2040	1234	268
cvWarpAffine	82	37	17
cvOpticalFlowPyrLK	9560	5240	344
cvMulSpecturm	104	69	11
cvHaarDetectObject	17500	8217	1180

Fig. 16. Operation time execution

Moreover, the parallelism due to the dual-core adds more velocity to the image processing (Fig. 17). And finally, we use pipeline architecture for an efficient use of the CPU thanks to the multiple controller included in the DSP. The first controller used is the direct memory access controller that allows to record the frame from the FPGA to a ping-pong buffer without the use of the CPU. The ping-pong buffer allows to record the second frame to a different address. This enables to work on the first frame during the record of the second frame without the problem of the double use of a file.

OpenCV Function	ARM Cortex™-A8 with NEON (ms)	ARM Cortex-A8 with C674x DSP (ms)
cvAdaptiveThreshold	85.029	33.433
cvHoughLines2D	2405.844	684.367
cvCornerHarris	666.928	168.57
cvDFT	594.532	95.539

Fig. 17. Dual Core operation time execution

The second controller used is the SDRAM controller that controls two external 256 Mb SDRAM. The controller manages the priority of the use of the SDRAM, the refresh of the SDRAM and the signals control. The third controller used is the LCD controller that allows to display the frame at the end of the image processing in order to verify the result and presentation of the product. This architecture offers a use of the CPU exclusively dedicated to the image processing (Fig. 18).

[8] www.opencv.com
[9] www.ti.com

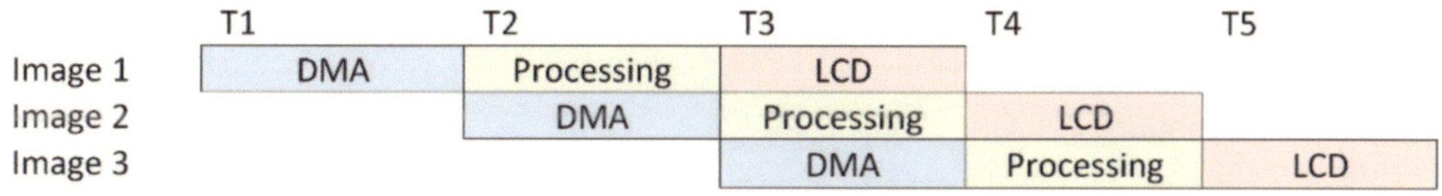

Fig. 18. Image processing

4.5 Electronic prototype

A prototype has been realized, as shown in Fig. 19. As introducted before, this prototype is based on : (i) a camera (ii) a FPGA card, (iii) a DSP card and (iv) a LCD screen.

Its associated size is 20*14*2cm. This size is due to the use of a development card. We choose respectively for the FPGA and DSP cards a Xilinx[10] Virtex 5 XC5VLX50 and a spectrum[11] digital evm omap l137. But on these two cards (FPGA, DSP), we just need the FPGA, DSP, memories and I/O ports. Indeed, the objective is to validate the software image processing. The LCD screen on the left of Fig19 is added to see the resulting image. This last one will not be present on the final product. For the test of the project, we choose a TFT sharp LQ043T3DX02.

So, the objective size for the final product is first of all a large reduction by removing the obsolete parts of these two cards (80%) and then by using integrated circuit solution. The support technology will be standard 0.35μm CMOS technology which provides low current leakage [Flandre (2011)] and so consumption reduction.

An other advantage of using this technology is the possibility to develop on the same wafer analog and digital circuits. In this case, it is possible to realize powerful functions with low consumption and size.

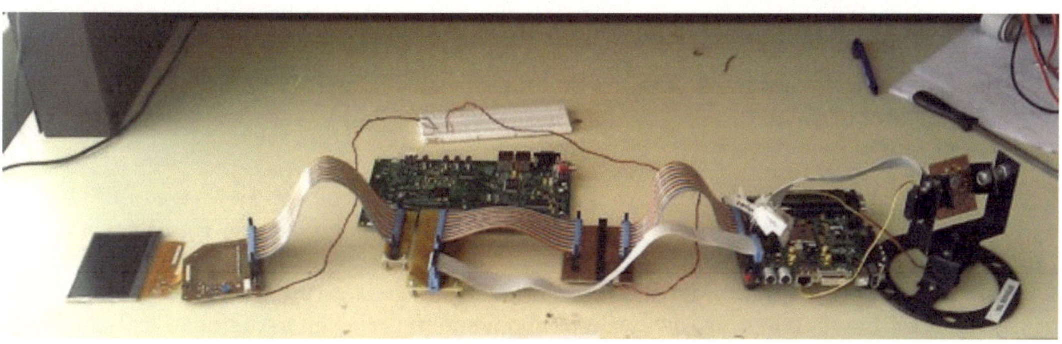

Fig. 19. Bionic Eye prototype

5. Image processing and analysis

The two main steps in HVS data processing that will be mimicked are focus of attention and detection of points of interest. Focus of attention enables to direct gaze at a particular point. In this way, the image around the focusing point is very clear (central vision) and becomes more and more blurred when the distance to the focusing point increases (peripheral vision).

[10] www.xilinx.com
[11] www.spectrumdigital.com

Detection of points of interest is the stage where a sequence of focusing points is determined in order to explore a scene.

5.1 Focus of attention

As a matter of fact, the role played by cones in diurnal vision is preponderant. Cones are much less numerous than rods in most parts of the retina, but greatly outnumber rods in the fovea. Furthermore cones are arranged in a concentric way inside the human retina [Marr (1982)]. In this way focus of attention may be modelized by representing cones in the fovea area and its surroundings. The general principle is the following. Firstly a focusing point is chosen as the fovea center (gaze center) and a foveal radius is defined as the radius of the central cell. Secondly an isotropic progression of concentric circles determines the blurring factor according to the distance to the focusing point. Thirdly integration sets are defined to represent cones and an integration method is selected in order to gather data over the integration set to obtain a single value. Integration methods can be chosen amongst averaging, median filtering, morphological filtering such as dilation, erosion, closing, opening, and so on. Then re-sampled data are stored in a rectangular image in polar coordinates. This gives the encoded image. This image is a compressed version of the original image, but the compression ratio varies according to the distance to the focusing point. The following step can be the reconstruction of the image from the encoded image. This step is not systematically achieved as there is no need of duplicating data to process them [Robert-Inacio (2010)]. When necessary it works by determining for each point of the reconstructed image the integration sets it belongs to. Then the dual method of the integration process is used to obtain the reconstructed value. When using directly the encoded image instead of the original or the reconstructed images, customized processing algorithms must be set up in order to take into account that data are arranged in a polar way. In this case a full pavement of the image is defined with hexagonal cells [Robert (1999)]. The hexagons are chosen so that they do not overlap each others and so that they are as regular as possible. A radius sequence is also defined as follows:

This hexagonal pavement is as close as possible to the biological cone distribution in the fovea. Furthermore data are taken into account only once in the encoded image because of non-overlapping.

Fig. 21 illustrates the type of results provided by previous methods on an image of the Kodak database[12] (Fig. 21). Firstly Fig. 21 shows the encoded image (on the right) for a foveal radius of 25 pixels and with hexagonal cells. The focusing point is chosen at (414, 228), ie: at the central flower heart. Secondly the reconstructed image is given after re-sampling of the original image. In the following, the hexagonal pavement is chosen to define foveated images as it is the closest one to the cone distribution in the fovea.

5.2 Detection of points of interest

The detection of points of interest is achieved by using the Harris detector [Harris (1988)]. Fig. 22 shows the images with the detected points of interest. Points of interest detected as corners are highlighted in red whereas those detected as edges are in green. Fig. 22 illustrates the Harris method when using a regular image (a), in other words, an image sampled in a rectangular way, and a foveated image (b).

[12] http://r0k.us/graphics/kodak/

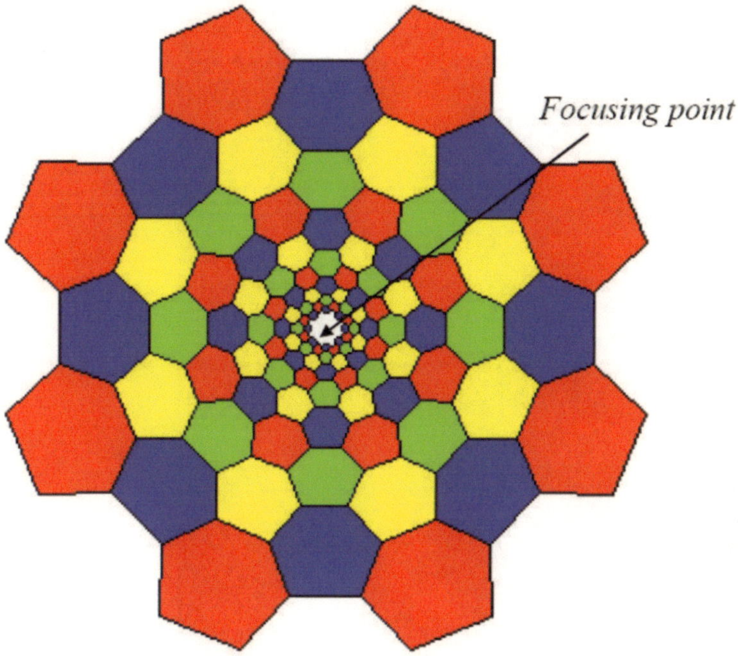

Fig. 20. Hexagonal cell distribution.

5.3 Sequence of points of interest

Short sequences of points of interest are studied: the first one has been computed and the second one is the result observed on a set of 7 people. Fig. 23 shows the sequences of points of interest on the original image of Fig. 21a and Table 1 gives the point coordinates. Sequences are made of points numbered from 1 to 4. The observer sequence in white goes from the pink flower heart to the bottom left plant, whereas the computed sequence in cyan goes from the pink flower heart to the end of the branch. Another difference concerns the point in the red flower. The observers chose to look at the flower heart whereas the detector focused at the border between the petal and the leaf. This is explained by the visual cortex behavior. Actually the detector is attracted by color differences whereas the human visual system is also sensitive to geometrical features such as symmetry. In this case the petals around the heart are quite arranged in a symmetrical way aroud the flower heart. That is why the observers chose to gaze at this point. In this example the computed sequence is determined without computing again a new foveated image for each point of interest, but by considering each significant point from the foveated image with the central point as focusing point. Furthermore for equivalent points of interest the distance between two consecutive points is chosen as great as possible in order to cover a maximal area of the scene with a minimal number of eye movements.

Table 1 gives the distance between two equivalent points from the two sequences. This distance varies from 8 to 32.249 with an average value of 18.214. This means that computed points are not so far from those of the observers. But the algorithm determining the sequence must be refined in order to prevent errors on point order.

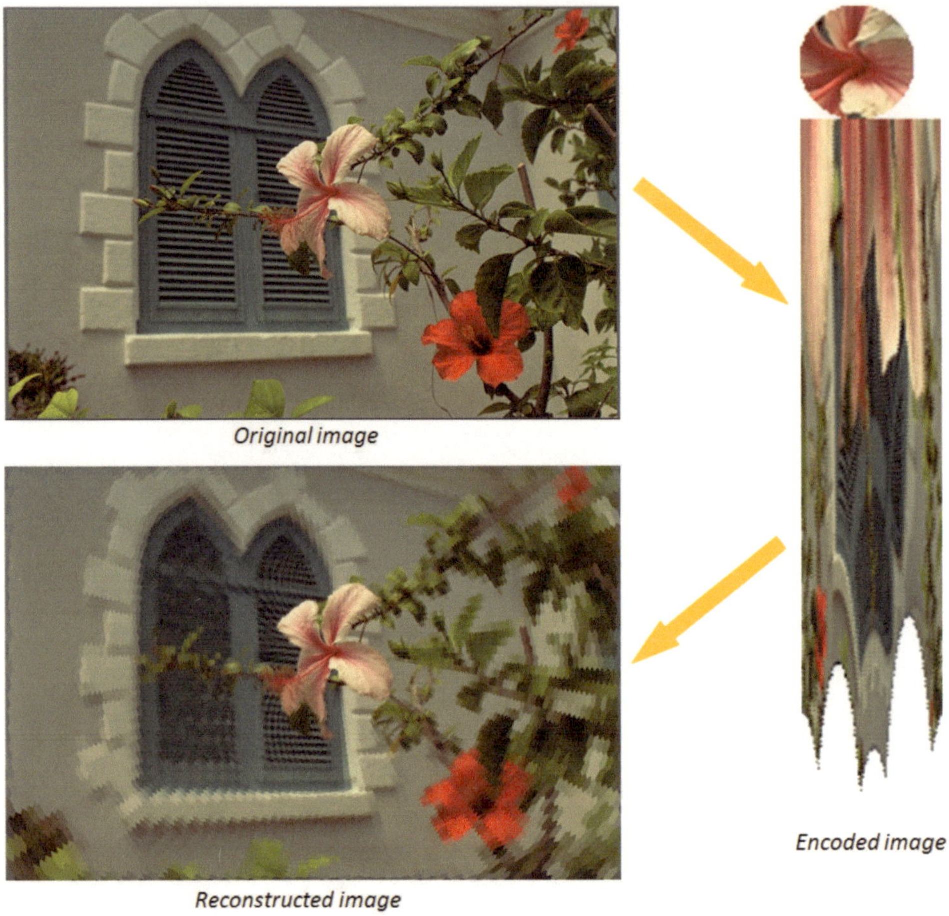

Fig. 21. Focus of attention on a particular image: from the original image to the reconstructed image, passing by the encoded image (foveated image)

Point Number	Regular Detection	Point Number	Foveated Detection	Distance
1	(191, 106)	1	(194, 114)	8.544
2	(279, 196)	2	(275, 164)	32.249
3	(99, 118)	4	(109, 103)	18.028
4	(24, 214)	3	(38, 215)	14.036

Table 1. Distances between points of interest.

6. Applications

There exist two great families of applications: on the one hand, applications in the biomedical and health field, and on the other hand, applications in robotics.

In the biomedical field, a system such as the bionic eye can be very helpful at different tasks:

- light perception,
- color perception,

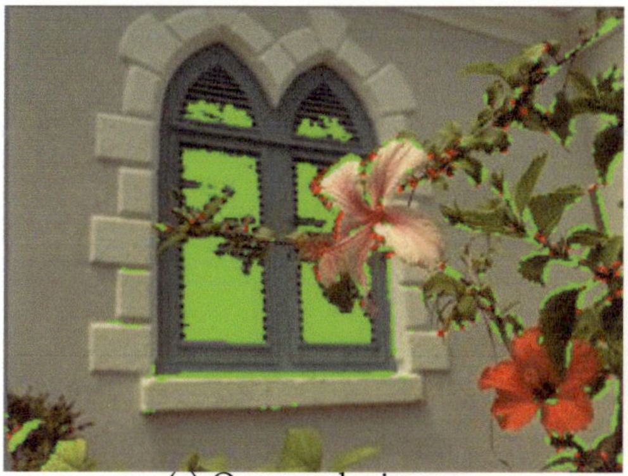
(a) On a regular image

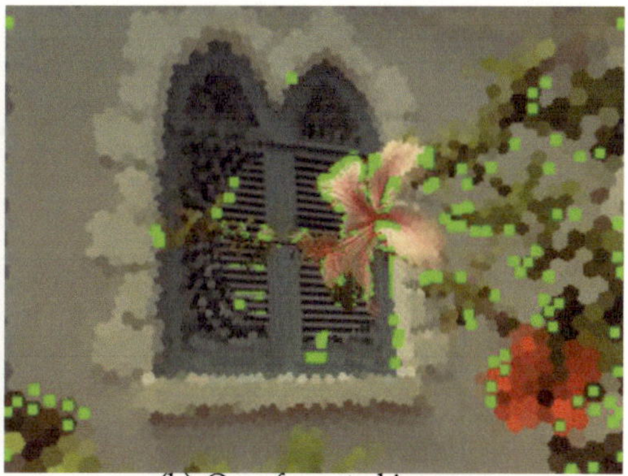
(b) On a foveated image

Fig. 22. Detection of points of interest

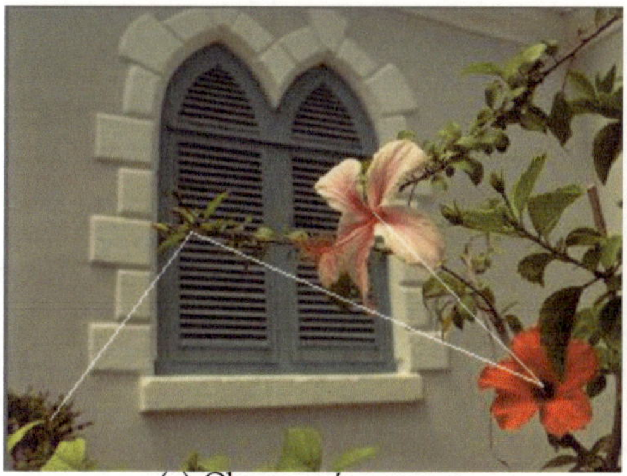
(a) Observers' sequence

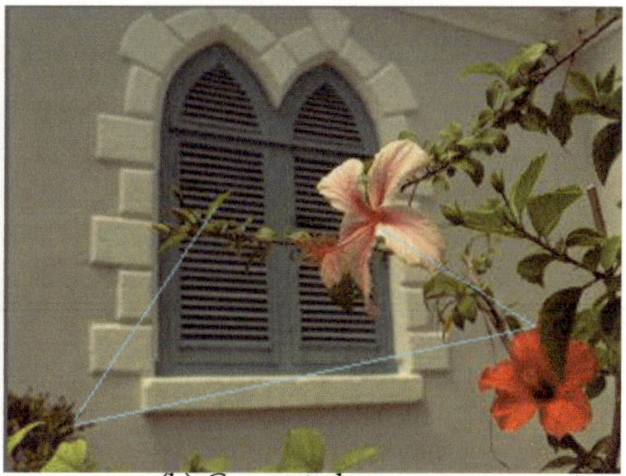
(b) Computed sequence

Fig. 23. Sequences of points of interest

- contextual environment perception,
- reading,
- pattern recognition,
- face recognition,
- autonomous moving,
- etc.

These different tasks are achieved very easily for sighted people, but they can be impossible for visually impaired people. For example, color perception cannot be operated by touch, by hearing, by the taste or smell. It is a pure visual sensation, unreachable to blind people. That is why the bionic eye must be able to replace the human visual system for such tasks.

In robotics, such a system able to explore an unknown scene by itself can be of a great help for autonomous robots. For example AUV (Autonomous Underwater Vehicles) can be even more autonomous by being able to decide by themselves what path to follow. Actually, by mimicking detection of points of interest, the bionic eye can determine obstacle position and then it can compute a path avoiding them. Furthermore, application fields are numerous:

- in archaeology and exploration in environments inaccessible to humans,
- in environmental protection and monitoring,
- in ship hull and infrastructure inspection,
- in infrastructure inspection of nuclear power plants,
- in military applications,
- etc.

Each time it is impossible for humans to reach a place, the bionic eye can be used to make decision or help making decision in order to drive a robot.

7. Conclusion

In this chapter, the bionic eye principle has been presented in order to demonstrate how powerful such a system is. Different approaches can be considered to stimulate either the retina or the primary visual cortex, but all the presented systems use a separate system for image acquisition. Images are then processed and data are turned into electrical pulses stimulating either retinal cells or cortical neurons.

The originality of our system lays in the fact that images are not only processed but analyzed in order to determine a sequence of focusing points. This sequence allows to explore automatically a complex scene. This principle is directly inspired by the human visual system behavior. Furthermore foveated images are used instead of classical images (sampled at a constant step in two orthogonal directions). In this way, every image processing algorithm even basic has to be redefined to fit to foveated images.

In particular, an algorithm for detection of points of interest on foveated images has been set up in order to determine sequences of points of interest. These sequences are compared to those obtained from a human observer by eye-tracking in order to validate the computational process. A comparison between detection of points of interest on regular images and foveated images has also been made. Results show that detection on foveated images is more efficient because it suppresses noise that is far enough from the focusing point while detecting as well significant points of interest. This is particularly interesting as the amount of data to process is greatly decreased by the radial re-sampling step.

In future works the two sequences of points of interest must be compared more accurately and their differences analyzed. Furthermore the computed sequence is the basis for the animation of the bionic eye in order to discover dynamically the new scene. Such a process assumes that the bionic eye is servo-controlled in several directions.

8. References

Archambeau C.; Delbeke J.; Veraart C. & Verleysen M. (2004). Prediction of visual perceptions with artificial neural networks in a visual prosthesis for the blind. *Artificial Intelligence in Medicine*, 32(3), pp 183-194

Chun DW.; Heier JS. & Raizman MB. (2005). Visual prosthetic device for bilateral end-stage macular degeneration. *Expert Rev Med Devices*, 2 (6), pp 657-665

Coulombe J.; Sawan M.& Gervais J. (2007). A highly flexible system for microstimulation of the visual cortex: Design and implementation. *IEEE Transaction on Biomedical Circuits and Systems*, Vol.14, No.4, (Dec.2007), pp 258-269, ISSN 1932-4545

Djilas M.; Oles C.; Lorach H.; Bendali A.; Degardin J.; Dubus E.; Lissorgues-Bazin G.; Rousseau L.; Benosman R.; Ieng SH.; Joucla S.; Yvert B.; Bergonzo P.; Sahel J. & Picaud S. (2011). Three-dimensional electrode arrays for retinal prostheses: modeling, geometry optimization and experimental validation. *J Neural Eng*, 8(4)

Dobelle WH. (2000). Artificial vision for the blind by connecting a television camera to visual cortex. *ASAIO Journal*, 46, pp 3-9

Faria, J.; Lopes, S.; Fernandes, H.; Martins, P. & Barroso, J. (2010). Electronic white cane for blind people navigation assistance. *World Automation Congress (WAC'10)*, 19-23 Sept, pp 1-7, Kobe , Japan

Flandre D. , Bulteel O., Gosset G. , Rue B. & Bol D. (2011). Disruptive ultra-low-leakage design techniques for ultra-low-power mixed-signal microsystems, *Faible Tension Faible Consommation (FTFC)*, pp 1-4

Harris C. & Stephens M. , (1998). A combined corner and edge detector,. *Proceedings of the 4th Alvey Vision Conference*, pp 147-151, England, Aug-Sept. 1988, Manchester, UK

Hernandez T.; Levitan, C.; Banks M. & Schor C. (2008). How does saccade adaptation affect visual perception?. *Journal of Vision*, Vol. 8, No. 3, Jan -2008, pp 1-16

Horsager A.; Greenberg RJ. & Fine I. (2010). Spatiotemporal interactions in retinal prosthesis subjects. *Invest Ophthalmol Vis Sci* 51, pp 1223-1233.

Hub A.; Hartter T. & Ertl T. (2006). Interactive tracking of movable objects for the blind on the basis of environment models and perception-oriented object recognition methods. *Proceedings of the 8th international ACM SIGACCESS conference on Computers and accessibility*, Assets '06, Portland, Oregon, USA, pp 111-118, ACM, New York, NY, USA

Ings S. (2007). Making eyes to see. *The Eye: a natural history*, London: Bloomsbury, pp 276-283

Kim D.-H.; Viventi, J & al (2010). Dissolvable films of silk fibroin for ultrathin conformal bio-integrated electronics, *Journal of Nature Materials*, Vol. 9, Apr-2010, pp 511-517

Lane SS.; Kuppermann BD.; Fine IH.; Hamill MB.; Gordon JF.; Chuck RS.; Hoffman RS.; Packer M. & Koch DD. (2004). A prospective multicenter clinical trial to evaluate the safety and effectiveness of the implantable miniature telescope. *Am J Ophthalmol*, 137 (6), pp 993-1001

Lane SS. & Kuppermann BD. (2006) The Implantable Miniature Telescope for macular degeneration. *Curr Opin Ophthalmol*, 17 (1), pp 94-98

Larson A. & Loschky, L. (2009). The contributions of central versus peripheral vision to scene gist recognition. *Journal of Vision*, Vol. 9, No. 6, Jan 2009, pp 1-6

Loudin J.; Simanovskii D.; Vijayraghavan K.; Sramek C.; Butterwick A.; Huie P.; McLean G. & Palanker D. (2007). Optoelectronic retinal prosthesis: system design and performance. *J Neural Engineering* 4 (1), pp 572-584

Marr D. (1982). *Vision: A Computational Investigation into the Human Representation and Processing of Visual Information*, eds. W.H. Freeman, San Francisco.

Parikh N.; Itti L. & Weiland J. (2010). Saliency-based image processing for retinal prostheses. *J Neural Eng*, 7.

Piedade, M.; Gerald, J.; Sousa, L.A.; Tavares, G.& Tomas, P.; (2005). Visual neuroprosthesis: a non invasive system for stimulating the cortex. *IEEE Transaction on Circuits and Systems I* , Vol.52, No.12, (Dec.2005), pp 2648-2662, ISSN 1549-8328

Robert F. & Dinet E., (1999). Biologically inspired pavement of the plane for image encoding,. *Proceedings of International Conference on Computational Intelligence for Modelling, Control and Automation (CIMCA'99)*, pp 1-6, Austria, Feb. 1999, Vienna

Robert-Inacio F.; Stainer Q.; Scaramuzzino R. & Kussener E. (2010). Visual attention simulation in rgb and hsv color spaces. *Proceedings of of 4th IS&T International Conference on Colour in Graphics, Imaging and Vision (CGIV 2010)*, pp 19-26, Finland, Joensuu

Sarpeshkar, R. (2010). *Ultra Low Power Bioelectronics: Fundamentals, Biomedical Applications and Bio-inspired Systems*, Cambridge, ISBN 978-0-521-85727-7

Sawan M.; Gosselin B. & Coulombe J. (2008). Learning from the primary visual cortex to recover vision for the blind by microstimulation,. *Proceedings of Norchip conference*, pp 1-4, ISBN 978-1-4244-2492-4 , Estony, Tallinn

Tong, F. (2003). Primary visual cortex and visual awareness, *Nature reviews: neuroscience*, 4, pp 219-229.

Troyk, P., Bak, M., Berg, J., Bradley, D., Cogan, S., Erickson, R., Kufta, C., McCreery, D., Schmidt, E. & Towle, V. (2003). A Model for Intracortical Visual Prosthesis Research, *Artificial Organs*, 27, 11, pp 1005-1015.

Wyatt, J. (2011). The retinal implant project, *Research Laboratory of Electronics (RLE) report at the Massachussetts Institute of Technology, Chapter 19*, 20 March, pp 1-11.

Yagi, T. (2005). Vision prosthesis (artificial retina), *The Cell*, 37, 2, pp 18-21.

Zrenner E. (2008). Visual sensations mediated by subretinal microelectrode arrays implanted into blind retinitis pigmentosa patients. *Proc. 13th Ann. Conf. of the IFESS*, Freiburg, Germany

2

Methods of Measurement and Evaluation of Eye, Head and Shoulders Position in Neurological Practice

Patrik Kutilek[1], Jiri Hozman[1], Rudolf Cerny[2] and Jan Hejda[1]
[1]*Czech Technical University in Prague, Faculty of Biomedical Engineering*
[2]*Charles University in Prague, Department of Neurology, 2nd Faculty of Medicine*
Czech Republic

1. Introduction

The position of the eye, head and shoulders can be negatively influenced by many diseases of the nervous system, (particularly by visual and vestibular disorders) (Cerny R. et al, 2006). Disturbances of the cervical vertebral column are another frequent cause of abnormal head position. In this chapter we describe advanced methods of measuring the precise position of the eye, head and shoulders in space. The systems and methods are designed for use in neurology to discover relationships between some neurological disorders (such as disorders of vestibular system) and postural head alignment. We have designed a system and a set of procedures for evaluating the inclination (roll), flexion (pitch) and rotation (yaw) of the head and the inclination (roll) and rotation (yaw) of the shoulders with resolution and accuracy from 1° to 2° (Hozman et al, 2007). We will also deal with systems designed for parallel measurement of eye and head positions and a new portable system for studying eye and head movements at the same time is described as well (Charfreitag et al, 2008). The main goal of this study is to describe new systems and possibilities of the present methods determined for diagnostics and therapy support in clinical neurology. Furthermore, we describe the benefits of each method for diagnosis in neurology.

2. Background and related works

The measurement of eye position is an important diagnostic instrument in both clinical and experimental examination of human vestibular system (Cerny R. et al, 2006). Also, the simultaneous measurement of head (Murphy et al, 1991) and shoulders position (Raine et al, 1997) could contribute to better definition of diseases affecting the vestibular system (labyrinthine) function in man.

2.1 Clinical significance of head posture measurement

Abnormal head posture (AHP) is an important clinical sign of disease in many medical specialities. AHP is a consequence of dysfunction of musculoskeletal, visual and vestibular systems (Brandt et al, 2003). AHP is of particular importance in childhood, when developmental abnormalities of different origin can manifest with AHP as a main clinical symptom. The differential diagnosis is broad and quantitative assessment of head position in space it is important for both treatment and evaluation of disease evolution. In an Italian study 73 children referred by paediatricians the most common cause of AHP was orthopaedic disease (congenital muscular torticollis, 35 cases) followed by ocular motor palsy (mostly superior oblique palsy, 25 cases). Neurological disease was found in 5 cases, in 8 cases no underlying disease was indentified (Nucci et al, 2005).

Most peculiar forms of AHP are due to cervical dystonia, a movement disorder due to the disturbance of motor control of cervical muscles. Exact pathophysiology of this disabling and hard to treat condition is not known and includes local, suprasegmental and psychological factors. It can be classified according to the abnormal positioning of the head and spine into ante/retrocollis (sagittal plane), laterocollis (frontal plane) and rotatocollis (horizontal plane), pure forms are rare, typical is combination (torticollis). The pattern of muscles involved in generation of the AHP can be inferred from the head position. Objective and quantitative measurement of head position is of great importance, as treatment with botulotoxin (nowadays first choice) requires exact identification of muscles involved in AHP generation and follow up of treatment efficacy with objective head positions recordings is important for choosing optimal long term treatment strategy. Standard assessment scales for torticollis use semiquantative clinical scores or simple goniometers with low precision (Galardi et al, 2003; Novak et al, 2010).

Blockades and disease of cervical spine due to spondylosis or trauma are very common cause of AHP in clinical practice. Here the quantitative head posture measurement is not imperative, but simple objective recording of abnormality evolution can be useful in chronic cases and when cervical spine surgery is considered.

AHP is a frequent and important sign in ophthalmology, particularly in childhood. It represents compensation of abnormal eye position and/or motility. Paralyses of eye muscles are compensated by a tilt of the head in direction of the weakened muscle. In congenital nystagmus the AHP tends to shift gaze direction in the null zone of the nystagmus. As a result of the compensatory head position, the vision acuity is enhanced or restored, but unbalanced muscle activation can lead to cervical spine disorders in the long term. Surgical procedures aimed at correction of the eyeball position are effective in repairing the AHP and are considered treatment of choice (artificial divergence, Kestenbaum surgery). The dosage of ocular muscle retroposition/resection depends on the angle of AHP with fixation of distant target. The reduction of abnormal head turn with 1mm muscle resection was 1.4° head turn on average in one study (Gräf et al, 2001).

Ocular tilt reaction is a well established symptom of dysfunction of the graviceptive pathways starting from the otholithic maculae of the inner ear to the vestibular nuclei and paramedian thalamus. This syndrome is defined by the triad of signs - head tilt, ocular globe rotation a deviation of the subjective visual vertical. All deviations directs towards the weak labyrinth, or to the contralateral side after crossing at the pontine level, in the case of brain stem lesions. Head tilt in the frontal plane is usually quickly compensated, after the acute phase is over, but more subtle signs (ocular rotation and subjective vertical) can last for weeks and months. Horizontal eyes alignment is precisely regulated within narrow range of several degrees (Halmagyi et al, 1991), (Brandt & Dieterich, 1994). Deviations in the horizontal plane are also easily appreciated even by naked eye during examination. Little is known about head turn in vestibular syndromes. This type of deviation is hard to assess by observation only, indeed, only gross deviations in cases of ocular torticollis are used in clinical practice and regularly cited in literature. Vestibular imbalance due to unilateral labyrinthine failure causes vestibulospinal deviations towards the weaker labyrinth (Hautant reaction, Romberg deviation in standing with closed eyes etc.). It is reasonable to expect head turns of several degrees due to the functional imbalance between the activity horizontal channels. In contrast to the tilt reaction such a finding was not well described until now. Probably, this type of vestibular rotatocollis is compensated by spatial visual clues with open eyes and can be easily overlooked. In this situation, precise technique for head rotation measurement would be of paramount importance.

Last, but not least, precise 3D head position measurement has many potential implications for physical medicine and rehabilitation, particularly in the management and diagnosis of disorders affecting cervical spine. Head position in the sagittal plane is very variable and influenced by many factors, particularly habitual holding of the spine as a whole. Habitual head anteflexion with chronic overload of cervical and upper thoracic spine and muscle imbalance is typical consequence of uncompensated sedentary way of life, starting already in school age. Main reference for sagittal plane is so called Frankfort horizontal (line connecting meatus acusticus with the orbital floor or line connecting tragus with the outer eye canthus), see Figure 1. In most subjects this line is inclined forward bellow the space horizontal, in the extensor type of cervical positions is reclined backwards. The real position of Frankfort horizontal can vary more than 20° in the normative population, in comparison, the position of the eyes in frontal plane is held tightly within several degrees only (Harrison & Wojtowicz, 1996).

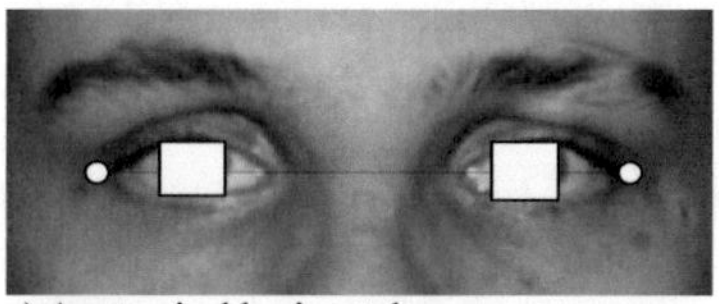
a) Anatomical horizontal

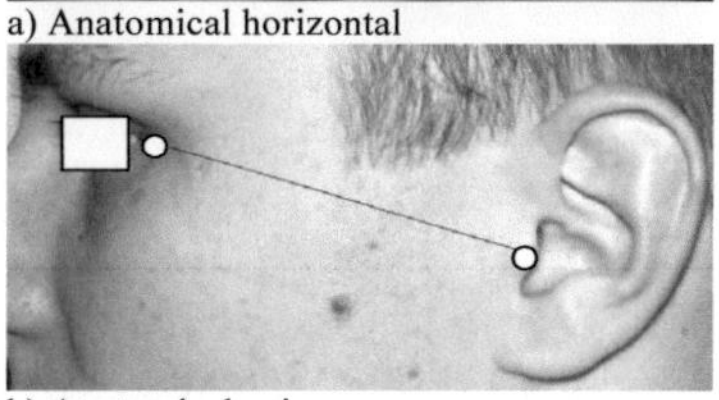
b) Anatomical axis

Fig. 1. Anatomical Frankfort horizontal and axis.

Precise measurement of head position in rehabilitation and physical medicine is important not only for objective diagnosis of the cervical spine abnormalities, but also as a means of cervical kinesthesia assessment. In this test the ability of the tested subject to assume exact position in space without visual clues is examined (Palmgren et al, 2009). Normal subjects are able to attain desired position with precision of several degrees. Again, these differences are below the discrimination capacity of simple observation or protractor measurement. It is hypothesized, that abnormal setting of cervical proprioception can play important role in many conditions like whiplash injury syndrome, chronic tension headache, cervicogennic vertigo, anteflexion headache etc. (Raine & Twomey, 1997). Evidence of abnormal cervical proprioception would be an important step in better understanding of these common clinical problems.

2.2 Monitoring head and shoulders movements

At present, an orthopedic goniometer is the widely used and standard way to simply and rapidly measure angles in clinical practice. However, there are some limitations, especially in case of head and shoulder posture measurement. Due to the combination of three movement components (in the three dimensional space), the measurement using only one goniometer is clearly insufficient. The following overview serves as enumeration of the applications related to the technology available during the last years. This enumeration is not exhaustive but the most important works in the area are included. The methods are typical by using some tools or technology.

Young, 1988, designeda new method to study head position by mirrors. The main principle of new approach is based on using three mirrors and special head markers. The resulting images are taken by one camera. After this, a set of vertical or horizontal lines is drawn with respect to the reference points i.e. markers. The last step is measurement of the relevant angles by a protractor. Head tilt (inclination), head turn (rotation) and chin elevation or depression (flexion/extension) is evaluated. One drawback is the evaluation method based on vertical or horizontal lines defined by reference points, i.e. markers and thus wide variation in cranial configuration found between patients and associated with age.

Murphy et al, 1991, described a system for measuring and recording cranial posture in a dynamic manner. Measurement of the declination and inclination was performed by inclinometers. Inclinometers are widely used instruments for measuring angles of elevation or inclination of an object with respect to gravity based on the accelerometers. Inclinometer was attached to the spectacle rims. Processing of the inclinometer voltages was performed by a modified universal data logger. The inclinometer was calibrated by plastic visor and a perpendicular spirit level. However, principle of the inclinometer does not provide measurement of head rotation.

Ferrario et al, 1994, integrated a method based on the photographic technique, radiographic technique, cephalometric measurements and photographic measurements. The measured subjects were photographed and X-rayed in the same room. The set of standardized marks was traced on all the records. On all photographs, the soft tissues were traced, and the angle between the soft tissue marks and true vertical was calculated. The same angle was calculated on the cephalometric films, and the difference between the two measurements was used to compute the position of the soft and hard tissues. These new values were compared with the values previously observed. The main drawback is exposition of patients to X-ray and relatively time consuming procedures.

Ferrario et al, 1995, developed a new method based on television technology that was faster than conventional analysis. Subject's body and face were identified by 12 points. All subjects were pictured using a standardized technique for frontal views of the total body and lateral views of the neck and face. After 20 seconds of standing, two 2-second films were taken of each subject. On the basis of an image analysis program, the specified angles were calculated after digitizing the recorded films.

Galardi et al, 2003, developed an objective method for measuring posture and voluntary movements in patients with cervical dystonia using Fastrack. Fastrack is commercial widely used electromagnetic system consisting of a stationary transmitter station and four sensors placed on patient's head. The head position in space was reconstructed based on sensor signals and exact values of angles were observed from the axial, sagittal and coronal planes. The drawback is its inaccuracy in determining the exact position in space because of relatively large sensors placed on the patient's head and therefore inaccurate determination of the anatomical axes. Second drawback is the negatively affected accuracy of an electromagnetic system by other laboratory systems.

Hozman et al, 2004, proposed a new method based on the application of three digital cameras placed on a stand and appropriate image processing software. The method was designed for use in neurology to discover relationships between some neurological disorders (such as disorders of vestibular system) and postural head alignment. The objective was to develop a technique for precise head posture measurement or, in other words, for measuring the native position of the head in 3D space. The technique was aimed at determining differences between the anatomical coordinate system (ACS) and the physical coordinate system (PCS). Pictures of the head marked on tragus and outer eye canthus are taken simultaneously by three digital cameras aligned by laser beam. Head position was measured with precision of 0.5° in three planes (rotation-yaw, flexion-pitch and inclination-roll). Hozman et al, 2005, described the new modified system and results are shown and measured on normal subjects. The disadvantage is complicated calibration and the impossibility of a frontal view of the measured subject (Hozman et al, 2007).

Cerny et al, 2006, described second advanced generation of the system. Head position was measured with precision of 0.5° in three planes. Mean values of the head position (100 healthy controls) are : retro flexion 21.7°; inclination to the right 0.2°; head rotation to the left 1.7°.

Meers et al, 2008, developed accurate methods for pinpointing the position of infrared LEDs using an inexpensive USB camera and low-cost algorithms for estimating the 3D coordinates of the LEDs based on known geometry. LEDs are implemented in the frame of eye-glasses. The system is accurate low-cost head-pose tracking system. Experimental results are provided demonstrating a head pose tracking accuracy of less than 0.5° when the user is within one meter from the camera. However, the system does not define the anatomical axis of the head and the adaptation of the system is impossible for measurement of anatomical angles.

Recently a number of instruments and tools based on commercial systems have been developed for evaluating the position of the head and shoulders. An example is Zebris motion analysis system (zebris Medical GmbH). Special instruments primarily allow studying ranges of motion of the head, ranges of motion of the spine and coordination of movement. The modified Zebris also allows studying the movement of the jaw. Zebris detects small misalignment of the lower jaw. The three-dimensional measuring coordinates of the ultrasonic markers can be recorded with an overall scanning rate of 200 measurements per second. The modified system consists of a face bow with integrated receiver module and an optimally balanced mandible which measures sensor close to the mandible joint. Unfortunately, the system also does not define the anatomical axis of the head and the adaptation of the system is complicated.

There are other modified commercial diagnostic systems based on ultrasonic measurement method (sonoSens Monitor), a camera method (Vicon motion systems, LUKOtronic AS100/AS200), a gyro-accelerometer sensors (Xsens motion trackers), etc. But the systems have the similar disadvantages such as complex preparation, very large sensors or the inability to accurately define the anatomical coordinate system.

2.3 Monitoring eye and head movements

Monitoring eye movements and plotting their trajectories have a long tradition in medical practice. The measurement of eye position is an important examination tool in understanding human vestibular system. It is used as a diagnostic tool in neurology and psychology (Brandt et al, 2003). Eye tracking is a widely used method of measuring the point of gaze or the motion of an eye relative to the head. An eye tracker is a device for measuring eye position and movement. There are number of methods of measuring eye movement. Eye trackers fall into three categories:

One type uses an attachment to the eye, such as a special contact lens with an embedded mirror or magnetic field sensor. Measurements with contact lenses have provided extremely sensitive recordings of eye movement. However, mechanical elements attached to the eye can negatively influence patient's eye.

The second category uses electric potentials measured by electrodes placed around the eyes. The eyes are the origin of a steady electric potential field. The electric signal that can be derived using two pairs of contact electrodes placed on the skin around eye is called Electrooculogram (EOG). This EOG is sensitive to the saccadic spike potentials from the ocular muscles. The electric potential field can also be detected in total darkness and if the eyes are closed.

The third category uses non-contact, optical method for measuring eye motion. The method is called Videooculography (VOG). Optical methods are widely used for gaze tracking and are favoured for being non-invasive and inexpensive. By looking to the eye we can see its elements - outer filamentous layer with title sclera, further is cornea, iris and eye pupilla. Light, typically infrared, is reflected from the eye and sensed by a camera. Video based eye trackers usually use the corneal reflection and the centre of the pupil as subjects to track over time. The videooculography based on IR spectrum usually uses the infrared light created by a LED (light emitting diode) diode with a wavelength approximately λ=880-940nm. The VOG method in the IR spectrum detects the pupil using an appropriate light that makes it completely black. The Advantage of this method is relatively easy pupil detection and good quality reflection, most often using an IR LED diode. Disadvantage and limitation is a need to make measurements without access of visible light, i.e. in conditions that do not correspond with patient's real situation.

Eye analysis in the visible light spectrum is far more complicated. The method is called passive, because the eye is scanned in the visible light spectrum due to the diffused visible light. The method without the IR supplementary light is not only safer for the patient (undesirably warms up the eye), but also much more preferable, because it does not necessarily need suppression of background light. Detection can be done due to the sclera and iris interface. Disadvantages of these methods are the uncontrolled lighting from scattered sources, considerable luminous artefacts and high computational power. Also accuracy of these methods is rather poor, because in contrast to the pupil of the eye which is visible during measuring, the interface between sclera and iris is often hidden.

For parallel measurement of head and eye position (Eui et al, 2007) the best way is to use a VOG method that is based on the principle of scanning the eye (Ruian et al, 2006) using a mobile set of video cameras and consequent data post-processing to a different result in IR (infra red) or visible light spectrum (e.g. nystagmogram, fixing the eye to the projected area etc.). The mobile set is then attached to the head position measurement system based, for example, on gyro-accelerometer sensors. This new parallel measurement method has not been systematically studied and bothmentioned measurement methods have been examined only separately.

3. Precise advanced eye, head and shoulders position measurement

Numerous systems for evaluation of eye and upper body parts positions are currently offered on the market, but their wider application is impeded by high financial demands and inaccuracy, because these universal systems are not usually designed for application to study a particular body part - head and shoulders. In the following part of the chapter we will describe the specialized systems designed at CTU Prague and the other labs, to precisely measure the eye, head and shoulders posture at the same time.

3.1 Precise head and shoulders posture measurement

Our new non-invasive head position measurement method was designed for use in neurology to discover relationships between some neurological disorders and postural alignment. The objective was to develop a technique for precise and non-invasive head posture measurement in 3D space. The technique is aimed at determining differences between the anatomical coordinate system and the physical coordinate system with accuracy from one to two degrees for inclination and rotation (Harrison & Wojtowicz, 1996). Pictures or recordings of the head marked on the tragus and the outer eye canthus, see Figure 1, and the shoulders marked on acromions are taken simultaneously by cameras aligned by a laser beam, magnetometers or inertial systems.

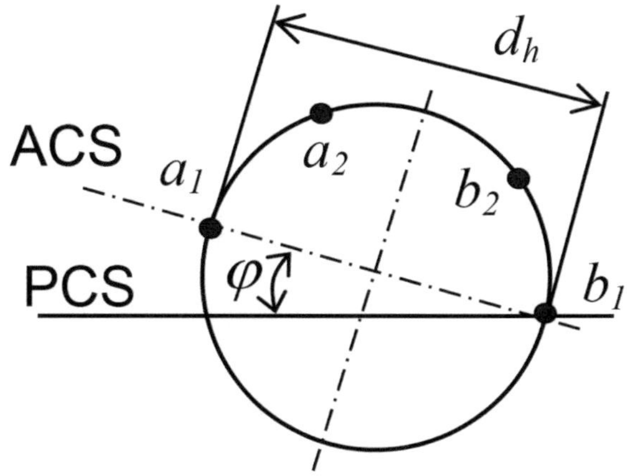

Fig. 2. Geometry used for measuring the head position (top view).

In our recent method for studying only head position (Kutilek & Hozman, 2009), only two cameras are required for determining head positions i.e. anatomical coordinate system in the physical coordinate system. The rotation and inclination of the head is calculated from the difference between the tragus coordinates in the left-profile and right-profile image or eventually in the frontal picture and top view picture of head. The coordinates of the left and right tragus are evaluated by finding the centre of the rounded mark attached to the tragus. After evaluating the coordinates of the tragus in the captured images, the angles of head rotation and inclination are calculated. The images are captured simultaneously, using two cameras, which are calibrated. The adjustment of the camera system defines the position of the head in the instrument coordinate system. The position of the head in the physical coordinate system is determined by special software and the exactly known adjustment of the camera system.

Generally, the angles of rotation and inclination can be determined by vector v and vector u, which represent the coordinates of the points evaluated in the image, see Figure 2. The angle (for example rotation φ) is calculated as follows (1):

$$\varphi = arctg\left(\frac{a_{1y}[px] - b_{1y}[px]}{a_{1x}[px] - b_{1x}[px]}\right) \tag{1}$$

where

$$u = \left(a_{1x}[px], a_{1y}[px]\right), \tag{2}$$

$$v = \left(b_{1x}[px], b_{1y}[px]\right). \tag{3}$$

The a_{1x} is the x-axis coordinate and a_{1y} is the y-axis coordinate of the left tragus in the top view image. The b_{1x} is the x-axis coordinate and b_{1y} is the y-axis coordinate of the right tragus in top view image. We can determine the angle of inclination σ in the similar way in the frontal view image. After calculation of the angles in the instrument coordinate system, the angles in physical coordinate system are derived by mathematical transformation.

If we use profile photographs (side shots) and want to evaluate the elevation/depression of the head in the instrument coordinate system and sagittal plane, it is also a mathematically simple problem. The flexion value is measured relatively as the inclination of the connecting line between the coordinates of tragus and the exterior eye corner. The coordinates are evaluated by finding the centre of the rounded mark attached to the tragus and outer eye canthus of the patient. The angle between the anatomical and physical or instrument horizontal (depends on adjustment of instrument) is determined by the angle between vector v (horizontal vector), here given by the camera position, and vector u, which here represents the coordinates of the points (corresponding to the tragus marker and exterior eye corner marker) evaluated in the image. The angle is calculated as follows (4):

$$\omega = \arccos\left(\frac{\vec{u} \cdot \vec{v}}{|\vec{u}| \cdot |\vec{v}|}\right) = \arccos\left(\frac{u_x \cdot v_x + u_y \cdot v_y}{\sqrt{u_x^2 + u_y^2} \cdot \sqrt{v_x^2 + v_y^2}}\right) \tag{4}$$

where

$$u = \left(a_{1x}\left[px\right] - a_{2x}\left[px\right], a_{1y}\left[px\right] - a_{2y}\left[px\right]\right), \tag{5}$$

$$v = (1,0). \tag{6}$$

a_{1x} is the x-axis coordinate and a_{1y} is the y-axis coordinate of the tragus in the profile image, and a_{2x} is the x-axis coordinate and a_{2y} is the y-axis coordinate of the outer eye canthus in the profile image.

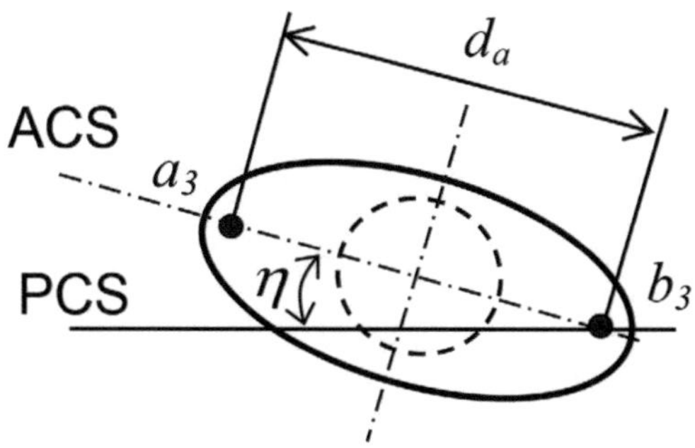

Fig. 3. Geometry used for measuring the shoulder position (top view).

For evaluating shoulder inclination and shoulder rotation, we use a method similar to the method that we use for evaluating head position. Picture of acromions on shoulders is taken by cameras. A medical doctor indicates acromions with marks for easy location of these anatomical points in the pictures. If the clinical investigation is carried out by an experienced medical doctor, it is not necessary to apply coloured marks to the anatomical parts of the body before making an examination using camera system. The software can also determine the angular displacement of the head to the shoulders for rotation, using the formula

$$\kappa = \eta - \varphi \tag{7}$$

where the η is angle of shoulders rotation (Figure 3) and φ is angle of head rotation (Figure 2). The angular displacement of the head to the shoulders for inclination

$$\lambda = \zeta - \sigma \tag{8}$$

where the ζ is angle of shoulders inclination and σ is angle of head inclination.

In the way described above, based on identifying anatomical points with the use of two cameras (Figure 4) we can avoid influencing patients while we are measuring the inclination (roll), flexion (pitch) and rotation (yaw) of the head and shoulders.

The last proposed system is a combination of camera and gyroscope-accelerometer system. One camera is placed vertically above the patient's head. The second camera is positioned behind the patient in order not to impede the frontal view of the patient during the examination. Shoulders are marked in 3D space by a two IR diodes. Position of the two anatomical points (acromions) on the shoulders is defined by the two IR diodes. Diodes are placed on patient's shoulders by the physician before the examination. The position of head's anatomical coordinate system is defined by a special instrument, see Figure 5. A physician puts the instrument on patient's head. The physician defines the position of the anatomical axes of the head by a special ruler on the instrument. Position of the head is defined by the two IR light diodes mounted on the instrument and gyroscope-accelerometer system. Rotation and inclination is then determined from the position of two infrared diodes mounted on the instrument and by two cameras. Flexion/extension is determined by accurate gyroscope-accelerometer system made by the company TRIVISIO, which is also part of the special instrument. The proposed special instrument is in Figure 5.

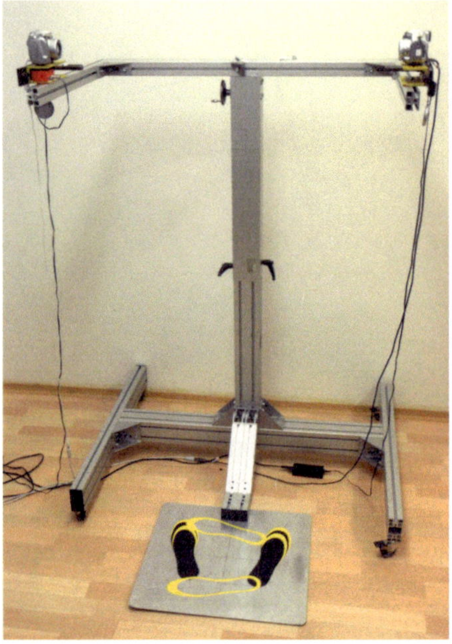

Fig. 4. The two-arm stand with fixed two cameras and laser collimators designed for the precise adjustment of the system.

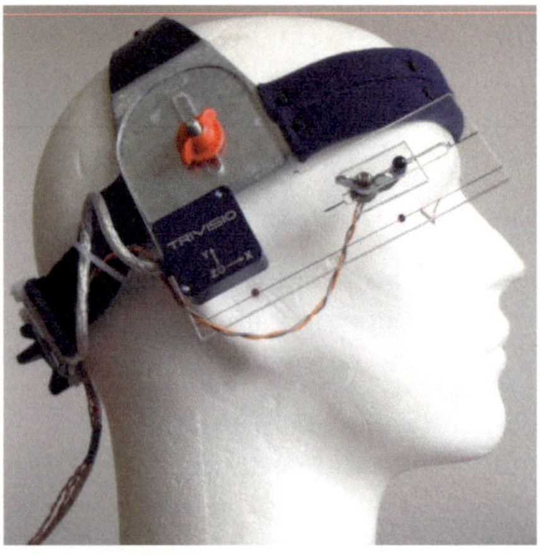

Fig. 5. Combined inertial system with infrared marker for detecting the position by IR camera system.

3.2 Measurement of eye and head position

Despite the fact that an accurate method for measuring the head position and the eye position could contribute to diagnosis of vestibular system, this issue has not been systematically studied (Hozman et al, 2008).

Horizontal and vertical eye movements can be measured by an image of the eye (Moore et al, 2006) by detecting the edges of the pupil (iris) and fitting them into an ellipse (Li, 2006). The main aim of the analysis of eye movements is to obtain the centre of the pupil or the iris. The torsion measurement needs high quality iris description. The video system PAL (NTSC) record video with frequency 50 Hz (60 Hz) non-interlace. These video systems are too slow to capture images of the eye movements, e.g. torsion iris description. In medical practice documented eye movements were with frequency approximately 200–250 Hz. These movements present angular change approximately 400 - 450 °/s.

We used the detection method which searches interface points between the pupil and the iris or between the iris and the sclera. The points are base of the mathematical function (e.g. circle or ellipse). Goal of our solution is to use eye movements' detection in comparison with the stimulation scene. The scene can be showed on the LCD screen or through the special HMD display unit in 2D or 3D space.

We used a new system based on finding the outline pupil of the eye. We applied modified Starburst (Duchowski et al, 2009) algorithm (Ruian et al, 2006), which we used in the IR spectrum or in the visible spectrum. The system and algorithm was first published by Iowa University in 2006 (Li, 2006). Thanks to the special 3D HMD projection displays we used Starburst algorithm for measuring in the IR spectrum and appropriate LED diode to illuminate the eye. The method is called active, because the eye is scanned in the infra red spectrum. Goal of eye movements' measurement was location of the centre of the pupil area. Method of finding the margins of the pupil (IR spectrum) or the iris (visible spectrum) is limited by quantity of the rays. The starting point shoots the rays to generate candidate pupil points. The candidate pupil points shoot rays back towards the start point to detect more candidate pupil points. This two-stage detection method takes advantage of the elliptical profile of the pupil contour to preferentially detect features on the pupil contour.

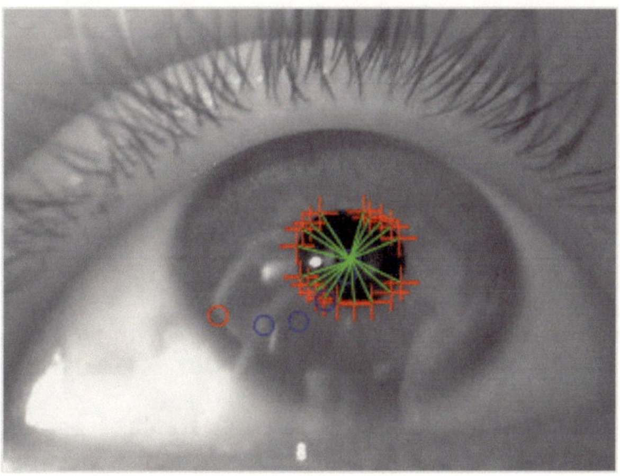

Fig. 6. Location of the pupil center with the rays.

The circle (see Figure 6) shows the centre of the pupil after the second iteration (and after the next iteration) and includes determined points. The iteration to find the centre of the pupil was stopped when the detected centre of the new points turned less than d=10 pixels. Thanks to exponential calculation the error of the pupil centre is about ±10 pixels of the whole circle bearings and it is important from the point of view of the found points´ fit resulting ellipse. At the end, we can find centre of the pupil from the resulting ellipse.

There are more possible methods how we can put together the resulting ellipse. We chose method (Ruian et al, 2006) Random Sample Consensus (RANSAC) to solve the problem with large error points (Lee & Park, 2009). The method RANSAC is an efficient technique for completion of the model in the presence of large, but unknown percentage outlines in sample measurement. In our case all internal found points are probable points that correspond with outline of the pupil. RANSAC algorithm was used to estimate parameters of the mathematical model from a set of observed data which contains outliers. On the basis of the MATLAB documentation we used optimal mathematical model to create the ellipse - Nelder-Mead's algorithm.

For the eye stimulation we used commercial HMD system eMagin Z800 3DVisor personal display with integrated head tracker which can measure head position in the 3D space. The Z800 3DVisor is the personal display system to combine two OLED (organic light-emitting diode) micro displays with stereovision 3D capabilities. Stereo vision refers to the human ability to see in three dimensions and most often refers to depth perception (the ability to determine the approximate distance of objects). Stereovision 3D provides this experience by delivering two distinct images simultaneously on two separate screens, one for each eye. The Z800 3DVisor personal display is used to stimulate the eye in 2D or 3D space. The position of eye and the position of head can be recorded simultaneously by the video camera and integrated head tracker to the laptop.

The HMD displays eMagin Z800 3DVisor's integrated head tracker uses MEMS (micro-electro-mechanical system) accelerometers and gyroscopes to detect motion. The head tracker features three gyroscopes, one each for the x-, y-, and z-axis. In addition, the head tracker contains corresponding compasses and accelerometers to ensure performance over varying forms of motion. Such equipment has not been used before in medical practice. From the point of view of contemporary technology there is a possibility to use more accurate miniature 3D inertial measurement unit/motion sensors (IMU) with accelerometer, magnetometer and gyroscope (for example Xsens motion technologies) and custom made Head Mounted Display (HMD). We used the head tracker for the measurement of head position.

For acquisition of the head motion we programmed special software based on Z800 3DVisor SDK 2.2. The software retrieves position of the head from the build-in head tracker through the USB connection and saves the measured results in to the CSV (comma-separated values) file. The result of measurement can be presented graphically as a graph of the head position. By this set we are able to measure eye and head movements continuously and simultaneously.

During the measurement problematic parts had to be solved before the next biomedical tests. The problems were with weight, sharp edges on the semi-permeable mirrors and minimal place between personal display Z800 3DVisor and the eyes.

On the previous base type we made the new projection displays, which allowed tracing projection on the LCD monitor or the projection screen in visible spectrum. Detection algorithm can measure the eye position and the scene position. The video files of positions are merged into the date file. The second version of projection displays has lower weight, does not contain any sharp edges and includes the cameras, which are connected with the help of USB (Universal Serial Bus) interface and does not use any special recorder. Power supply is solved over the USB port. We used record software TVideoGrabber. The software TVideoGrabber can set capture parameters (30 FPS – Frames Per Second, 640 x 480 pixels, RGB24, data format AVI). We used an external flash from photographic apparatus for synchronisation between two cameras (In the future we will use the TVideoGrabber component with more threads. The threads will start recording from several video sources at the same time).

The next type of our projection displays is designated for measuring in the IR spectrum. The third projection displays use the IR USB cameras which record eye movements. The type of these projection displays must use cameras which support eye movements scans in the IR spectrum because lighting is already poor. This type of projection displays combines a unique system for measuring eye movements and head position with 2D or 3D stimulation.

The specialized glasses - projection displays for neurological examination can be used without the LCD monitor thanks to build-in HMD 3D projections displays eMagin Z800 3DVisor. These projections displays can be used as a mobile system as well.. We use experimental systems for monitoring eye movements with different luminous conditions (in the visible spectrum or in the IR spectrum) or using different stimulation sources (e.g. record eye movements at specific activities - „eye Holter", long time eye movements record, 2D and 3D stimulation et al.).

4. Interpretation and evaluation of eye, head and shoulders position

For analysis of the positions we use simple methods based on combination of the basic methods of evaluation of individual body parts. Below we describe methods for accurate interpretation of the measured data. Given that the systems provide the processed data, the assessment is simple for physicians. Physicians only need to observe the conditions of measurement, such as the precise adjustment of the system before the measurement. They also need to respect the maximum certified accuracy of systems.

4.1 Evaluation of head and shoulders position

It is mathematically a simple problem to determine the inclination, rotation and flexion/extension of the head from photographs and by gyro-accelerometer sensor. The angle values are measured and transformed automatically to physical coordinate system. The measurement process is usually carried out according to a predefined procedure to be followed, see Figure 7. The process is based on two main steps/parts of measurement and computational algorithm. First part of algorithm is designed for the precise adjustment of the system. The second part is intended to measure patient's body segments and to calculate of the angles in physical coordinate system.

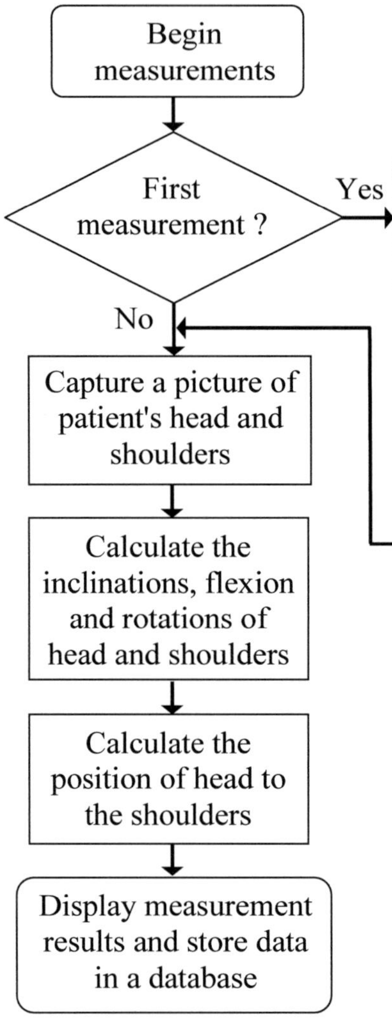

Fig. 7. Flowchart of clinical measurements using designed camera system.

The described systems provide direct information for physicians on the current position of the patient's head and patient's shoulders represented by the angles. There is no further information processing and the physician may use the data to evaluate patient's health. The designed systems measure head position with precision of 0,5° (Hozman et al, 2008) in three planes (rotation -yaw, flexion-pitch and inclination-roll). Our experimental measurement of the head position was completed with measurement of subjective perception of vertical (SPV). The subject tried to align a needle to vertical position when peering into white sphere. Final angle of the needle was measured. The measured data shows that healthy subject holds his head aligned with physical coordinate system in the range of ±5 degrees for inclination. The set of data was measured on recruited volunteers. The results also predict that there is a correlation between values of inclination and SPV.

4.2 Eye and head movement analysis

The Goal of our new designed methods is to use eye movements' detection together with the stimulation scene. Thanks to the special 3D HMD projection displays, we used Starburst algorithm for measuring in the IR spectrum and appropriate LED diode for illumination of the eye (Charfreitag et al, 2008). The Goal of the eye movements' measurement was to locate the centre of the pupil area (Stampe, 1993). We used a new system based on finding the contour line of the pupil of the eye. Finally, at the end, we can find the centre of the pupil from the resulting ellipse at the camera coordinate system i.e. shots, see Figure 8.

The second part was to use the headtracker to measure the head position. The first measured values were used as initial, i.e. zero and were used as correction for all subsequent values. The new systems provide direct information for physicians on the current position of the pupil centre represented by pixels or millimetres and patient's head represented by three angles, see Figure 9. There is no further information processing and the physician may use the data to evaluate patient's health. The head position was measured by modified 3D HMD (Z800 3DVisor) with precision of 1.0° in three planes (Charfreitag et al, 2009). Thus, we can study the three dimensional motion of head defined by three angles - inclination, rotation and flexion/extension. By this method we can also study, analyze and measure eye and head movements continuously and simultaneously.

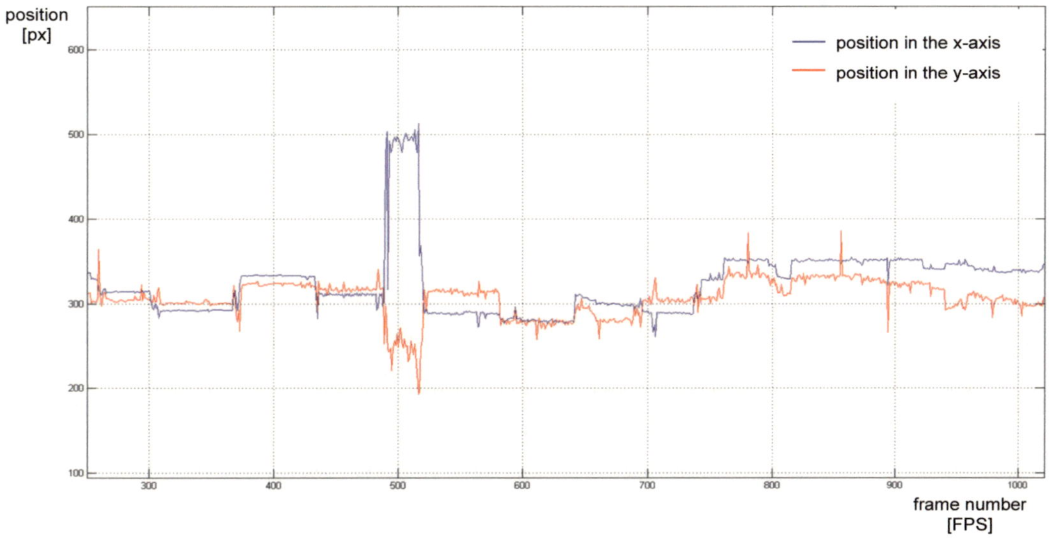

Fig. 8. Example of graph of pupil center movements

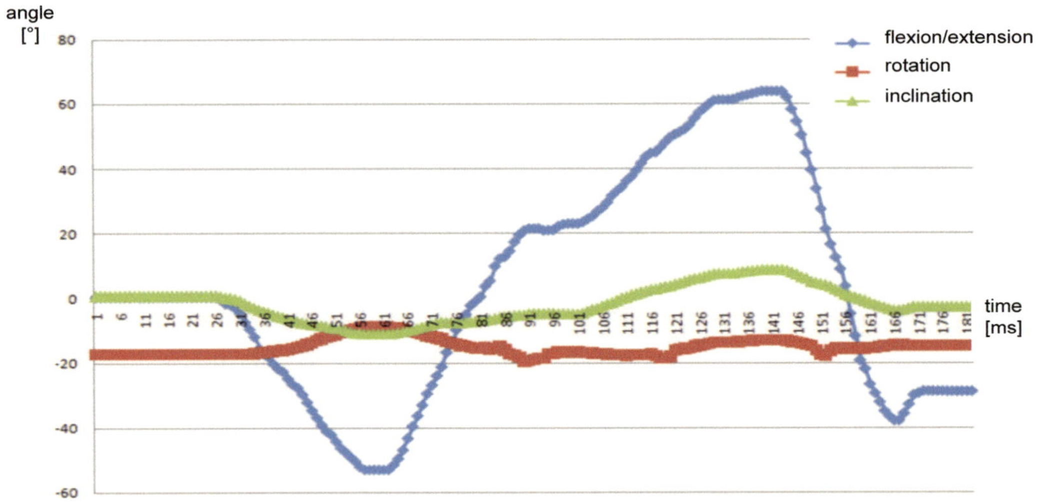

Fig. 9. Example of graph of head movements

5. Conclusion

In this chapter we have described related works and designed special equipment and measurement methods for very accurate evaluation of eye, head and shoulder position in neurological practice. Possible applications and perspectives for clinical practice are also described in the chapter.

We have described systems and sets of procedures for evaluation of the inclination, flexion and rotation of the head and the inclination and rotation of the shoulders with resolution and accuracy to 2°. This accuracy is the minimum accuracy required in clinical practice. The described ways of measuring and evaluating eye, head and shoulder positions could also be applied in other areas of medicine and science.

Our designed systems are based on cameras or/ possibly on gyro-accelerometer (inertial) sensors. The new two or three camera equipment designed to measure the head and shoulders positions is cheaper and more accurate than sophisticated systems which use accelerometers and magnetometers. The second advantage of our camera system over conventional and commercial systems such as Zebris motion analysis system (zebris Medical GmbH), LUKOtronic AS100/AS200 (Lukotronic Lutz-Kovacs-Electronics Oeg.) or sonoSens Monitor (sensomotion, Inc.) is that it can measure a patient without the influence of mechanical elements on patient's body segments or that the system allows direct detection of anatomical axes of patient's head and shoulders, which cannot be done when using current systems (Hozman et al, 2005). The systems based on two cameras have cameras placed on both sides (lateral profiles) or in front and above the patient. This is a very important advantage for medical doctors, because they can make various examinations which require open space in front of the face. Our systems based on combination of infrared cameras and inertial systems are also sufficient and more accurate and cheaper than commercial systems for broader use than just to analyze the position of the head and shoulders.

The measurement results of mean values of the head position being (100 healthy controls): retro flexion 21.7°; inclination to the right 0.2°; head rotation to the left 1.7°. The rotation measurement has a greater error in comparison with the inclination and flexion/extension measurement (Kutilek & Hozman, 2009).

We have also described related systems and designed system for monitoring eye movements. Our equipment designed for measurement of the eye and head movements is based on display units - specialized glasses with eMagin 3DVisor. We modified the specialized projection displays for neurological examination which can perform measurements using a variable set of visual stimuli and active head movements. The solution combines system for measurement of the eye movements and the head posture in the 3D space with 2D or 3D eye stimulation. We came to the conclusion that it is possible to join together the two important and closely related methods for the measurement of the human vestibular system.

A result of this study is the recommendation to use the video cameras with higher frequency (approximately 200 Hz) for the measurement of eye movements and the head tracker with lower dynamic error (less than 0.3°/s) for the measurement of head position. The overall accuracy of our designed system could increase significantly because the accuracy of the method alone is in eights of degree per the ten measurements. This is the dynamic error due to the low-cost head tracker which needs long time to stabilise after the previous measurement.

Above described and designed ways of measuring eye, head and shoulder position and motion could also be applied in other areas of engineering, medicine and science. Our systems can be used anywhere to study the posture of a person.

6. Acknowledgment

The work presented here was carried out at the Czech Technical University in Prague, Faculty of Biomedical Engineering within the framework of research program No. MSM 6840770012 "Transdisciplinary Biomedical Engineering Research II" of the Czech Technical University, sponsored by the Ministry of Education, Youth and Sports of the Czech Republic.

7. References

Brandt, T., Cohen, B., Siebold, Ch. (2003). *The Oculomotor and Vestibular Systems: Their Function and Disorders*, Vol. 1004, Ann. N.Y. Acad. Sci.

Brandt T., Dieterich M. (1994). Vestibular Syndromes in the Roll Plane: Topographic Diagnosis from Brain Stem to Cortex, *Annals of Neurology*, Vol. 36, pp. 337–347.

Cerny R., Strohm K., Hozman J., Stoklasa J., Sturm D. (2006). Head in Space - Noninvasive Measurement of Head Posture, *The 11th Danube Symposium - International Otorhinolaryngological Congress*, Bled, pp. 39-42.

Cerny R., Hozman J., Charfreitag J., Kutílek P. (2009). Position of the head measured by digital photograph analysis, *World Congress on Medical Physics and Biomedical*

Engineering, September 7 - 12, 2009, Munich, Germany [CD-ROM]. Berlin: Springer Science+Business Media , p. 562-565. ISBN 978-3-642-03881-5.

Charfreitag J., Hozman J., Cerny R. (2009). Measurement of eye and head position in neurological practice, *World Congress on Medical Physics and Biomedical Engineering*, September 7 - 12, 2009, Munich, Germany [CD-ROM]. Berlin: Springer Science+Business Media, p. 57-60. ISBN 978-3-642-03881-5.

Charfreitag J., Hozman J., Černý R. (2008). Specialized glasses - projection displays for neurology investigation, *IFMBE Proceedings*, Berlin: Springer, 2008, Vol. 1, p. 97-101. ISBN 978-3-540-89207-6.

Duchowski A. T., Medlin E., Cournia N. A., Murphy H. A., Gramopadhye A. K., Nair S. N., Vorah J., Melloy B. J. (2002). 3D Eye Movement Analysis, *Behavior Research Methods, Instruments, & Computers*, Vol. 34, No. 4 , pp. 18.

Galardi G., Micera S., Carpaneto J., Scolari S., Gambini M., Dario P. (2003). Automated Assessment of Cervical Dystonia, *Movement Disorders*, Vol. 18, No. 11, pp. 1358-1367.

Gräf M., Droutsas K., Kaufmann H. (2001). Surgery for nystagmus related head turn: Kestenbaum procedure and artificial divergence, *Graefes Arch Clin Exp Ophthalmol*, Vol. 239, No. 5, pp. 334–341. doi:10.1007/s004170100270.

Harrison A., Wojtowicz G. (1996). Clinical Measurement of Head and Shoulder Posture Variables, *The Journal of Orthopaedic & Amp; Sports Physical Therapy (JOSPT)*, Vol. 23, pp. 353-361.

Hozman J., Sturm D., Stoklasa J. (2004). Measurement of Head Position in Neurological Practice, *Biomedical Engineering*, Zürich: Acta Press, p. 586-589. ISBN 0-88986-379-2.

Hozman J., Kutílek P., Szabó Z., Krupička R., Jiřina M. (2008). Digital Wireless Craniocorpography with Sidelong Scanning by TV Fisheye Camera, *IFMBE Proceedings*, Berlin: Springer, Vol. 1, pp. 102-105. ISBN 978-3-540-89207-6.

Hozman J., Sturm D., Stoklasa J., Cerny R. (2005). Measurement of Postural Head Alignment in Neurological Practice, *The 3rd European Medical and Biological Engineering Conference - EMBEC´05*, Society of Biomedical Engineering and Medical Informatics of the Czech Medical Association JEP, Vol. 11, Prague, pp. 4229-4232.

Hozman J., Zanchi V., Cerny R., Marsalek P., Szabo Z. (2007). Precise Advanced Head Posture Measurement, *The 3rd WSEAS International Conference on Remote Sensing (REMOTE´07)*, WSEAS Press, pp. 18-26.

Eui C. L., Kang R. P. (2007). *A robust eye gaze tracking method based on a virtual eyeball model*, Soul: Electronic Engineering of Yonsei University

Ferrario V., Sforza C., Germann D., Dalloca L., Miani A. (1994). Head Posture and Cephalometric Analyses: An Integrated Photographic/ Radiographic Technique, *American Journal of Orthodontics & Dentofacial Orthopedics*, Vol. 106, pp. 257-264.

Ferrario V., Sforza C., Tartaglia G., Barbini E., Michielon G. (1995). New Television Technique for Natural Head and Body Posture Analysis, *Cranio*, Vol. 13, pp. 247-255.

Halmagyi M. G., Curthoys I. S., Brandt T., Dieterich M. (1991). Ocular Tilt Reaction: Clinical Sign of Vestibular Lesion, *Acta Otolaryngologica*, Suppl. 481, pp. 47-50.

Kutilek P., Hozman J. (2009). Non-contact method for measurement of head posture by two cameras and calibration means, *The 8th Czech-Slovak Conference on Trends in Biomedical Engineering*, Bratislava, pp. 51-54, ISBN 978-80-227-3105-8

Lee J. J., Park K. R., Kim J. H., (2003). Gaze detection system under HMD environment for user interface, *Joint International conference ICANN/ICONIP 2003*, Istanbul, pp. 512-515.

Lee E. C., Park K. R. (2009). A robust eye gaze tracking method based on a virtual eyeball model, *Machine Vision and Applications*, Vol. 20, No. 5, pp. 319-337.

Li D. (2006) *Low-cost eye-tracking for human computer interaction*, Master's thesis, Iowa: Iowa State University

Meers S., Ward K., Piper I. (2006). Robust and Accurate Head-Pose Tracking Using a Single Camera, *Mechatronics and Machine Vision in Practice*, Berlin: Springer Science + Business Media, pp. 111-122, ISBN 978-3-540-74026-1.

Moore S., Curthoys I., Haslwanter T., Halmagyi M. (2006). *Measuring Three-Dimensional Eye Position Using Image Processint – The VTM System*, Sydney: Department of Psychology, University of Sydney

Murphy K., Preston Ch., Evans W. (1991). The Development of Instrumentation for the Dynamic Measurement of Changing Head Posture, *American Journal of Orthodontics and Dentofacial Orthopedics*, Vol. 99, No. 6, pp. 520-526.

Novak I., Campbell L., Boyce M., Fung V. S. (2010). Botulinum Toxin Assessment, Intervention and Aftercare for Cervical Dystonia and other Causes of Hypertonia of the Neck : International Consensus Statement, *European Journal of Neurology*, Vol. 17, Suppl. 2, pp. 94-108.

Nucci P., Kushner J. B., Serafino M, Orzalesi N. (2005). A Multi-Disciplinary Study of the Ocular, Orthopedic, and Neurologic Causes of Abnormal Head Postures in Children, *American Journal of Ophthalmology*, Vol. 140, pp. 65-68.

Palmgren P.J., Andreasson D., Eriksson M., Hägglund A. (2009). Cervicocephalic Kinesthetic Sensibility and Postural Balance in Patients with Nontraumatic Chronic Neck Pain – a Pilot Study, *Chiropractic & Osteopathy*, Vol. 17, No. 6, doi:10.1186/1746-1340-17-6

Raine S., Twomey L.T. (1997). Head and Shoulder Posture Variations in 160 Asymptomatic Women and Men, *Archives of Physical Medicine and Rehabilitation*, Vol. 78, No. Nov., pp. 1215-1223.

Ruian L., Shijiu J., Xiaorong W. (2006). *Single Camera Remote Eye Gaze Tracking Under Natural Head Movements*, Tianjin: College of Physics and Electronic Information Science, Tianjin Normal University

Stampe D. M. (1993). Heuristic filtering and reliable calibration methods for video-based pupil tracking systems, *Behavior Research Methods, Instruments and Computers*, Vol. 25, No. 2, pp. 137-142.

Young, J. D. (1988). Head Posture Measurement, *Journal of Pediatric Ophthalmology and Strabismus*, Vol. 25, No.2, pp. 86-89.

3

Mesenchymal Stromal Cells to Treat Brain Injury

Ciara C. Tate and Casey C. Case
SanBio, Inc., Mountain View, California
USA

1. Introduction

Brain injury occurs from either a traumatic (mechanical), ischemic (decreased oxygen; accounts for 83% of stroke cases), or hemorrhagic (ruptured blood vessel; accounts for 17% of stroke cases) insult to the brain. Stroke and traumatic brain injury (TBI) are major contributors worldwide to both deaths and persistent disabilities. Stroke is the third leading cause of death (behind heart disease and cancer) in the United States, with 137,000 Americans dying from stroke each year (Heron *et al.*, 2009). Stroke is the leading cause of serious, long-term disability in the United States. Currently, 795,000 people have a stroke each year and 15-30% of survivors have a permanent disability (Roger *et al.*, 2011). Annually, 1.7 million people sustain a TBI in the United States, resulting in 52,000 deaths and over 124,000 permanent disabilities each year (Faul *et al.*, 2010). Annual direct (e.g., medical) and indirect (e.g., loss of productivity) costs to the United States are $41 billion and $60 billion for stroke and TBI, respectively (Finkelstein *et al.*, 2006; Roger *et al.*, 2011).

Though the etiology differs between traumatic and ischemic injury, there are many similarities in their pathology (Bramlett & Dietrich, 2004; Leker & Shohami, 2002). The primary insult initiates a cascade of secondary events such as edema, excitotoxicity, and increases in free radicals, which act to spread the injury to surrounding tissue (for reviews of the pathology, see Greve & Zink, 2009 for TBI and Mitsios *et al.*, 2006 for ischemic stroke). Note that ischemia is part of the secondary injury response for TBI (Coles, 2004; Garnett *et al.*, 2001). The brain attempts to repair and regenerate, but depending on such factors as injury severity, age of onset, and prior injuries, these endogenous attempts are often insufficient to restore normal function. A treatment that limits the spread of secondary damage and/or promotes repair and regeneration is needed. Current clinical treatment practices for TBI primarily aim to reduce intracranial pressure in an effort to minimize brain damage caused by swelling. For ischemic stroke, the only FDA-approved treatment is breaking down blood clots with tissue plasminogen activator. However, patients must meet strict criteria for receiving this therapy, including a 4 hour time window and no evidence of the following: bleeding, a severely elevated blood pressure or blood sugar, recent surgery, low platelet count, or end-stage liver or kidney disorders. Numerous pharmacological treatments that seemed promising in animal models have failed in clinical trials (Maas *et al.*, 2010; O'Collins *et al.*, 2006). Patients with brain injury vary widely with respect to demographics, severity of injury, location of injury, and co-morbidity factors making clinical trials challenging. Most treatments previously tested involved pathways that are both deleterious and beneficial, making the dosage and timing critical to not interfere with normal homeostasis or reparative mechanisms in the brain. Furthermore, these treatments targeted single mechanisms, which may not be enough in light of the multi-faceted pathology. Therapies that currently seem more promising, such as progesterone administration (Wright *et al.*, 2007) and cell transplantation, address multiple pathological events.

2. Mesenchymal stromal cells to treat brain injury

2.1 Mesenchymal stromal cells (MSCs)

Mesenchymal stem cells are multipotent cells that can differentiate into cells of the mesoderm germ layer. These cells can be isolated from adipose tissue, amniotic fluid, placenta and umbilical cord, though are most commonly and efficiently derived from adult bone marrow. Marrow-derived cells that adhere to tissue-culture plastic *in vitro* are a heterogeneous population of cells that contain mesenchymal stem cells, but the entire population is more correctly defined as mesenchymal stromal cells (Horwitz *et al.*, 2005). As we learn more about these cell populations, the terminology evolves and the acronym MSC is used (and sometimes misused) for mesenchymal stem cell, mesenchymal stromal cell, multipotent stromal cell, and marrow stromal cell. For the purposes of this chapter, we will not distinguish amongst these cell populations and use MSC as a general acronym.

2.2 Using MSCs to treat brain injury

MSCs are an attractive cell source for transplantation because they are relatively easy to obtain, expand, and manipulate *in vitro*. In addition, adult human MSCs do not have the tumorigenicity risks that pluripotent cells carry. Ample preclinical data demonstrate that MSC transplantation promotes functional recovery following experimental cerebral ischemic or TBI (for review, see Li & Chopp, 2009 or Parr *et al.*, 2007). Autologous MSC therapy has already shown promise for treating clinical stroke (Battistella *et al.*, 2011; Honmou *et al.*, 2011; Lee *et al.*, 2010; Suarez-Monteagudo *et al.*, 2009) and TBI (Cox *et al.*, 2011; Zhang *et al.*, 2008). Collectively, these trials demonstrate that transplanting MSCs either intra-arterially, intravenously, or intracerebrally is safe and no cell-related adverse events were reported. These groups also indicate that some patients receiving MSCs had improved functional outcome; however, these hints at efficacy must be cautiously interpreted because these were primarily safety trials and were not designed to show robust efficacy.

Important considerations for using MSCs in the clinic include timing (acute versus chronic), delivery route (most commonly intravenous, intra-arterial, or intracerebral), and donor source (autologous versus allogeneic). There are advantages and disadvantages for each of these issues, which are outlined in Table 1. According to www.clinicaltrials.gov (searched in August 2011; summarized in Table 2), there are 11 ongoing clinical trials worldwide using MSCs (either primary or derivatives) to treat stroke. Of these 11 studies, 5 are using autologous MSCs and the other 6 are using allogeneic MSCs from either bone marrow, placenta (1 study) or umbilical cord (1 study). Two of the trials are injecting cells directly into the injured brain (either into the injury cavity or the peri-infarct tissue), 1 trial is injecting cells into the carotid artery, and the other 8 are injecting MSCs intravenously. With regard to timing, 2 of the trials are delivering the cells during the acute phase (within 72 hours post-stroke), 7 trials during the sub-acute phase (between 4 days and 6 weeks post-stroke), and 2 studies are delivering cells during the chronic phase (over 6 months post-stroke). As trials more definitively reveal that MSCs transplantation is both safe and effective for treating brain injury in humans, issues of delivery timing and route and donor source, as well as dosage and the use of immunosuppression will need to be more carefully compared.

Issue	Options	Advantages	Disadvantages
Timing	**Acute phase**	supports neuroprotection	volatile environment
			strict timing may limit availability
	Chronic phase	supports regeneration	endogenous regeneration efforts are stabilized
		easier to distinguish between effects of cell therapy and normal recovery	
		targets larger patient population	
Delivery	**Intravenous or Intra-arterial**	less invasive	cells accumulate in the lungs and spleen
		cells home to site of injury	requires high cell numbers
			possible systemic effects
			requires blood brain barrier permeability (thus limits time window)
	Intracerebral	cells placed at site of injury	more invasive
			extent and location of injury is variable
Donor Source	**Autologous**	immunocompatible	patients undergo additional procedures
	Allogeneic	MSCs are immunoprivileged	may require immunosuppression
		more cost-effective	requires storage of cell product
		better for repeat dosing	
		off-the-shelf treatment	
		cells can be manipulated *ex vivo* without treatment delays	

Table 1. Clinical considerations for using MSCs to treat brain injury

Sponsor	Country	Start Date	Phase	# Px	Donor	Cell Description	Route	Timing (post-stroke)	Follow-up	clinicaltrials.gov ID
National Cardiovascular Center	Japan	2008-May	I/IIa	12	Auto	Bone marrow mononuclear cells	IV	7-10 days	30 days	NCT01028794
CellMed AG, a subsidiary of BTG plc.	Germany	2008-October	I/II	20	Allo	GLP-1 CellBeads: alginate microcapsules with mesenchymal cells transfected to secrete glucagon like peptide-1	IC	acute	6 months	NCT01298830
University of Texas Health Science Center	USA	2009-January	I	30	Auto	Bone marrow mononuclear cells	IV	24-72 hours	5 years	NCT00859014
University of California, Irvine	USA	2010-January	I	33	Auto	Bone marrow mononuclear cells OR Cultured marrow mesenchymal stromal cells	IV	Mononuclear: 4 days; Mesenchymal: 23 days	90 days	NCT00908856
University Hospital, Grenoble	France	2010-August	II	30	Auto	Mesenchymal stem cells	IV	Up to 6 weeks	24 months	NCT00875654
Stempeutics Research Pvt. Ltd.	Malaysia	2010-December	I/II	78	Allo	Cultured adult mesenchymal stem cells	IV	Up to 10 days	12 months	NCT01091701
SanBio, Inc.	USA	2011-January	I/IIa	18	Allo	SB623: modified marrow stromal cells	IC	6-24 months	24 months	NCT01287936
Stemedica Cell Technologies, Inc.	USA	2011-February	I/II	35	Allo	Adult mesenchymal bone marrow stem cells	IV	Beyond 6 months	12 months	NCT01297413
Celgene Corporation	USA	2011-March	IIa	44	Allo	Human placenta-derived cells PDA001-(cenplacel-L)	IV	1 OR 1 and 8 days	24 months	NCT01310114
Aldagen	USA	2011-March	II	100	Auto	ALD-401: derived from bone marrow	IA	13-19 days	12 months	NCT01273337
General Hospital of Chinese Armed Police Forces	China	2011-April	II	120	Allo	Umbilical cord mesenchymal stem cells	IV	1st TP: 10-21 days (hemorrhage) OR 7-24 days (ischemic); 2nd TP: lumbar puncture 7d after 1st TP	12 months	NCT01389453

Px= planned number of patients to enroll; Auto=autologous; Allo=allogeneic; IV=intravenously; IC=intracerebral (cavity or peri-infarct tissue); IA=intra-arterial (carotid); TP=transplant

Table 2. Ongoing clinical trials for using MSCs to treat stroke

3. Mechanisms of action underlying beneficial effects

Transplanting stem cells is attractive because they can potentially differentiate into multiple cell types and replace cells lost to injury or disease. MSCs normally give rise to cells along the mesodermal lineage (including bone, cartilage, and adipose tissue); however, there are reports suggesting that they can transdifferentiate into neural cells in certain *in vitro* (Sanchez-Ramos *et al.*, 2000; Woodbury *et al.*, 2000) and *in vivo* (Kopen *et al.*, 1999; Munoz-Elias *et al.*, 2004) environments. Though some studies show a small percentage of donor MSCs express neuronal markers in the injured brain, there is little evidence that these cells functionally incorporate into the endogenous neuronal circuitry. In fact, there is a decidedly lack of evidence that neuronal replacement is the primary mechanism of action for MSC therapy; moreover, there are data demonstrating artifacts associated with MSC to neuron transdifferentiation (Barnabe *et al.*, 2009; Lu *et al.*, 2004; Neuhuber *et al.*, 2004; Phinney & Prockop, 2007; Wells, 2002). There is also the possibility that MSCs replace supporting glial cells (astrocytes, oligodendrocytes, or microglia), which outnumber neurons 10:1 in the brain (reviewed in Boucherie & Hermans, 2009). However, ample evidence shows that benefits and functional recovery occur rapidly and persist long after the donor cells are gone, indicating permanent cell replacement is not required. The most likely governing mechanism is that MSCs provide trophic support to the injured brain, which augments endogenous repair and regeneration pathways. Trophic support, by definition, acts through secreted molecules called trophic factors. MSCs may act as mini-pumps delivering beneficial factors to their microenvironment. Using cells as pumps is preferred to actual engineered pumps because they can deliver a plethora of factors at the site of injury in physiologic concentrations and also respond to the needs of the injured tissue with appropriate feedback. Trophic factors can either directly or indirectly (via a mediator cell) promote neuroprotection (enhance cell survival through repair) or neuroregeneration. MSCs also secrete factors that augment angiogenesis - another important aspect of regeneration after brain injury. An additional likely mechanism of action contributing to the benefit of MSCs is immunosuppression. MSCs can affect immune cells via secreted factors, which would fall under trophic support. For the purposes of this chapter, we will treat it as a separate category since targeting immune functions indirectly promotes recovery compared to acting directly on neural or vascular cells. There is a great deal of overlap between these functions and these categories are fluid. Figure 1 summarizes hypothesized mechanisms of action for MSCs in the injured brain, which are mediated by secreted factors and direct cell-cell contacts.

3.1 Terminology

Trophic support classically means to provide nutrition, but the definition has been expanded to include promoting cellular growth, survival, differentiation, or migration. Similarly, the terms "trophic factor" and "growth factor" have also become more inclusive. Neurotrophic factors are trophic factors acting specifically on neural cells, i.e., promoting the growth, survival, differentiation, or migration of primarily neurons, but also glial cells (astrocytes, oligodendrocytes, microglia and Schwann cells). The name neurotrophin is sometimes used synonymously with neurotrophic factor; however neurotrophins specify a family of four structurally-related proteins: nerve growth factor (NGF), brain-derived neurotrophic factor (BDNF), neurotrophin-3 (NT-3), and neurotrophin-4/5 (NT-4/5). The term cytokines was initially used to distinguish factors that had specific immunomodulatory properties (produced by and act on immune cells), such as interleukins, lymphokines, and interferons. However, it is now known that many classic cytokines are also produced by and act on non-immune cells. Chemokines are a subclass of cytokines that promote chemotaxis (cell movement in response to a chemical concentration gradient). In general, as more functions are discovered about these proteins, definitions and classifications broaden and the terms are often used interchangeably. While trophic factors commonly refer to soluble proteins, extracellular matrix (ECM) proteins that are immobilized in the intercellular space also fall into this category since they direct cell growth, survival, differentiation, and migration.

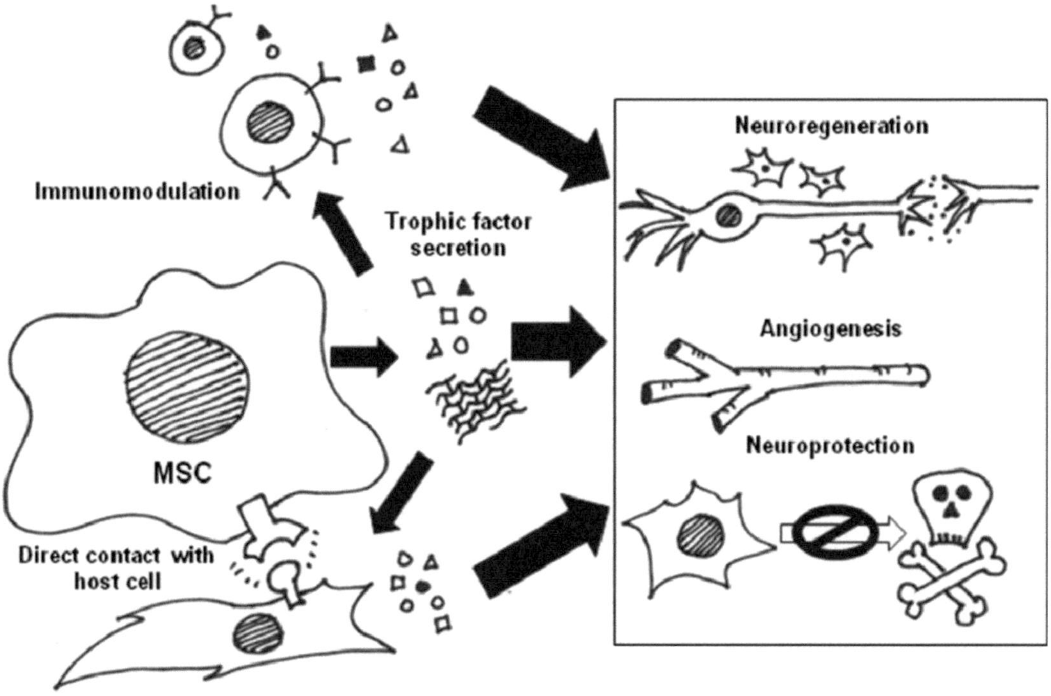

Fig. 1. Summary of likely mechanisms of action for MSCs in the injured brain, highlighting the interconnectivity.

3.2 Trophic support

Transplanted MSCs augment host repair and recovery primarily through direct and indirect trophic support. MSCs secrete a plethora of factors that are known to promote neural cell survival and regeneration through paracrine signaling to neural, vascular, and immune cells. An overview of relevant trophic factors found to be secreted by human bone marrow-derived MSCs *in vitro* is provided in Table 3. Which of these factors are secreted in the injured brain is under current investigation. Research is also ongoing to determine the exact or even the most critical mechanism(s) governing the beneficial effects of MSC transplantation. For now, we make a leap of knowledge based on existing evidence. There are numerous studies demonstrating that transplanted MSCs promote certain aspects of

Reference	Detection Method	Trophic Factors Found	Abbreviation
(Haynesworth *et al.*, 1996)	ELISA of Conditioned Medium	Granulocyte colony stimulating factor	G-CSF
		Granulocyte-macrophage colony stimulating factor	GM-CSF
		Interleukin-11	IL-11
		Interleukin-6	IL-6
		Leukemia inhibitory factor	LIF
		Macrophage colony stimulating factor	M-CSF
		Stem cell factor	SCF
(Potian *et al.*, 2003)	Cytokine Array of Conditioned Medium	Angiogenin	Angiogenin
		Granulocyte colony stimulating factor	G-CSF
		Granulocyte-macrophage colony stimulating factor	GM-CSF
		Growth related oncogene-α	GROα
		Interleukin-6	IL-6
		Interleukin-8	IL-8
		Monocyte chemoattractant protein-1	MCP-1
		Oncostatin M	OSM
		Transforming growth factor-β	TGFβ
(Kinnaird *et al.*, 2004)	ELISA or Immunoblotting of Conditioned Medium	Angiopoietin-1	ANG-1
		Fibroblast growth factor-2	FGF-2
		Interleukin-6	IL-6
		Monocyte chemoattractant protein-1	MCP-1
		Platelet derived growth factor	PDGF
		Placental growth factor	PlGF
		Vascular endothelial growth factor-A	VEGF-A
(Arnhold *et al.*, 2006)	ELISA of Conditioned Medium	Brain derived neurotrophic factor	BDNF
		Glial cell line-derived neurotrophic factor	GDNF
		Nerve growth factor	NGF
(Crigler *et al.*, 2006)	ELISA of Conditioned Medium	Brain derived neurotrophic factor	BDNF
		Interleukin-11	IL-11
		Nerve growth factor	NGF
		Stromal derived factor-1	SDF-1
(Wang *et al.*, 2006)	ELISA of Conditioned Medium	Hepatocyte growth factor	HGF
		Insulin-like growth factor-1	IGF-1
		Vascular endothelial growth factor	VEGF

Reference	Detection Method	Trophic Factors Found	Abbreviation
(Potapova *et al.*, 2007)	ELISA of Conditioned Medium	Angiogenin	Angiogenin
		Bone morphogenetic protein-2	BMP-2
		Interleukin-6	IL-6
		Interleukin-8	IL-8
		Interleukin-11	IL-11
		Monocyte chemoattractant protein-1	MCP-1
		Vascular endothelial growth factor	VEGF
(Schinkothe *et al.*, 2008)	Cytokine Array of Conditioned Medium	Angiopoietin-2	ANG-2
		Fibroblast growth factor-4	FGF-4
		Fibroblast growth factor-9	FGF-9
		Granulocyte colony stimulating factor	G-CSF
		Growth related oncogene	GRO
		Hepatocyte growth factor	HGF
		Interleukin-8	IL-8
		Interleukin-11	IL-11
		Interleukin-17	IL-17
		Monocyte chemoattractant protein-1	MCP-1
		Neurotrophin-4/5	NT-4/5
		Oncostatin M	OSM
		Placental growth factor	PlGF
		Tissue inhibitors of metalloproteinase-1	TIMP-1
		Vascular endothelial growth factor	VEGF
		Bone morphogenetic protein-4	BMP-4
(Tate *et al.*, 2010)	Cytokine Array of Conditioned Medium	Bone morphogenetic protein-7	BMP-7
		Dickkopf-1	DKK-1
		Fibroblast growth factor-7	FGF-7
		Heparin-binding epidermal growth factor-like growth factor	HB-EGF
		Hepatocyte growth factor	HGF
		Interleukin-6	IL-6
		Monocyte chemoattractant protein -1	MCP-1
		Platelet derived growth factor-AA	PDGF-AA
		Vascular endothelial growth factor	VEGF
		Collagen I	Collagen I
(Lai *et al.*, 2010)	Immunofluorescence of Extracellular Matrix	Decorin	Decorin
		Fibronectin	Fibronectin
		Laminin	Laminin
		Perlecan	Perlecan

Table 3. Factors secreted *in vitro* by human bone marrow MSCs that may affect neural recovery.

recovery (e.g., decrease apoptosis, increase neurogenesis, synaptogenesis, and angiogenesis) in the injured brain. Concurrently, there are other studies showing that factors known to be secreted by MSCs are involved in mechanisms that promote these same aspects of recovery. The assumption is that some combination of these pro-recovery mechanisms occurs when MSCs are transplanted into the injured brain and that MSC-secreted factors are essential for these effects. Table 4 reviews potential beneficial mechanisms of action for repair and regeneration of the injured brain provided by MSC-secreted factors. The table provides references that demonstrate that the protein of interest enhances either 1) neuroprotection, 2) neural stem/progenitor cell proliferation or migration, 3) neural stem/progenitor cell differentiation, 4) neuritogenesis or synaptogenesis, 5) angiogenesis, or 6) another mechanism involved in recovery (such as reducing inhibitory components of the glial scar). While these entries are based on a thorough search, it is not intended to be completely exhaustive. Also, only the beneficial aspects of the various growth factors are presented. Some factors that enhance one pathway act as inhibitors in another (e.g., the pro-inflammatory molecule interleukin-17 potentiates neuronal cell death but supports angiogenesis). Since these studies often examine pathways individually, it is not clear which are the primary mechanisms that occur when (if) the molecule is secreted by MSCs in the injured brain. Further, the exact timing and concentration of the trophic factor are likely critical in determining to which pathways they contribute.

			Promotes Neuroregeneration				
		Neuro-protection (↓Apoptosis)	**↑ NSC Proliferation or Migration**	**↑ NSC Differentiation**	**↑ Neurite Outgrowth or Synapse Formation**	**↑Angiogenesis**	**Additional**
Soluble Growth Factors	Angio-genin					(*Distler *et al.*, 2003)	
	ANG-1	(*Hansen *et al.*, 2008)	(*Ohab & Carmichael, 2008)		(*Hansen *et al.*, 2008)	(*Distler *et al.*, 2003)	Restore BBB (Nag *et al.*, 2011)
	ANG-2		(Liu *et al.*, 2009)	neuronal (Liu *et al.*, 2009)		in presence of VEGF (*Distler *et al.*, 2003)	
	BDNF	(*Lykissas *et al.*, 2007)	(*Bath & Lee, 2010; *Schabitz *et al.*, 2007)	neuronal (*Bath & Lee, 2010)	(Gascon *et al.*, 2005; *Lipsky & Marini, 2007; *Lykissas *et al.*, 2007)	(Qin *et al.*, 2011)	
	BMP-2	(Iantosca *et al.*, 1999)		astrocytic (*Sabo *et al.*, 2009)	(Gratacos *et al.*, 2001)		
	BMP-4	(Iantosca *et al.*, 1999)		astrocytic (*Sabo *et al.*, 2009)			
	BMP-7	(Yabe *et al.*, 2002)	(Chou *et al.*, 2006)	astrocytic (Gajavelli *et al.*, 2004)			

	Neuro-protection (↓Apoptosis)	Promotes Neuroregeneration			↑Angiogenesis	Additional
		↑ NSC Proliferation or Migration	↑ NSC Differentiation	↑ Neurite Outgrowth or Synapse Formation		
DKK-1				(Endo *et al.*, 2008)	(Smadja *et al.*, 2010)	
FGF-2	(*Alzheimer & Werner, 2002; *Zechel *et al.*, 2010)	(*Mudo *et al.*, 2009; *Zechel *et al.*, 2010)	(*Mudo *et al.*, 2009; *Zechel *et al.*, 2010)	(*Zechel *et al.*, 2010)	(*Distler *et al.*, 2003; Kumar *et al.*, 1998)	↑MSC homing (Schmidt *et al.*, 2006); Restore BBB (Bendfeldt *et al.*, 2007)
FGF-4		(Kosaka *et al.*, 2006)	neuronal (Kosaka *et al.*, 2006)		(*Fan & Yang, 2007)	
FGF-7	(Sadohara *et al.*, 2001)			(Terauchi *et al.*, 2010)	(Gillis *et al.*, 1999)	
FGF-9	(Lum *et al.*, 2009)	(Lum *et al.*, 2009)	neuronal (Lum *et al.*, 2009)		(Frontini *et al.*, 2011)	
G-CSF	(Schabitz *et al.*, 2003; Schneider *et al.*, 2005; Sehara *et al.*, 2007; Solaroglu *et al.*, 2006)	(Schneider *et al.*, 2005; Shyu *et al.*, 2004)	neuronal (Schneider *et al.*, 2005)		(Minamino *et al.*, 2005; Sehara *et al.*, 2007)	↑MSC homing (Deng *et al.*, 2011)
GM-CSF	(Huang *et al.*, 2007)			(Bouhy *et al.*, 2006)	(Buschmann *et al.*, 2003)	
GDNF	(Lu *et al.*, 2005; Shang *et al.*, 2011; Shirakura *et al.*, 2004)	(Dempsey *et al.*, 2003)		(Shirakura *et al.*, 2004)		
GROα			oligodendrocytic (Robinson *et al.*, 1998)		(Bechara *et al.*, 2007)	
HB-EGF	(Opanashuk *et al.*, 1999)	(Jin *et al.*, 2002)	neuronal (Jin *et al.*, 2004) and glial (Korblum 1999)			
HGF	(Honda *et al.*, 1995; Shang *et al.*, 2011)	(Shang *et al.*, 2011)	neuronal and glial (Shang *et al.*, 2011)	(Hamanoue *et al.*, 1996; Shang *et al.*, 2011; Shimamura *et al.*, 2006)	(*Distler *et al.*, 2003; Shang *et al.*, 2011; Shimamura *et al.*, 2006)	↑ MSC homing (Neuss *et al.*, 2004; Ponte *et al.*, 2007; Son *et al.*, 2006); ↓ glial scar (Shang *et al.*, 2011; Shimamura *et al.*, 2006)

	Neuro-protection (↓Apoptosis)	Promotes Neuroregeneration: ↑ NSC Proliferation or Migration	Promotes Neuroregeneration: ↑ NSC Differentiation	Promotes Neuroregeneration: ↑ Neurite Outgrowth or Synapse Formation	↑Angiogenesis	Additional
IGF-1	(Wilkins *et al.*, 2001; Yamada *et al.*, 2001)	(Dempsey *et al.*, 2003; *Joseph D'Ercole & Ye, 2008)	neuronal and glial (*Joseph D'Ercole & Ye, 2008)	(*Joseph D'Ercole & Ye, 2008)	(*Distler *et al.*, 2003; Lopez-Lopez *et al.*, 2004)	↑MSC homing (Ponte *et al.*, 2007)
IL-6	(Swartz *et al.*, 2001)		neuronal (Oh *et al.*, 2010) and astrocytic (Taga & Fukuda, 2005)	(Oh *et al.*, 2010)	(*Fan & Yang, 2007)	
IL-8	(Araujo & Cotman, 1993)				(*Fan & Yang, 2007)	↑MSC homing (Wang *et al.*, 2002)
IL-11			neuronal (Mehler *et al.*, 1993)			
IL-17					(Numasaki *et al.*, 2003)	
LIF	(Nobes & Tolkovsky, 1995)	(Bauer *et al.*, 2003; Shimazaki *et al.*, 2001)		(Blesch *et al.*, 1999)		↑cell homing (Sugiura *et al.*, 2000)
MCP-1		(Widera *et al.*, 2004; Yan *et al.*, 2007)				↑MSC homing (Wang *et al.*, 2002)
M-CSF	(Vincent *et al.*, 2002)				(Minamino *et al.*, 2005)	
NGF	(*Lykissas *et al.*, 2007; Shirakura *et al.*, 2004)		neuronal (Yung *et al.*, 2010; Zhu *et al.*, 2011)	(Gascon *et al.*, 2005; *Lykissas *et al.*, 2007)	(*Lazarovici *et al.*, 2006)	
NT-4/5	(*Lykissas *et al.*, 2007)		neuronal (Shen *et al.*, 2010)	(*Lykissas *et al.*, 2007)		
OSM	(Weiss *et al.*, 2006)		oligoendrocytic (Glezer & Rivest, 2010)		(Vasse *et al.*, 1999)	
PDGF	(Iihara *et al.*, 1997; Vana *et al.*, 2007)	(Forsberg-Nilsson *et al.*, 1998)	neuronal (Johe *et al.*, 1996)		(*Beck & Plate, 2009; *Fan & Yang, 2007)	↑MSC homing (Ponte *et al.*, 2007)
PlGF	(Du *et al.*, 2010)				(*Beck & Plate, 2009)	

		Neuro-protection (↓Apoptosis)	Promotes Neuroregeneration			↑Angiogenesis	Additional
			↑ NSC Proliferation or Migration	↑ NSC Differentiation	↑ Neurite Outgrowth or Synapse Formation		
	SCF	(Dhandapani *et al.*, 2005; Erlandsson *et al.*, 2004; Li *et al.*, 2009)	(Bantubungi *et al.*, 2008; Erlandsson *et al.*, 2004; Zhao *et al.*, 2007)			(Sun *et al.*, 2006)	↑MSC homing (Bantubungi *et al.*, 2008; Erlandsson *et al.*, 2004)
	SDF-1		(*Ohab & Carmichael, 2008; Thored *et al.*, 2006)				↑ MSC homing (Ponte *et al.*, 2007; Son *et al.*, 2006) and survival (Kortesidis *et al.*, 2005)
	TGFβ	(*Buisson *et al.*, 2003; Lu *et al.*, 2005)	(Ma *et al.*, 2008; Mathieu *et al.*, 2010)		(Yi *et al.*, 2010)	(*Beck & Plate, 2009; *Fan & Yang, 2007)	
	TIMP-1	(Tan *et al.*, 2003)					
	VEGF	(Jin *et al.*, 2000; Sun *et al.*, 2003)	(Sun *et al.*, 2003; Wang *et al.*, 2007a; Wang *et al.*, 2007b)		(Erskine *et al.*, 2011; Jin *et al.*, 2006)	(*Greenberg & Jin, 2005; *Shibuya, 2009)	
Matrix Proteins	Collagen I		(Ma *et al.*, 2004)	neuronal (Ma *et al.*, 2004)		(*Sottile, 2004)	
Matrix Proteins	Decorin				(Davies *et al.*, 2004)		↓ glial scar (Davies *et al.*, 2004)
Matrix Proteins	Fibro-nectin	(Sakai *et al.*, 2001; Tate *et al.*, 2007)	(*Henderson & Copp, 1997; Tate *et al.*, 2004; Testaz & Duband, 2001)	oligodendrocytic (Hu *et al.*, 2009)	(Einheber *et al.*, 1996; *Pires Neto *et al.*, 1999)	(*Sottile, 2004)	
Matrix Proteins	Laminin	(Hall *et al.*, 2008)	(Hall *et al.*, 2008; *Perris & Perissinotto, 2000; Tate *et al.*, 2004)	neuronal (Boote Jones & Mallapragada, 2007; Tate *et al.*, 2004)	(*Colognato and Yurchenco, 2000; *Pires-Neto 1999)	(*Sottile, 2004)	Restore BBB (Hunter *et al.*, 1992);↓glial scar (Hou *et al.*, 2005)
Matrix Proteins	Perlecan	(*Bix & Iozzo, 2008; Lee *et al.*, 2011)				(*Bix & Iozzo, 2008; Lee *et al.*, 2011)	

*Indicates review article; NSC=Neural stem/progenitor cell; Growth factor abbreviations are defined in Table 3

Table 4. Evidence of MSC-secreted factors promoting neuroprotection or regeneration.

3.2.1 Neuroprotection

Following the initial insult, secondary injury mechanisms persist and cause cell death to surrounding tissue. While the initial ischemic or mechanical insult causes immediate necrotic death, secondary cell death primarily occurs through apoptosis. MSCs secrete multiple factors known to promote neural cell survival (see Table 4). Human MSCs have been shown to rescue neural cells following *in vitro* injury (e.g., oxygen glucose deprivation, glutamate toxicity) via secreted soluble factors (Tate *et al.*, 2010; Zhong *et al.*, 2003) and ECM proteins (Aizman *et al.*, 2009). There are several reports of decreased apoptotic markers and enhanced preservation of neural cells in the injury penumbra when transplanting MSCs following experimental ischemic stroke (Li *et al.*, 2010; Li *et al.*, 2002; Xin *et al.*, 2010) or TBI (Kim *et al.*, 2010; Xiong *et al.*, 2009). For example, delivering human MSCs intravenously 1 day following experimental cerebral ischemia in rats led to significant reduction in apoptotic cell death in the injury penumbra as well as functional behavioral recovery (Li *et al.*, 2002). This study also found an increase in BDNF and NGF in the ipsilateral hemisphere of MSC-treated rats at 7 days post-stroke; however, they did not distinguish whether these trophic factors were produced by the donor or host cells. Li *et al.* (2010) show that transplanting human MSCs into the injury penumbra 1 week following experimental cerebral ischemia in monkeys decreased apoptotic cell death and the lesion volume. Human MSCs transplanted into the injury cavity 1 week following experimental TBI in rats lead to enhanced cell survival in the hippocampus and improved functional recovery, and this was further improved when the MSCs were delivered within a collagen I scaffold (Xiong *et al.*, 2009). Kim *et al.* (2010) found that delivering human MSCs intravenously 1 day post-TBI in rats improved functional recovery and enhanced host cell survival by increasing pAkt and decreasing caspace-3 cleavage. Further, this group reports increases in BDNF, NGF, and NT-3 in the MSC-treated brains, though they did not distinguish between donor or host origin. Clearly, exogenous MSCs provide neuroprotection following brain injury and this is one probable mechanism of action for their benefit.

3.2.2 Neuroregeneration

After brain injury, the brain attempts to regenerate by resorting to a developmental-like state with increased neurogenesis, neurite outgrowth, synaptogenesis, re-myelination, re-formation of the blood brain barrier, and angiogenesis. Once thought to be unable to regenerate, it is now known that neural stem cells persist in the normal adult brain (neurogenic zones include the subventricular zone in the lateral ventricles and the subgranular zone in the dentate gyrus of the hippocampus). After an ischemic or traumatic injury, endogenous neural stem cells proliferate, migrate to the site of injury, and differentiate into neurons and glia (Kernie & Parent, 2010). Neuroplasticity is the reorganization of neuronal circuitry by changing the number and/or strength of neurites and synapses. Such remapping occurs throughout life for learning and memory formation, and compensatory plasticity occurs in the spared tissue following brain injury (Nishibe *et al.*, 2010). Neuroregeneration collectively includes neural stem/progenitor cell proliferation, migration and differentiation, neurite outgrowth, and synapse formation.

There are multiple *in vitro* studies showing that MSCs direct neuroregenerative processes. Bai *et al.* (2007) show that mouse neural stem cells had increased migration and neuronal and oligodendrocytic differentiation when they were cultured with either human MSCs or MSC-conditioned medium, indicating that soluble proteins are responsible for these effects. In related work, co-culture of human MSCs with rat neural stem cells revealed that MSCs promote differentiation into primarily astrocytes and oligodendrocytes (Robinson *et al.*, 2011). However MSC-conditioned media promoted primarily oligodendrocytic differentiation (Robinson *et al.*, 2011), indicating that matrix components or direct cell-cell contact also account for the effects of MSCs on neural stem cell differentiation. Indeed, Aizman *et al.* (2009) demonstrate that human MSC-derived ECM promotes differentiation of cortical cells into neurons, astrocytes and oligodendrocytes and also enhances neuronal neurite networks compared to single ECM proteins. Transplantation of MSCs augments endogenous regeneration following experimental ischemic stroke (Bao *et al.*, 2011; Li *et al.*, 2010; Li *et al.*, 2002; Xin *et al.*, 2010; Yoo *et al.*, 2008) and TBI (Mahmood *et al.*, 2004; Xiong *et al.*, 2009). For example, both Bao *et al.* (2011) and Yoo *et al.* (2008) show that intracerebral transplantation of human MSCs 3 days following experimental cerebral ischemia in rats increases proliferation and migration of host neural stem cells and also decreases their apoptosis, thus enhancing neurogenesis. They also report enhanced behavioral recovery, and Bao *et al.* demonstrate increases in BDNF, NT-3, and VEGF in the brains of MSC-treated rats, though they do not identify the source of these cytokines. Xin *et al.* (2010) found that intravenous delivery of mouse MSCs 1 day following experimental stroke in mice lead to increases in axon fiber density, synaptogenesis and myelination. Following experimental TBI in rats, transplanted rat MSCs promoted increased proliferation and neuronal differentiation in neurogenic zones along with improved motor and sensory recovery (Mahmood *et al.*, 2004). Xiong *et al.* (2009) also report that transplanting human MSCs intracerebrally 1 week post-TBI in rats leads to increased axonal fiber length and that the fiber length was directly proportional to performance on the behavior tasks. Multiple trophic factors secreted by MSCs may contribute to enhancing neuroregeneration (see Table 4).

The glial scar that forms following brain injury acutely acts to sequester the injury. Cellular components of the glial scar include reactive astrocytes, which help buffer excess glutamate and secrete neurotrophic factors, and activated microglia/macrophages which clear out dead tissue and secrete neurotrophic factors. However, extracellular components of the glial scar that persists adjacent to the injury site have been found to inhibit neurite extension (e.g., neurocan, Nogo protein), thus limiting regeneration (for review, see Properzi *et al.*, 2003). Transplantation of MSCs helps overcome this glial scar limitation following experimental stroke (Li *et al.*, 2010; Li *et al.*, 2005; Pavlichenko *et al.*, 2008; Shen *et al.*, 2008) and TBI (Zanier *et al.*, 2011). Following ischemic stroke, rats treated with rat MSCs transplanted intravenously had decreased glial scar thickness at both the acute (3 and 6 days post-stroke; Pavlichenko *et al.*, 2008) and chronic (4 months post-stroke; Li *et al.*, 2005) phases. Along with decreased glial scar thickness, these studies report decreased lesion volume, enhanced regeneration, and functional recovery for animals treated with MSCs. Shen *et al.* (2008) show a decrease in neurocan (an inhibitory chondroitin sulphate proteoglycan) and enhanced axonal outgrowth in the injury penumbra when ischemic rats were treated with rat MSCs. Zanier *et al.* (2011) transplanted human umbilical cord blood-derived MSCs MSCs into the traumatically injured mouse brain and observed a decrease in reactive astrocytes in the glial scar region along with decreased lesion volume and functional recovery. Collectively, these data illustrate that exogenous MSCs promote neuroregeneration following brain injury by directly affecting neural stem/progenitor cells and neurons and/or by reducing inhibitory glial scar components.

3.2.3 Angiogenesis

Another important aspect of regeneration is angiogenesis, which is the formation of new blood vessels from existing vasculature. In the adult, angiogenesis occurs after injury to help supply the damaged tissue with oxygen and nutrients. The process includes basement membrane disruption, endothelial cell migration and proliferation, three-dimensional tube formation, maturation, and stabilization by vascular smooth muscle cells. Each step is regulated by multiple cytokines and ECM molecules (for review, see Distler *et al.*, 2003 or Fan & Yang 2007). Studies show that MSC-conditioned medium enhances endothelial cell proliferation (Kaigler *et al.*, 2003) and promotes angiogenesis *in vitro* and *in vivo* (Kinnaird *et al.*, 2004). Transplanting MSCs increases angiogenesis following experimental ischemic stroke (Omori *et al.*, 2008; Onda *et al.*, 2008; Pavlichenko *et al.*, 2008) and TBI (Xiong *et al.*, 2009). Potential pro-angiogenic factors secreted by MSCs are provided in Table 4. Notably, there is overlap between factors that promote angiogenesis and neurogenesis/neuritogenesis (reviewed in Emanueli *et al.*, 2003 and Lazarovici *et al.*, 2006). A unique feature of brain vasculature is the existence of the blood-brain barrier (BBB), formed by astrocyte end-feet surrounding specialized capillary endothelial cells in order to tightly regulate brain homeostasis. After injury, there is increased permeability of the BBB leading to edema (reviewed in Nag *et al.*, 2011). Part of the repair process includes restoring the BBB, and regeneration includes formation of the BBB for new vasculature. Specific MSC-secreted factors such as ANG-1, FGF-2, and laminin may be involved in reforming the BBB following injury.

3.3 Immunomodulation

There is a potent immune response following ischemic and traumatic brain injury. The innate immune response is a part of the normal wound healing process; however, persistent inflammation can become cytotoxic. In addition to interacting with neural and vascular cells, MSCs communicate with immune cells and are now known to be immnosuppressive. Examining the interactions of MSCs with immune cells *in vitro* reveals that MSCs suppress T cell proliferation and activation, inhibit B cell proliferation and IgG production, prevent dendritic cell differentiation and migration, and shift the cytokine secretion profile of dendritic cells, helper T cells, and natural killer cells towards anti-inflammatory (reviewed in Mezey *et al.*, 2010 and Nauta & Fibbe, 2007). Interestingly, studies that separate the MSCs from the immune cells using semi-permeable membranes indicate that soluble factors are critical for these effects. Candidate immunomodulatory factors secreted by MSCs include interleukin-6 (IL-6), transforming growth factor β (TGFβ), prostaglandin E2, hepatocyte growth factor (HGF), indoleamine 2,3-dioxygenase (IDO), and monocyte colony stimulating factor (M-CSF) (reviewed in Mezey *et al.*, 2010 and Nauta & Fibbe, 2007). Moreover, ECM proteins, such as fibronectin, also interact with immune cells (Mosesson, 1984; Nasu-Tada *et al.*, 2005). Since shifting to a less inflammatory environment may facilitate neural repair and regeneration, immunomodulation is another feasible therapeutic mechanism of action for transplanted MSCs. Note that many immunomodulatory factors also have potential roles for directly promoting neural cell survival and regeneration (see Table 4). Likewise, NGF, the prototypic neurotrophic factor, has been shown to be anti-inflammatory (Villoslada & Genain, 2004). The interaction between angiogenesis and inflammation is also well-documented (for review, see Jackson *et al.*, 1997 or Noonan *et al.*, 2008), which further underscores the complexity and interrelatedness of these recovery mechanisms.

3.4 Challenges of identifying critical factors and mechanisms

Cell transplantation is a dynamic treatment that can target multiple therapeutic mechanisms. Advantages of transplanting cells compared to pharmaceutical treatments include the ability to 1) easily localize the treatment to the affected tissue, 2) supply a variety of trophic factors at physiologic concentrations, 3) persist long enough to alter the microenvironment of the injured brain tissue; and 4) interact with host cells. The beneficial effects of transplanted MSCs have been corraborated *in vitro* and *in vivo* and some potential pathways have been identified as described above. It is probable that a combination of multiple mechanisms of action synergistically contribute to improve functional recovery. While this ability to intervene along multiple pathways is desirable for a robust treatment, it makes identifying key mechanisms and factors challenging. Clarifying critical mechanisms of action would allow for treatments to be optimized to best facilitate these roles. Furthermore, difficulty pinpointing key mechanisms is a hurdle for developing potency assays for the clinical use of MSCs. Potency assays are critical for ranking and qualifying different cell lots on their ability to promote recovery. Another complication for determining potency of cells *ex vivo* is that transplanted cells interact with the host cells via paracrine signaling and possibly direct cell-cell contact. MSCs alter the secretion profile of host neural and immune cells, such as astrocytes and microglia (Gao *et al.*, 2005; Xin *et al.*, 2010), which further acts to promote repair and regeneration. Additionally, the secretion profile of MSCs is a function of the microenvironment and changes in the presence of injured brain tissue (Chen *et al.*, 2002a, 2002b). Thus, there is a complex and dynamic web of players involved in MSC-mediated effects. Ideally, potency assays would be easily reproducible *in vitro* assays, however the interplay between donor cells and the host environment is difficult to model *in vitro*. Elucidating critical aspects of this therapy will be the focus of intense research for years to come.

4. Conclusion

Stroke and TBI are major contributors to death and persistent disability, and treatments that effectively promote repair and regeneration are desired. Cell transplantation is a promising treatment for brain injury, and MSCs are an attractive cell source due to their technical and safety advantages. Pre-clinical *in vivo* data show that transplanting MSCs enhances neuroprotection, promotes regeneration and/or suppresses inflammation. MSCs secrete numerous soluble and insoluble factors that are known to benefit the injured brain, which are likely crucial to the mechanisms of action governing MSC-mediated recovery. MSCs aid injured brain tissue by targeting multiple, non-mutually exclusive pathways, which is an advantage for a potential treatment, but a challenge for elucidating critical mechanisms and factors.

5. References

Aizman, I., Tate, C.C., McGrogan, M. & Case, C.C. (2009). Extracellular Matrix Produced by Bone Marrow Stromal Cells and by their Derivative, SB623 Cells, Supports Neural Cell Growth. *Journal of Neuroscience Research,* Vol.87, No.14, pp. 3198-3206, ISSN 1097-4547

Alzheimer, C. & Werner, S. (2002). Fibroblast Growth Factors and Neuroprotection. *Advances in Experimental Medicine and Biology,* Vol.513, pp. 335-351, ISSN 0065-2598

Araujo, D.M. & Cotman, C.W. (1993). Trophic Effects of Interleukin-4, -7 and -8 on Hippocampal Neuronal Cultures: Potential Involvement of Glial-Derived Factors. *Brain Research,* Vol.600, No.1, pp. 49-55, ISSN 0006-8993

Arnhold, S., Klein, H., Klinz, F.J., Absenger, Y., Schmidt, A., Schinkothe, T., Brixius, K., Kozlowski, J., Desai, B., Bloch, W. & Addicks, K. (2006). Human Bone Marrow Stroma Cells Display Certain Neural Characteristics and Integrate in the Subventricular Compartment After Injection into the Liquor System. *European Journal of Cell Biology,* Vol.85, No.6, pp. 551-565, ISSN 0171-9335

Bai, L., Caplan, A., Lennon, D. & Miller, R.H. (2007). Human Mesenchymal Stem Cells Signals Regulate Neural Stem Cell Fate. *Neurochemical Research,* Vol.32, No.2, pp. 353-362, ISSN 0364-3190

Bantubungi, K., Blum, D., Cuvelier, L., Wislet-Gendebien, S., Rogister, B., Brouillet, E. & Schiffmann, S.N. (2008). Stem Cell Factor and Mesenchymal and Neural Stem Cell Transplantation in a Rat Model of Huntington's Disease. *Molecular and Cellular Neurosciences,* Vol.37, No.3, pp. 454-470, ISSN 1095-9327; 1044-7431

Bao, X., Wei, J., Feng, M., Lu, S., Li, G., Dou, W., Ma, W., Ma, S., An, Y., Qin, C., Zhao, R.C. & Wang, R. (2011). Transplantation of Human Bone Marrow-Derived Mesenchymal Stem Cells Promotes Behavioral Recovery and Endogenous Neurogenesis After Cerebral Ischemia in Rats. *Brain Research,* Vol.1367, pp. 103-113, ISSN 1872-6240; 0006-8993

Barnabe, G.F., Schwindt, T.T., Calcagnotto, M.E., Motta, F.L., Martinez, G.,Jr, de Oliveira, A.C., Keim, L.M., D'Almeida, V., Mendez-Otero, R. & Mello, L.E. (2009). Chemically-Induced RAT Mesenchymal Stem Cells Adopt Molecular Properties of Neuronal-Like Cells but do Not have Basic Neuronal Functional Properties. *PloS One,* Vol.4, No.4, pp. e5222, ISSN 1932-6203; 1932-6203

Bath, K.G. & Lee, F.S. (2010). Neurotrophic Factor Control of Adult SVZ Neurogenesis. *Developmental Neurobiology,* Vol.70, No.5, pp. 339-349, ISSN 1932-846X; 1932-8451

Battistella, V., de Freitas, G.R., da Fonseca, L.M., Mercante, D., Gutfilen, B., Goldenberg, R.C., Dias, J.V., Kasai-Brunswick, T.H., Wajnberg, E., Rosado-de-Castro, P.H., Alves-Leon, S.V., Mendez-Otero, R. & Andre, C. (2011). Safety of Autologous Bone Marrow Mononuclear Cell Transplantation in Patients with Nonacute Ischemic Stroke. *Regenerative Medicine,* Vol.6, No.1, pp. 45-52, ISSN 1746-076X; 1746-0751

Bauer, S., Rasika, S., Han, J., Mauduit, C., Raccurt, M., Morel, G., Jourdan, F., Benahmed, M., Moyse, E. & Patterson, P.H. (2003). Leukemia Inhibitory Factor is a Key Signal for Injury-Induced Neurogenesis in the Adult Mouse Olfactory Epithelium. *The Journal of Neuroscience : The Official Journal of the Society for Neuroscience,* Vol.23, No.5, pp. 1792-1803, ISSN 1529-2401; 0270-6474

Bechara, C., Chai, H., Lin, P.H., Yao, Q. & Chen, C. (2007). Growth Related Oncogene-Alpha (GRO-Alpha): Roles in Atherosclerosis, Angiogenesis and Other Inflammatory Conditions. *Medical Science Monitor: International Medical Journal of Experimental and Clinical Research,* Vol.13, No.6, pp. RA87-90, ISSN 1234-1010

Beck, H. & Plate, K.H. (2009). Angiogenesis After Cerebral Ischemia. *Acta Neuropathologica,* Vol.117, No.5, pp. 481-496, ISSN 1432-0533; 0001-6322

Bendfeldt, K., Radojevic, V., Kapfhammer, J. & Nitsch, C. (2007). Basic Fibroblast Growth Factor Modulates Density of Blood Vessels and Preserves Tight Junctions in Organotypic Cortical Cultures of Mice: A New in Vitro Model of the Blood-Brain Barrier. *The Journal of Neuroscience,* Vol.27, No.12, pp. 3260-3267, ISSN 1529-2401; 0270-6474

Bix, G. & Iozzo, R.V. (2008). Novel Interactions of Perlecan: Unraveling Perlecan's Role in Angiogenesis. *Microscopy Research and Technique,* Vol.71, No.5, pp. 339-348, ISSN 1059-910X

Boote Jones, E.N. & Mallapragada, S.K. (2007). Directed Growth and Differentiation of Stem Cells Towards Neural Cell Fates using Soluble and Surface-Mediated Cues. *Journal of Biomaterials Science.Polymer Edition,* Vol.18, No.8, pp. 999-1015, ISSN 0920-5063

Boucherie, C. & Hermans, E. (2009). Adult Stem Cell Therapies for Neurological Disorders: Benefits Beyond Neuronal Replacement? *Journal of Neuroscience Research,* Vol.87, No.7, pp. 1509-1521, ISSN 1097-4547; 0360-4012

Bouhy, D., Malgrange, B., Multon, S., Poirrier, A.L., Scholtes, F., Schoenen, J. & Franzen, R. (2006). Delayed GM-CSF Treatment Stimulates Axonal Regeneration and Functional Recovery in Paraplegic Rats Via an Increased BDNF Expression by Endogenous Macrophages. *The FASEB Journal,* Vol.20, No.8, pp. 1239-1241, ISSN 1530-6860; 0892-6638

Bramlett, H.M. & Dietrich, W.D. (2004). Pathophysiology of Cerebral Ischemia and Brain Trauma: Similarities and Differences. *Journal of Cerebral Blood Flow and Metabolism,* Vol.24, No.2, pp. 133-150, ISSN 0271-678X

Buisson, A., Lesne, S., Docagne, F., Ali, C., Nicole, O., MacKenzie, E.T. & Vivien, D. (2003). Transforming Growth Factor-Beta and Ischemic Brain Injury. *Cellular and Molecular Neurobiology,* Vol.23, No.4-5, pp. 539-550, ISSN 0272-4340

Buschmann, I.R., Busch, H.J., Mies, G. & Hossmann, K.A. (2003). Therapeutic Induction of Arteriogenesis in Hypoperfused Rat Brain Via Granulocyte-Macrophage Colony-Stimulating Factor. *Circulation,* Vol.108, No.5, pp. 610-615, ISSN 1524-4539; 0009-7322

Chen, X., Katakowski, M., Li, Y., Lu, D., Wang, L., Zhang, L., Chen, J., Xu, Y., Gautam, S., Mahmood, A. & Chopp, M. (2002a). Human Bone Marrow Stromal Cell Cultures Conditioned by Traumatic Brain Tissue Extracts: Growth Factor Production. *Journal of Neuroscience Research,* Vol.69, No.5, pp. 687-691, ISSN 0360-4012

Chen, X., Li, Y., Wang, L., Katakowski, M., Zhang, L., Chen, J., Xu, Y., Gautam, S.C. & Chopp, M. (2002b). Ischemic Rat Brain Extracts Induce Human Marrow Stromal Cell Growth Factor Production. *Neuropathology,* Vol.22, No.4, pp. 275-279, ISSN 0919-6544

Chou, J., Harvey, B.K., Chang, C.F., Shen, H., Morales, M. & Wang, Y. (2006). Neuroregenerative Effects of BMP7 After Stroke in Rats. *Journal of the Neurological Sciences,* Vol.240, No.1-2, pp. 21-29, ISSN 0022-510X

Coles, J.P. (2004). Regional Ischemia After Head Injury. *Current Opinion in Critical Care,* Vol.10, No.2, pp. 120-125, ISSN 1070-5295

Cox, C.S.,Jr, Baumgartner, J.E., Harting, M.T., Worth, L.L., Walker, P.A., Shah, S.K., Ewing-Cobbs, L., Hasan, K.M., Day, M.C., Lee, D., Jimenez, F. & Gee, A. (2011). Autologous Bone Marrow Mononuclear Cell Therapy for Severe Traumatic Brain Injury in Children. *Neurosurgery,* Vol.68, No.3, pp. 588-600, ISSN 1524-4040; 0148-396X

Crigler, L., Robey, R.C., Asawachaicharn, A., Gaupp, D. & Phinney, D.G. (2006). Human Mesenchymal Stem Cell Subpopulations Express a Variety of Neuro-Regulatory Molecules and Promote Neuronal Cell Survival and Neuritogenesis. *Experimental Neurology,* Vol.198, No.1, pp. 54-64, ISSN 0014-4886

Davies, J.E., Tang, X., Denning, J.W., Archibald, S.J. & Davies, S.J. (2004). Decorin Suppresses Neurocan, Brevican, Phosphacan and NG2 Expression and Promotes Axon Growth Across Adult Rat Spinal Cord Injuries. *The European Journal of Neuroscience,* Vol.19, No.5, pp. 1226-1242, ISSN 0953-816X

Dempsey, R.J., Sailor, K.A., Bowen, K.K., Tureyen, K. & Vemuganti, R. (2003). Stroke-Induced Progenitor Cell Proliferation in Adult Spontaneously Hypertensive Rat Brain: Effect of Exogenous IGF-1 and GDNF. *Journal of Neurochemistry,* Vol.87, No.3, pp. 586-597, ISSN 0022-3042

Deng, J., Zou, Z.M., Zhou, T.L., Su, Y.P., Ai, G.P., Wang, J.P., Xu, H. & Dong, S.W. (2011). Bone Marrow Mesenchymal Stem Cells can be Mobilized into Peripheral Blood by G-CSF in Vivo and Integrate into Traumatically Injured Cerebral Tissue. *Neurological Sciences,* Vol.32, No.4, pp. 641-651, ISSN 1590-3478; 1590-1874

Dhandapani, K.M., Wade, F.M., Wakade, C., Mahesh, V.B. & Brann, D.W. (2005). Neuroprotection by Stem Cell Factor in Rat Cortical Neurons Involves AKT and NFkappaB. *Journal of Neurochemistry,* Vol.95, No.1, pp. 9-19, 0022-3042; 0022-3042

Distler, J.H., Hirth, A., Kurowska-Stolarska, M., Gay, R.E., Gay, S. & Distler, O. (2003). Angiogenic and Angiostatic Factors in the Molecular Control of Angiogenesis. *The Quarterly Journal of Nuclear Medicine,* Vol.47, No.3, pp. 149-161, ISSN 1125-0135

Du, H., Li, P., Pan, Y., Li, W., Hou, J., Chen, H., Wang, J. & Tang, H. (2010). Vascular Endothelial Growth Factor Signaling Implicated in Neuroprotective Effects of Placental Growth Factor in an in Vitro Ischemic Model. *Brain Research,* Vol.1357, pp. 1-8, ISSN 1872-6240; 0006-8993

Einheber, S., Schnapp, L.M., Salzer, J.L., Cappiello, Z.B. & Milner, T.A. (1996). Regional and Ultrastructural Distribution of the Alpha 8 Integrin Subunit in Developing and Adult Rat Brain Suggests a Role in Synaptic Function. *Journal of Comparative Neurology,* Vol.370, No.1, pp. 105-34, ISSN 1096-9861; 0021-9967

Emanueli, C., Schratzberger, P., Kirchmair, R. & Madeddu, P. (2003). Paracrine Control of Vascularization and Neurogenesis by Neurotrophins. *British Journal of Pharmacology,* Vol.140, No.4, pp. 614-619, ISSN 0007-1188

Endo, Y., Beauchamp, E., Woods, D., Taylor, W.G., Toretsky, J.A., Uren, A. & Rubin, J.S. (2008). Wnt-3a and Dickkopf-1 Stimulate Neurite Outgrowth in Ewing Tumor Cells

Via a Frizzled3- and c-Jun N-Terminal Kinase-Dependent Mechanism. *Molecular and Cellular Biology,* Vol.28, No.7, pp. 2368-2379, ISSN 1098-5549; 0270-7306

Erlandsson, A., Larsson, J. & Forsberg-Nilsson, K. (2004). Stem Cell Factor is a Chemoattractant and a Survival Factor for CNS Stem Cells. *Experimental Cell Research,* Vol.301, No.2, pp. 201-210, ISSN 0014-4827

Erskine, L., Reijntjes, S., Pratt, T., Denti, L., Schwarz, Q., Vieira, J.M., Alakakone, B., Shewan, D. & Ruhrberg, C. (2011). VEGF Signaling through Neuropilin 1 Guides Commissural Axon Crossing at the Optic Chiasm. *Neuron,* Vol.70, No.5, pp. 951-965, ISSN 1097-4199; 0896-6273

Fan, Y. & Yang, G.Y. (2007). Therapeutic Angiogenesis for Brain Ischemia: A Brief Review. *Journal of Neuroimmune Pharmacology,* Vol.2, No.3, pp. 284-289, ISSN 1557-1904; 1557-1890

Faul, M., Xu, L., Wald, M.M. & Coronado, V.G. (2010). *Traumatic brain injury in the United States: emergency department visits, hospitalizations, and deaths 2002-2006*. Centers for Disease Control and Prevention, National Center for Injury Prevention and Control, Atlanta, GA

Finkelstein EA, Corso PS, Miller TR. 2006. *The Incidence and Economic Burden of Injuries in the United States*. Oxford University Press, New York, NY

Forsberg-Nilsson, K., Behar, T.N., Afrakhte, M., Barker, J.L. & McKay, R.D. (1998). Platelet-Derived Growth Factor Induces Chemotaxis of Neuroepithelial Stem Cells. *J Neurosci Res,* Vol.53, No.5, pp. 521-530, ISSN 1097-4547; 0360-4012

Frontini, M.J., Nong, Z., Gros, R., Drangova, M., O'Neil, C., Rahman, M.N., Akawi, O., Yin, H., Ellis, C.G. & Pickering, J.G. (2011). Fibroblast growth factor 9 delivery during angiogenesis produces durable, vasoresponsive microvessels wrapped by smooth muscle cells. *Nature Biotechnology,* Vol.29, No.5, pp. 421-427, ISSN 1546-1696; 1087-0156

Gajavelli, S., Wood, P.M., Pennica, D., Whittemore, S.R. & Tsoulfas, P. (2004). BMP Signaling Initiates a Neural Crest Differentiation Program in Embryonic Rat CNS Stem Cells. *Experimental Neurology,* Vol.188, No.2, pp. 205-223, ISSN 0014-4886

Gao, Q., Li, Y. & Chopp, M. (2005). Bone Marrow Stromal Cells Increase Astrocyte Survival via Upregulation of Phosphoinositide 3-kinase/threonine Protein Kinase and Mitogen-Activated Protein Kinase kinase/extracellular Signal-Regulated Kinase Pathways and Stimulate Astrocyte Trophic Factor Gene Expression After Anaerobic Insult. *Neuroscience,* Vol.136, No.1, pp. 123-134, ISSN 0306-4522

Garnett, M.R., Blamire, A.M., Corkill, R.G., Rajagopalan, B., Young, J.D., Cadoux-Hudson, T.A. & Styles, P. (2001). Abnormal Cerebral Blood Volume in Regions of Contused and Normal Appearing Brain Following Traumatic Brain Injury using Perfusion Magnetic Resonance Imaging. *Journal of Neurotrauma,* Vol.18, No.6, pp. 585-593, ISSN 0897-7151

Gascon, E., Vutskits, L., Zhang, H., Barral-Moran, M.J., Kiss, P.J., Mas, C. & Kiss, J.Z. (2005). Sequential Activation of p75 and TrkB is Involved in Dendritic Development of Subventricular Zone-Derived Neuronal Progenitors in Vitro. *The European Journal of Neuroscience,* Vol.21, No.1, pp. 69-80, ISSN 0953-816X

Gillis, P., Savla, U., Volpert, O.V., Jimenez, B., Waters, C.M., Panos, R.J. & Bouck, N.P. (1999). Keratinocyte Growth Factor Induces Angiogenesis and Protects Endothelial

Barrier Function. *Journal of Cell Science,* Vol.112, Pt 12, pp. 2049-2057, ISSN 0021-9533

Glezer, I. & Rivest, S. (2010). Oncostatin M is a Novel Glucocorticoid-Dependent Neuroinflammatory Factor that Enhances Oligodendrocyte Precursor Cell Activity in Demyelinated Sites. *Brain, Behavior, and Immunity,* Vol.24, No.5, pp. 695-704, ISSN 1090-2139; 0889-1591

Gratacos, E., Checa, N., Perez-Navarro, E. & Alberch, J. (2001). Brain-Derived Neurotrophic Factor (BDNF) Mediates Bone Morphogenetic Protein-2 (BMP-2) Effects on Cultured Striatal Neurones. *Journal of Neurochemistry,* Vol.79, No.4, pp. 747-755, ISSN 0022-3042

Greenberg, D.A. & Jin, K. (2005). From Angiogenesis to Neuropathology. *Nature,* Vol.438, No.7070, pp. 954-959, ISSN 1476-4687; 0028-0836

Greve, M.W. & Zink, B.J. (2009). Pathophysiology of Traumatic Brain Injury. *The Mount Sinai Journal of Medicine, New York,* Vol.76, No.2, pp. 97-104, ISSN 1931-7581; 0027-2507

Hall, P.E., Lathia, J.D., Caldwell, M.A. & Ffrench-Constant, C. (2008). Laminin Enhances the Growth of Human Neural Stem Cells in Defined Culture Media. *BMC Neuroscience,* Vol.9, pp. 71, ISSN 1471-2202

Hamanoue, M., Takemoto, N., Matsumoto, K., Nakamura, T., Nakajima, K. & Kohsaka, S. (1996). Neurotrophic Effect of Hepatocyte Growth Factor on Central Nervous System Neurons in Vitro. *Journal of Neuroscience Research,* Vol.43, No.5, pp. 554-564, ISSN 0360-4012

Hansen, T.M., Moss, A.J. & Brindle, N.P. (2008). Vascular Endothelial Growth Factor and Angiopoietins in Neurovascular Regeneration and Protection Following Stroke. *Current Neurovascular Research,* Vol.5, No.4, pp. 236-245, ISSN 1875-5739; 1567-2026

Haynesworth, S.E., Baber, M.A. & Caplan, A.I. (1996). Cytokine Expression by Human Marrow-Derived Mesenchymal Progenitor Cells in Vitro: Effects of Dexamethasone and IL-1 Alpha. *Journal of Cellular Physiology,* Vol.166, No.3, pp. 585-592, ISSN 0021-9541

Henderson, D.J. & Copp, A.J. (1997). Role of the Extracellular Matrix in Neural Crest Cell Migration. *Journal of Anatomy,* Vol.191, Pt.4, pp. 507-515, ISSN 1469-7580; 0021-8782

Heron, M., Hoyert, D.L., Murphy, S.L., Xu, J., Kochanek, K.D. & Tejada-Vera, B. (2009). Deaths: Final Data for 2006. *National Vital Statistics Reports : From the Centers for Disease Control and Prevention, National Center for Health Statistics, National Vital Statistics System,* Vol.57, No.14, pp. 1-134, ISSN 1551-8922

Honda, S., Kagoshima, M., Wanaka, A., Tohyama, M., Matsumoto, K. & Nakamura, T. (1995). Localization and Functional Coupling of HGF and c-Met/HGF Receptor in Rat Brain: Implication as Neurotrophic Factor. *Brain Research.Molecular Brain Research,* Vol.32, No.2, pp. 197-210, ISSN 0169-328X

Honmou, O., Houkin, K., Matsunaga, T., Niitsu, Y., Ishiai, S., Onodera, R., Waxman, S.G. & Kocsis, J.D. (2011). Intravenous Administration of Auto Serum-Expanded Autologous Mesenchymal Stem Cells in Stroke. *Brain,* Vol.134, No.Pt 6, pp. 1790-1807, ISSN 1460-2156; 0006-8950

Horwitz, E.M., Le Blanc, K., Dominici, M., Mueller, I., Slaper-Cortenbach, I., Marini, F.C., Deans, R.J., Krause, D.S., Keating, A. & International Society for Cellular Therapy.

(2005). Clarification of the Nomenclature for MSC: The International Society for Cellular Therapy Position Statement. *Cytotherapy,* Vol.7, No.5, pp. 393-395, ISSN 1465-3249

Hou, S., Xu, Q., Tian, W., Cui, F., Cai, Q., Ma, J. & Lee, I.S. (2005). The Repair of Brain Lesion by Implantation of Hyaluronic Acid Hydrogels Modified with Laminin. *Journal of Neuroscience Methods,* Vol.148, No.1, pp. 60-70, ISSN 0165-0270

Hu, J., Deng, L., Wang, X. & Xu, X.M. (2009). Effects of Extracellular Matrix Molecules on the Growth Properties of Oligodendrocyte Progenitor Cells in Vitro. *Journal of Neuroscience Research,* Vol.87, No.13, pp. 2854-2862, ISSN 1097-4547; 0360-4012

Huang, X., Choi, J.K., Park, S.R., Ha, Y., Park, H., Yoon, S.H., Park, H.C., Park, J.O. & Choi, B.H. (2007). GM-CSF Inhibits Apoptosis of Neural Cells Via Regulating the Expression of Apoptosis-Related Proteins. *Neuroscience Research,* Vol.58, No.1, pp. 50-57, ISSN 0168-0102

Hunter, D.D., Llinas, R., Ard, M., Merlie, J.P. & Sanes, J.R. (1992). Expression of s-Laminin and Laminin in the Developing Rat Central Nervous System. *The Journal of Comparative Neurology,* Vol.323, No.2, pp. 238-251, ISSN 0021-9967

Iantosca, M.R., McPherson, C.E., Ho, S.Y. & Maxwell, G.D. (1999). Bone Morphogenetic Proteins-2 and -4 Attenuate Apoptosis in a Cerebellar Primitive Neuroectodermal Tumor Cell Line. *Journal of Neuroscience Research,* Vol.56, No.3, pp. 248-258, ISSN 0360-4012

Iihara, K., Hashimoto, N., Tsukahara, T., Sakata, M., Yanamoto, H. & Taniguchi, T. (1997). Platelet-Derived Growth Factor-BB, but Not -AA, Prevents Delayed Neuronal Death After Forebrain Ischemia in Rats. *Journal of Cerebral Blood Flow and Metabolism,* Vol.17, No.10, pp. 1097-1106, ISSN 0271-678X

Jackson, J.R., Seed, M.P., Kircher, C.H., Willoughby, D.A. & Winkler, J.D. (1997). The Codependence of Angiogenesis and Chronic Inflammation. *The FASEB Journal,* Vol.11, No.6, pp. 457-465, ISSN 0892-6638

Jin, K., Mao, X.O. & Greenberg, D.A. (2006). Vascular Endothelial Growth Factor Stimulates Neurite Outgrowth from Cerebral Cortical Neurons Via Rho Kinase Signaling. *Journal of Neurobiology,* Vol.66, No.3, pp. 236-242, ISSN 0022-3034

Jin, K., Mao, X.O., Sun, Y., Xie, L., Jin, L., Nishi, E., Klagsbrun, M. & Greenberg, D.A. (2002). Heparin-Binding Epidermal Growth Factor-Like Growth Factor: Hypoxia-Inducible Expression in Vitro and Stimulation of Neurogenesis in Vitro and in Vivo. *The Journal of Neuroscience,* Vol.22, No.13, pp. 5365-5373, ISSN 1529-2401; 0270-6474

Jin, K., Sun, Y., Xie, L., Childs, J., Mao, X.O. & Greenberg, D.A. (2004). Post-Ischemic Administration of Heparin-Binding Epidermal Growth Factor-Like Growth Factor (HB-EGF) Reduces Infarct Size and Modifies Neurogenesis After Focal Cerebral Ischemia in the Rat. *Journal of Cerebral Blood Flow and Metabolism,* Vol.24, No.4, pp. 399-408, ISSN 0271-678X

Jin, K.L., Mao, X.O. & Greenberg, D.A. (2000). Vascular Endothelial Growth Factor: Direct Neuroprotective Effect in in Vitro Ischemia. *Proceedings of the National Academy of Sciences of the United States of America,* Vol.97, No.18, pp. 10242-10247, ISSN 0027-8424

Johe, K.K., Hazel, T.G., Muller, T., Dugich-Djordjevic, M.M. & McKay, R.D. (1996). Single Factors Direct the Differentiation of Stem Cells from the Fetal and Adult Central Nervous System. *Genes & Development,* Vol.10, No.24, pp. 3129-3140, ISSN 0890-9369

Joseph D'Ercole, A. & Ye, P. (2008). Expanding the Mind: Insulin-Like Growth Factor I and Brain Development. *Endocrinology,* Vol.149, No.12, pp. 5958-5962, ISSN 0013-7227

Kaigler, D., Krebsbach, P.H., Polverini, P.J. & Mooney, D.J. (2003). Role of Vascular Endothelial Growth Factor in Bone Marrow Stromal Cell Modulation of Endothelial Cells. *Tissue Engineering,* Vol.9, No.1, pp. 95-103, ISSN 1076-3279

Kernie, S.G. & Parent, J.M. (2010). Forebrain Neurogenesis After Focal Ischemic and Traumatic Brain Injury. *Neurobiology of Disease,* Vol.37, No.2, pp. 267-274, ISSN 1095-953X; 0969-9961

Kim, H.J., Lee, J.H. & Kim, S.H. (2010). Therapeutic Effects of Human Mesenchymal Stem Cells on Traumatic Brain Injury in Rats: Secretion of Neurotrophic Factors and Inhibition of Apoptosis. *Journal of Neurotrauma,* Vol.27, No.1, pp. 131-138, ISSN 1557-9042; 0897-7151

Kinnaird, T., Stabile, E., Burnett, M.S., Lee, C.W., Barr, S., Fuchs, S. & Epstein, S.E. (2004). Marrow-Derived Stromal Cells Express Genes Encoding a Broad Spectrum of Arteriogenic Cytokines and Promote in Vitro and in Vivo Arteriogenesis through Paracrine Mechanisms. *Circulation Research,* Vol.94, No.5, pp. 678-685, ISSN 1524-4571

Kopen, G.C., Prockop, D.J. & Phinney, D.G. (1999). Marrow Stromal Cells Migrate Throughout Forebrain and Cerebellum, and they Differentiate into Astrocytes After Injection into Neonatal Mouse Brains. *Proceedings of the National Academy of Sciences of the United States of America,* Vol.96, No.19, pp. 10711-10716, ISSN 0027-8424

Kortesidis, A., Zannettino, A., Isenmann, S., Shi, S., Lapidot, T. & Gronthos, S. (2005). Stromal-Derived Factor-1 Promotes the Growth, Survival, and Development of Human Bone Marrow Stromal Stem Cells. *Blood,* Vol.105, No.10, pp. 3793-3801, ISSN 0006-4971

Kosaka, N., Kodama, M., Sasaki, H., Yamamoto, Y., Takeshita, F., Takahama, Y., Sakamoto, H., Kato, T., Terada, M. & Ochiya, T. (2006). FGF-4 Regulates Neural Progenitor Cell Proliferation and Neuronal Differentiation. *The FASEB Journal,* Vol.20, No.9, pp. 1484-1485, ISSN 1530-6860; 0892-6638

Kumar, R., Yoneda, J., Bucana, C.D. & Fidler, I.J. (1998). Regulation of Distinct Steps of Angiogenesis by Different Angiogenic Molecules. *International Journal of Oncology,* Vol.12, No.4, pp. 749-757, ISSN 1019-6439

Lai, Y., Sun, Y., Skinner, C.M., Son, E.L., Lu, Z., Tuan, R.S., Jilka, R.L., Ling, J. & Chen, X.D. (2010). Reconstitution of Marrow-Derived Extracellular Matrix Ex Vivo: A Robust Culture System for Expanding Large-Scale Highly Functional Human Mesenchymal Stem Cells. *Stem Cells and Development,* Vol.19, No.7, pp. 1095-1107, ISSN 1557-8534; 1547-3287

Lazarovici, P., Marcinkiewicz, C. & Lelkes, P.I. (2006). Cross Talk between the Cardiovascular and Nervous Systems: Neurotrophic Effects of Vascular Endothelial Growth Factor (VEGF) and Angiogenic Effects of Nerve Growth Factor

(NGF)-Implications in Drug Development. *Current Pharmaceutical Design,* Vol.12, No.21, pp. 2609-2622, ISSN 1381-6128

Lee, B., Clarke, D., Al Ahmad, A., Kahle, M., Parham, C., Auckland, L., Shaw, C., Fidanboylu, M., Orr, A.W., Ogunshola, O., Fertala, A., Thomas, S.A. & Bix, G.J. (2011). Perlecan Domain V is Neuroprotective and Proangiogenic Following Ischemic Stroke in Rodents. *The Journal of Clinical Investigation,* Vol.121, No.8, pp. 3005-3023, ISSN 1558-8238; 0021-9738

Lee, J.S., Hong, J.M., Moon, G.J., Lee, P.H., Ahn, Y.H., Bang, O.Y. & STARTING collaborators. (2010). A Long-Term Follow-Up Study of Intravenous Autologous Mesenchymal Stem Cell Transplantation in Patients with Ischemic Stroke. *Stem Cells (Dayton, Ohio),* Vol.28, No.6, pp. 1099-1106, ISSN 1549-4918; 1066-5099

Leker, R.R. & Shohami, E. (2002). Cerebral Ischemia and Trauma-Different Etiologies Yet Similar Mechanisms: Neuroprotective Opportunities. *Brain Research.Brain Research Reviews,* Vol.39, No.1, pp. 55-73, ISSN 0165-0173

Li, J., Zhu, H., Liu, Y., Li, Q., Lu, S., Feng, M., Xu, Y., Huang, L., Ma, C., An, Y., Zhao, R.C., Wang, R. & Qin, C. (2010). Human Mesenchymal Stem Cell Transplantation Protects Against Cerebral Ischemic Injury and Upregulates Interleukin-10 Expression in Macacafascicularis. *Brain Research,* Vol.1334, pp. 65-72, ISSN 1872-6240; 0006-8993

Li, J.W., Li, L.L., Chang, L.L., Wang, Z.Y. & Xu, Y. (2009). Stem Cell Factor Protects Against Neuronal Apoptosis by Activating AKT/ERK in Diabetic Mice. *Brazilian Journal of Medical and Biological Research,* Vol.42, No.11, pp. 1044-1049, ISSN 1414-431X; 0100-879X

Li, Y., Chen, J., Chen, X.G., Wang, L., Gautam, S.C., Xu, Y.X., Katakowski, M., Zhang, L.J., Lu, M., Janakiraman, N. & Chopp, M. (2002). Human Marrow Stromal Cell Therapy for Stroke in Rat: Neurotrophins and Functional Recovery. *Neurology,* Vol.59, No.4, pp. 514-523, ISSN 0028-3878

Li, Y., Chen, J., Zhang, C.L., Wang, L., Lu, D., Katakowski, M., Gao, Q., Shen, L.H., Zhang, J., Lu, M. & Chopp, M. (2005). Gliosis and Brain Remodeling After Treatment of Stroke in Rats with Marrow Stromal Cells. *Glia,* Vol.49, No.3, pp. 407-417, ISSN 0894-1491

Li, Y. & Chopp, M. (2009). Marrow Stromal Cell Transplantation in Stroke and Traumatic Brain Injury. *Neuroscience Letters,* Vol.456, No.3, pp. 120-123, ISSN 1872-7972; 0304-3940

Lipsky, R.H. & Marini, A.M. (2007). Brain-Derived Neurotrophic Factor in Neuronal Survival and Behavior-Related Plasticity. *Annals of the New York Academy of Sciences,* Vol.1122, pp. 130-143, ISSN 0077-8923

Liu, X.S., Chopp, M., Zhang, R.L., Hozeska-Solgot, A., Gregg, S.C., Buller, B., Lu, M. & Zhang, Z.G. (2009). Angiopoietin 2 Mediates the Differentiation and Migration of Neural Progenitor Cells in the Subventricular Zone After Stroke. *The Journal of Biological Chemistry,* Vol.284, No.34, pp. 22680-22689, ISSN 1083-351X; 0021-9258

Lopez-Lopez, C., LeRoith, D. & Torres-Aleman, I. (2004). Insulin-Like Growth Factor I is Required for Vessel Remodeling in the Adult Brain. *Proceedings of the National Academy of Sciences of the United States of America,* Vol.101, No.26, pp. 9833-9838, ISSN 0027-8424

Lu, P., Blesch, A. & Tuszynski, M.H. (2004). Induction of Bone Marrow Stromal Cells to Neurons: Differentiation, Transdifferentiation, Or Artifact? *Journal of Neuroscience Research,* Vol.77, No.2, pp. 174-191, ISSN 0360-4012

Lu, Y.Z., Lin, C.H., Cheng, F.C. & Hsueh, C.M. (2005). Molecular Mechanisms Responsible for Microglia-Derived Protection of Sprague-Dawley Rat Brain Cells during in Vitro Ischemia. *Neuroscience Letters,* Vol.373, No.2, pp. 159-164, ISSN 0304-3940

Lum, M., Turbic, A., Mitrovic, B. & Turnley, A.M. (2009). Fibroblast Growth Factor-9 Inhibits Astrocyte Differentiation of Adult Mouse Neural Progenitor Cells. *Journal of Neuroscience Research,* Vol.87, No.10, pp. 2201-2210, ISSN 1097-4547; 0360-4012

Lykissas, M.G., Batistatou, A.K., Charalabopoulos, K.A. & Beris, A.E. (2007). The Role of Neurotrophins in Axonal Growth, Guidance, and Regeneration. *Current Neurovascular Research,* Vol.4, No.2, pp. 143-151, ISSN 1567-2026

Ma, M., Ma, Y., Yi, X., Guo, R., Zhu, W., Fan, X., Xu, G., Frey, W.H.,2nd & Liu, X. (2008). Intranasal Delivery of Transforming Growth Factor-beta1 in Mice After Stroke Reduces Infarct Volume and Increases Neurogenesis in the Subventricular Zone. *BMC Neuroscience,* Vol.9, pp. 117, ISSN 1471-2202

Ma, W., Fitzgerald, W., Liu, Q.Y., O'Shaughnessy, T.J., Maric, D., Lin, H.J., Alkon, D.L. & Barker, J.L. (2004). CNS Stem and Progenitor Cell Differentiation into Functional Neuronal Circuits in Three-Dimensional Collagen Gels. *Experimental Neurology,* Vol.190, No.2, pp. 276-288, ISSN 0014-4886

Maas, A.I., Roozenbeek, B. & Manley, G.T. (2010). Clinical Trials in Traumatic Brain Injury: Past Experience and Current Developments. *Neurotherapeutics,* Vol.7, No.1, pp. 115-126, ISSN 1878-7479

Mahmood, A., Lu, D. & Chopp, M. (2004). Marrow Stromal Cell Transplantation After Traumatic Brain Injury Promotes Cellular Proliferation within the Brain. *Neurosurgery,* Vol.55, No.5, pp. 1185-1193, ISSN 1524-4040; 0148-396X

Mathieu, P., Piantanida, A.P. & Pitossi, F. (2010). Chronic Expression of Transforming Growth Factor-Beta Enhances Adult Neurogenesis. *Neuroimmunomodulation,* Vol.17, No.3, pp. 200-201, ISSN 1423-0216; 1021-7401

Mehler, M.F., Rozental, R., Dougherty, M., Spray, D.C. & Kessler, J.A. (1993). Cytokine Regulation of Neuronal Differentiation of Hippocampal Progenitor Cells. *Nature,* Vol.362, No.6415, pp. 62-65, ISSN 0028-0836

Mezey, E., Mayer, B. & Nemeth, K. (2010). Unexpected Roles for Bone Marrow Stromal Cells (Or MSCs): A Real Promise for Cellular, but Not Replacement, Therapy. *Oral Diseases,* Vol.16, No.2, pp. 129-135, ISSN 1601-0825; 1354-523X

Minamino, K., Adachi, Y., Okigaki, M., Ito, H., Togawa, Y., Fujita, K., Tomita, M., Suzuki, Y., Zhang, Y., Iwasaki, M., Nakano, K., Koike, Y., Matsubara, H., Iwasaka, T., Matsumura, M. & Ikehara, S. (2005). Macrophage Colony-Stimulating Factor (M-CSF), as Well as Granulocyte Colony-Stimulating Factor (G-CSF), Accelerates Neovascularization. *Stem Cells,* Vol.23, No.3, pp. 347-354, ISSN 1066-5099

Mitsios, N., Gaffney, J., Kumar, P., Krupinski, J., Kumar, S. & Slevin, M. (2006). Pathophysiology of Acute Ischaemic Stroke: An Analysis of Common Signalling Mechanisms and Identification of New Molecular Targets. *Pathobiology : Journal of Immunopathology, Molecular and Cellular Biology,* Vol.73, No.4, pp. 159-175, ISSN 1015-2008

Mosesson, M.W. (1984). The Role of Fibronectin in monocyte/macrophage Function. *Progress in Clinical and Biological Research,* Vol.154, pp. 155-175, ISSN 0361-7742

Mudo, G., Bonomo, A., Di Liberto, V., Frinchi, M., Fuxe, K. & Belluardo, N. (2009). The FGF-2/FGFRs Neurotrophic System Promotes Neurogenesis in the Adult Brain. *Journal of Neural Transmission,* Vol.116, No.8, pp. 995-1005, ISSN 1435-1463; 0300-9564

Munoz-Elias, G., Marcus, A.J., Coyne, T.M., Woodbury, D. & Black, I.B. (2004). Adult Bone Marrow Stromal Cells in the Embryonic Brain: Engraftment, Migration, Differentiation, and Long-Term Survival. *The Journal of Neuroscience,* Vol.24, No.19, pp. 4585-4595, 1529-2401

Nag, S., Kapadia, A. & Stewart, D.J. (2011). Review: Molecular Pathogenesis of Blood-Brain Barrier Breakdown in Acute Brain Injury. *Neuropathology and Applied Neurobiology,* Vol.37, No.1, pp. 3-23, 1365-2990; 0305-1846

Nasu-Tada, K., Koizumi, S. & Inoue, K. (2005). Involvement of beta1 Integrin in Microglial Chemotaxis and Proliferation on Fibronectin: Different Regulations by ADP through PKA. *Glia,* Vol.52, No.2, pp. 98-107, ISSN 1098-1136; 0894-1491

Nauta, A.J. & Fibbe, W.E. (2007). Immunomodulatory Properties of Mesenchymal Stromal Cells. *Blood,* Vol.110, No.10, pp. 3499-3506, ISSN 0006-4971

Neuhuber, B., Gallo, G., Howard, L., Kostura, L., Mackay, A. & Fischer, I. (2004). Reevaluation of in Vitro Differentiation Protocols for Bone Marrow Stromal Cells: Disruption of Actin Cytoskeleton Induces Rapid Morphological Changes and Mimics Neuronal Phenotype. *Journal of Neuroscience Research,* Vol.77, No.2, pp. 192-204, ISSN 0360-4012

Neuss, S., Becher, E., Woltje, M., Tietze, L. & Jahnen-Dechent, W. (2004). Functional Expression of HGF and HGF receptor/c-Met in Adult Human Mesenchymal Stem Cells Suggests a Role in Cell Mobilization, Tissue Repair, and Wound Healing. *Stem Cells,* Vol.22, No.3, pp. 405-414, ISSN 1066-5099

Nishibe, M., Barbay, S., Guggenmos, D. & Nudo, R.J. (2010). Reorganization of Motor Cortex After Controlled Cortical Impact in Rats and Implications for Functional Recovery. *Journal of Neurotrauma,* Vol.27, No.12, pp. 2221-2232, ISSN 1557-9042; 0897-7151

Nobes, C.D. & Tolkovsky, A.M. (1995). Neutralizing Anti-p21ras Fabs Suppress Rat Sympathetic Neuron Survival Induced by NGF, LIF, CNTF and cAMP. *The European Journal of Neuroscience,* Vol.7, No.2, pp. 344-350, ISSN 0953-816X

Noonan, D.M., De Lerma Barbaro, A., Vannini, N., Mortara, L. & Albini, A. (2008). Inflammation, Inflammatory Cells and Angiogenesis: Decisions and Indecisions. *Cancer Metastasis Reviews,* Vol.27, No.1, pp. 31-40, ISSN 0167-7659

Numasaki, M., Fukushi, J., Ono, M., Narula, S.K., Zavodny, P.J., Kudo, T., Robbins, P.D., Tahara, H. & Lotze, M.T. (2003). Interleukin-17 Promotes Angiogenesis and Tumor Growth. *Blood,* Vol.101, No.7, pp. 2620-2627, 0006-4971; 0006-4971

O'Collins, V.E., Macleod, M.R., Donnan, G.A., Horky, L.L., van der Worp, B.H. & Howells, D.W. (2006). 1,026 Experimental Treatments in Acute Stroke. *Annals of Neurology,* Vol.59, No.3, pp. 467-477, ISSN 0364-5134

Oh, J., McCloskey, M.A., Blong, C.C., Bendickson, L., Nilsen-Hamilton, M. & Sakaguchi, D.S. (2010). Astrocyte-Derived Interleukin-6 Promotes Specific Neuronal Differentiation of Neural Progenitor Cells from Adult Hippocampus. *Journal of Neuroscience Research,* Vol.88, No.13, pp. 2798-2809, ISSN 1097-4547; 0360-4012

Ohab, J.J. & Carmichael, S.T. (2008). Poststroke Neurogenesis: Emerging Principles of Migration and Localization of Immature Neurons. *The Neuroscientist,* Vol.14, No.4, pp. 369-380, ISSN 1073-8584

Omori, Y., Honmou, O., Harada, K., Suzuki, J., Houkin, K. & Kocsis, J.D. (2008). Optimization of a Therapeutic Protocol for Intravenous Injection of Human Mesenchymal Stem Cells After Cerebral Ischemia in Adult Rats. *Brain Research,* Vol.1236, pp. 30-38, ISSN 0006-8993

Onda, T., Honmou, O., Harada, K., Houkin, K., Hamada, H. & Kocsis, J.D. (2008). Therapeutic Benefits by Human Mesenchymal Stem Cells (hMSCs) and Ang-1 Gene-Modified hMSCs After Cerebral Ischemia. *Journal of Cerebral Blood Flow and Metabolism,* Vol.28, No.2, pp. 329-340, ISSN 0271-678X

Opanashuk, L.A., Mark, R.J., Porter, J., Damm, D., Mattson, M.P. & Seroogy, K.B. (1999). Heparin-Binding Epidermal Growth Factor-Like Growth Factor in Hippocampus: Modulation of Expression by Seizures and Anti-Excitotoxic Action. *The Journal of Neuroscience,* Vol.19, No.1, pp. 133-146, ISSN 0270-6474

Parr, A.M., Tator, C.H. & Keating, A. (2007). Bone Marrow-Derived Mesenchymal Stromal Cells for the Repair of Central Nervous System Injury. *Bone Marrow Transplantation,* Vol.40, No.7, pp. 609-619, ISSN 0268-3369

Pavlichenko, N., Sokolova, I., Vijde, S., Shvedova, E., Alexandrov, G., Krouglyakov, P., Fedotova, O., Gilerovich, E.G., Polyntsev, D.G. & Otellin, V.A. (2008). Mesenchymal Stem Cells Transplantation could be Beneficial for Treatment of Experimental Ischemic Stroke in Rats. *Brain Research,* Vol.1233, pp. 203-213, ISSN 0006-8993

Perris, R. & Perissinotto, D. (2000). Role of the Extracellular Matrix during Neural Crest Cell Migration. *Mechanisms of Development,* Vol.95, No.1-2, pp. 3-21, ISSN 0925-4773

Phinney, D.G. & Prockop, D.J. (2007). Concise Review: Mesenchymal stem/multipotent Stromal Cells: The State of Transdifferentiation and Modes of Tissue Repair--Current Views. *Stem Cells,* Vol.25, No.11, pp. 2896-2902, ISSN 1549-4918; 1066-5099

Pires Neto, M.A., Braga-de-Souza, S. & Lent, R. (1999). Extracellular Matrix Molecules Play Diverse Roles in the Growth and Guidance of Central Nervous System Axons. *Brazilian Journal of Medical and Biological Research,* Vol.32, No.5, pp. 633-638, ISSN 0100-879X

Ponte, A.L., Marais, E., Gallay, N., Langonne, A., Delorme, B., Herault, O., Charbord, P. & Domenech, J. (2007). The in Vitro Migration Capacity of Human Bone Marrow Mesenchymal Stem Cells: Comparison of Chemokine and Growth Factor Chemotactic Activities. *Stem Cells,* Vol.25, No.7, pp. 1737-1745, ISSN 1066-5099

Potapova, I.A., Gaudette, G.R., Brink, P.R., Robinson, R.B., Rosen, M.R., Cohen, I.S. & Doronin, S.V. (2007). Mesenchymal Stem Cells Support Migration, Extracellular Matrix Invasion, Proliferation, and Survival of Endothelial Cells in Vitro. *Stem Cells,* Vol.25, No.7, pp. 1761-1768, ISSN 1066-5099

Potian, J.A., Aviv, H., Ponzio, N.M., Harrison, J.S. & Rameshwar, P. (2003). Veto-Like Activity of Mesenchymal Stem Cells: Functional Discrimination between Cellular Responses to Alloantigens and Recall Antigens. *Journal of Immunology,* Vol.171, No.7, pp. 3426-3434, ISSN 0022-1767

Properzi, F., Asher, R.A. & Fawcett, J.W. (2003). Chondroitin Sulphate Proteoglycans in the Central Nervous System: Changes and Synthesis After Injury. *Biochemical Society Transactions,* Vol.31, No.2, pp. 335-336, ISSN 1470-8752; 0300-5127

Qin, L., Kim, E., Ratan, R., Lee, F.S. & Cho, S. (2011). Genetic Variant of BDNF (Val66Met) Polymorphism Attenuates Stroke-Induced Angiogenic Responses by Enhancing Anti-Angiogenic Mediator CD36 Expression. *The Journal of Neuroscience,* Vol.31, No.2, pp. 775-783, ISSN 1529-2401; 0270-6474

Robinson, A.P., Foraker, J.E., Ylostalo, J. & Prockop, D.J. (2011). Human stem/progenitor Cells from Bone Marrow Enhance Glial Differentiation of Rat Neural Stem Cells: A Role for Transforming Growth Factor Beta and Notch Signaling. *Stem Cells and Development,* Vol.20, No.2, pp. 289-300, ISSN 1557-8534; 1547-3287

Robinson, S., Tani, M., Strieter, R.M., Ransohoff, R.M. & Miller, R.H. (1998). The Chemokine Growth-Regulated Oncogene-Alpha Promotes Spinal Cord Oligodendrocyte Precursor Proliferation. *The Journal of Neuroscience,* Vol.18, No.24, pp. 10457-10463, ISSN 0270-6474

Roger, V.L., Go, A.S., Lloyd-Jones, D.M., Adams, R.J., Berry, J.D., Brown, T.M., Carnethon, M.R., Dai, S., de Simone, G., Ford, E.S., Fox, C.S., Fullerton, H.J., Gillespie, C., Greenlund, K.J., Hailpern, S.M., Heit, J.A., Ho, P.M., Howard, V.J., Kissela, B.M., Kittner, S.J., Lackland, D.T., Lichtman, J.H., Lisabeth, L.D., Makuc, D.M., Marcus, G.M., Marelli, A., Matchar, D.B., McDermott, M.M., Meigs, J.B., Moy, C.S., Mozaffarian, D., Mussolino, M.E., Nichol, G., Paynter, N.P., Rosamond, W.D., Sorlie, P.D., Stafford, R.S., Turan, T.N., Turner, M.B., Wong, N.D., Wylie-Rosett, J. & American Heart Association Statistics Committee and Stroke Statistics Subcommittee. (2011). Heart Disease and Stroke Statistics--2011 Update: A Report from the American Heart Association. *Circulation,* Vol.123, No.4, pp. e18-e209, ISSN 1524-4539; 0009-7322

Sabo, J.K., Kilpatrick, T.J. & Cate, H.S. (2009). Effects of Bone Morphogenic Proteins on Neural Precursor Cells and Regulation during Central Nervous System Injury. *Neuro-Signals,* Vol.17, No.4, pp. 255-264, ISSN 1424-8638; 1424-862X

Sadohara, T., Sugahara, K., Urashima, Y., Terasaki, H. & Lyama, K. (2001). Keratinocyte Growth Factor Prevents Ischemia-Induced Delayed Neuronal Death in the Hippocampal CA1 Field of the Gerbil Brain. *Neuroreport,* Vol.12, No.1, pp. 71-76, ISSN 0959-4965

Sakai, T., Johnson, K.J., Murozono, M., Sakai, K., Magnuson, M.A., Wieloch, T., Cronberg, T., Isshiki, A., Erickson, H.P. & Fassler, R. (2001). Plasma Fibronectin Supports Neuronal Survival and Reduces Brain Injury Following Transient Focal Cerebral Ischemia but is Not Essential for Skin-Wound Healing and Hemostasis. *Nature Medicine,* Vol.7, No.3, pp. 324-30., ISSN 1546-170X; 1078-8956

Sanchez-Ramos, J., Song, S., Cardozo-Pelaez, F., Hazzi, C., Stedeford, T., Willing, A., Freeman, T.B., Saporta, S., Janssen, W., Patel, N., Cooper, D.R. & Sanberg, P.R. (2000). Adult Bone Marrow Stromal Cells Differentiate into Neural Cells in Vitro. *Experimental Neurology,* Vol.164, No.2, pp. 247-256, ISSN 0014-4886

Schabitz, W.R., Kollmar, R., Schwaninger, M., Juettler, E., Bardutzky, J., Scholzke, M.N., Sommer, C. & Schwab, S. (2003). Neuroprotective Effect of Granulocyte Colony-

Stimulating Factor After Focal Cerebral Ischemia. *Stroke,* Vol.34, No.3, pp. 745-751, ISSN 1524-4628; 0039-2499

Schabitz, W.R., Steigleder, T., Cooper-Kuhn, C.M., Schwab, S., Sommer, C., Schneider, A. & Kuhn, H.G. (2007). Intravenous Brain-Derived Neurotrophic Factor Enhances Poststroke Sensorimotor Recovery and Stimulates Neurogenesis. *Stroke,* Vol.38, No.7, pp. 2165-2172, ISSN 1524-4628; 0039-2499

Schinkothe, T., Bloch, W. & Schmidt, A. (2008). In Vitro Secreting Profile of Human Mesenchymal Stem Cells. *Stem Cells and Development,* Vol.17, No.1, pp. 199-206, ISSN 1547-3287

Schmidt, A., Ladage, D., Schinkothe, T., Klausmann, U., Ulrichs, C., Klinz, F.J., Brixius, K., Arnhold, S., Desai, B., Mehlhorn, U., Schwinger, R.H., Staib, P., Addicks, K. & Bloch, W. (2006). Basic Fibroblast Growth Factor Controls Migration in Human Mesenchymal Stem Cells. *Stem Cells,* Vol.24, No.7, pp. 1750-1758, ISSN 1066-5099

Schneider, A., Kruger, C., Steigleder, T., Weber, D., Pitzer, C., Laage, R., Aronowski, J., Maurer, M.H., Gassler, N., Mier, W., Hasselblatt, M., Kollmar, R., Schwab, S., Sommer, C., Bach, A., Kuhn, H.G. & Schabitz, W.R. (2005). The Hematopoietic Factor G-CSF is a Neuronal Ligand that Counteracts Programmed Cell Death and Drives Neurogenesis. *The Journal of Clinical Investigation,* Vol.115, No.8, pp. 2083-2098, ISSN 0021-9738

Sehara, Y., Hayashi, T., Deguchi, K., Zhang, H., Tsuchiya, A., Yamashita, T., Lukic, V., Nagai, M., Kamiya, T. & Abe, K. (2007). Potentiation of Neurogenesis and Angiogenesis by G-CSF After Focal Cerebral Ischemia in Rats. *Brain Research,* Vol.1151, pp. 142-149, ISSN 0006-8993

Shang, J., Deguchi, K., Ohta, Y., Liu, N., Zhang, X., Tian, F., Yamashita, T., Ikeda, Y., Matsuura, T., Funakoshi, H., Nakamura, T. & Abe, K. (2011). Strong Neurogenesis, Angiogenesis, Synaptogenesis, and Antifibrosis of Hepatocyte Growth Factor in Rats Brain After Transient Middle Cerebral Artery Occlusion. *Journal of Neuroscience Research,* Vol.89, No.1, pp. 86-95, ISSN 1097-4547; 0360-4012

Shen, L.H., Li, Y., Gao, Q., Savant-Bhonsale, S. & Chopp, M. (2008). Down-Regulation of Neurocan Expression in Reactive Astrocytes Promotes Axonal Regeneration and Facilitates the Neurorestorative Effects of Bone Marrow Stromal Cells in the Ischemic Rat Brain. *Glia,* Vol.56, No.16, pp. 1747-1754, ISSN 1098-1136; 0894-1491

Shen, Y., Inoue, N. & Heese, K. (2010). Neurotrophin-4 (ntf4) Mediates Neurogenesis in Mouse Embryonic Neural Stem Cells through the Inhibition of the Signal Transducer and Activator of Transcription-3 (stat3) and the Modulation of the Activity of Protein Kinase B. *Cellular and Molecular Neurobiology,* Vol.30, No.6, pp. 909-916, ISSN 1573-6830; 0272-4340

Shibuya, M. (2009). Brain Angiogenesis in Developmental and Pathological Processes: Therapeutic Aspects of Vascular Endothelial Growth Factor. *The FEBS Journal,* Vol.276, No.17, pp. 4636-4643, ISSN 1742-4658; 1742-464X

Shimamura, M., Sato, N., Waguri, S., Uchiyama, Y., Hayashi, T., Iida, H., Nakamura, T., Ogihara, T., Kaneda, Y. & Morishita, R. (2006). Gene Transfer of Hepatocyte Growth Factor Gene Improves Learning and Memory in the Chronic Stage of Cerebral Infarction. *Hypertension,* Vol.47, No.4, pp. 742-751, ISSN 1524-4563

Shimazaki, T., Shingo, T. & Weiss, S. (2001). The Ciliary Neurotrophic factor/leukemia Inhibitory factor/gp130 Receptor Complex Operates in the Maintenance of Mammalian Forebrain Neural Stem Cells. *The Journal of Neuroscience,* Vol.21, No.19, pp. 7642-7653, ISSN 1529-2401; 0270-6474

Shirakura, M., Inoue, M., Fujikawa, S., Washizawa, K., Komaba, S., Maeda, M., Watabe, K., Yoshikawa, Y. & Hasegawa, M. (2004). Postischemic Administration of Sendai Virus Vector Carrying Neurotrophic Factor Genes Prevents Delayed Neuronal Death in Gerbils. *Gene Therapy,* Vol.11, No.9, pp. 784-790, ISSN 0969-7128

Shyu, W.C., Lin, S.Z., Yang, H.I., Tzeng, Y.S., Pang, C.Y., Yen, P.S. & Li, H. (2004). Functional Recovery of Stroke Rats Induced by Granulocyte Colony-Stimulating Factor-Stimulated Stem Cells. *Circulation,* Vol.110, No.13, pp. 1847-1854, ISSN 1524-4539; 0009-7322

Smadja, D.M., d'Audigier, C., Weiswald, L.B., Badoual, C., Dangles-Marie, V., Mauge, L., Evrard, S., Laurendeau, I., Lallemand, F., Germain, S., Grelac, F., Dizier, B., Vidaud, M., Bièche, I. & Gaussem, P. (2010). The Wnt Antagonist Dickkopf-1 Increases Endothelial Progenitor Cell Angiogenic Potential. *Arteriosclerosis, thrombosis, and vascular biology,* Vol.30, No.12, pp. 2544-2552, ISSN 1079-5642; 1524-4636

Solaroglu, I., Tsubokawa, T., Cahill, J. & Zhang, J.H. (2006). Anti-Apoptotic Effect of Granulocyte-Colony Stimulating Factor After Focal Cerebral Ischemia in the Rat. *Neuroscience,* Vol.143, No.4, pp. 965-974, ISSN 0306-4522

Son, B.R., Marquez-Curtis, L.A., Kucia, M., Wysoczynski, M., Turner, A.R., Ratajczak, J., Ratajczak, M.Z. & Janowska-Wieczorek, A. (2006). Migration of Bone Marrow and Cord Blood Mesenchymal Stem Cells in Vitro is Regulated by Stromal-Derived Factor-1-CXCR4 and Hepatocyte Growth Factor-c-Met Axes and Involves Matrix Metalloproteinases. *Stem Cells,* Vol.24, No.5, pp. 1254-1264, ISSN 1066-5099

Sottile, J. (2004). Regulation of Angiogenesis by Extracellular Matrix. *Biochimica Et Biophysica Acta,* Vol.1654, No.1, pp. 13-22, ISSN 0006-3002

Suarez-Monteagudo, C., Hernandez-Ramirez, P., Alvarez-Gonzalez, L., Garcia-Maeso, I., de la Cuetara-Bernal, K., Castillo-Diaz, L., Bringas-Vega, M.L., Martinez-Aching, G., Morales-Chacon, L.M., Baez-Martin, M.M., Sanchez-Catasus, C., Carballo-Barreda, M., Rodriguez-Rojas, R., Gomez-Fernandez, L., Alberti-Amador, E., Macias-Abraham, C., Balea, E.D., Rosales, L.C., Del Valle Perez, L., Ferrer, B.B., Gonzalez, R.M. & Bergado, J.A. (2009). Autologous Bone Marrow Stem Cell Neurotransplantation in Stroke Patients. an Open Study. *Restorative Neurology and Neuroscience,* Vol.27, No.3, pp. 151-161, ISSN 0922-6028

Sugiura, S., Lahav, R., Han, J., Kou, S.Y., Banner, L.R., de Pablo, F. & Patterson, P.H. (2000). Leukaemia Inhibitory Factor is Required for Normal Inflammatory Responses to Injury in the Peripheral and Central Nervous Systems in Vivo and is Chemotactic for Macrophages in Vitro. *The European Journal of Neuroscience,* Vol.12, No.2, pp. 457-466, ISSN 0953-816X

Sun, L., Hui, A.M., Su, Q., Vortmeyer, A., Kotliarov, Y., Pastorino, S., Passaniti, A., Menon, J., Walling, J., Bailey, R., Rosenblum, M., Mikkelsen, T. & Fine, H.A. (2006). Neuronal and Glioma-Derived Stem Cell Factor Induces Angiogenesis within the Brain. *Cancer Cell,* Vol.9, No.4, pp. 287-300, ISSN 1535-6108

Sun, Y., Jin, K., Xie, L., Childs, J., Mao, X.O., Logvinova, A. & Greenberg, D.A. (2003). VEGF-Induced Neuroprotection, Neurogenesis, and Angiogenesis After Focal Cerebral Ischemia. *The Journal of Clinical Investigation,* Vol.111, No.12, pp. 1843-1851, ISSN 0021-9738

Swartz, K.R., Liu, F., Sewell, D., Schochet, T., Campbell, I., Sandor, M. & Fabry, Z. (2001). Interleukin-6 Promotes Post-Traumatic Healing in the Central Nervous System. *Brain Research,* Vol.896, No.1-2, pp. 86-95, ISSN 0006-8993

Taga, T. & Fukuda, S. (2005). Role of IL-6 in the Neural Stem Cell Differentiation. *Clinical Reviews in Allergy & Immunology,* Vol.28, No.3, pp. 249-256, ISSN 1080-0549

Tan, H.K., Heywood, D., Ralph, G.S., Bienemann, A., Baker, A.H. & Uney, J.B. (2003). Tissue Inhibitor of Metalloproteinase 1 Inhibits Excitotoxic Cell Death in Neurons. *Molecular and Cellular Neurosciences,* Vol.22, No.1, pp. 98-106, ISSN 1044-7431

Tate, C.C., Fonck, C., McGrogan, M. & Case, C.C. (2010). Human Mesenchymal Stromal Cells and their Derivative, SB623 Cells, Rescue Neural Cells via Trophic Support Following in Vitro Ischemia. *Cell Transplantation,* Vol.19, No.8, pp. 973-984, ISSN 1555-3892; 0963-6897

Tate, C.C., Garcia, A.J. & LaPlaca, M.C. (2007). Plasma Fibronectin is Neuroprotective Following Traumatic Brain Injury. *Experimental Neurology,* Vol.207, No.1, pp. 13-22, ISSN 0014-4886

Tate, M.C., Garcia, A.J., Keselowsky, B.G., Schumm, M.A., Archer, D.R. & LaPlaca, M.C. (2004). Specific beta1 Integrins Mediate Adhesion, Migration, and Differentiation of Neural Progenitors Derived from the Embryonic Striatum. *Molecular and Cellular Neuroscience,* Vol.27, No.1, pp. 22-31, ISSN 1095-9327; 1044-7431

Terauchi, A., Johnson-Venkatesh, E.M., Toth, A.B., Javed, D., Sutton, M.A. & Umemori, H. (2010). Distinct FGFs Promote Differentiation of Excitatory and Inhibitory Synapses. *Nature,* Vol.465, No.7299, pp. 783-787, ISSN 1476-4687; 0028-0836

Testaz, S. & Duband, J.L. (2001). Central Role of the alpha4beta1 Integrin in the Coordination of Avian Truncal Neural Crest Cell Adhesion, Migration, and Survival. *Developmental dynamics,* Vol.222, No.2, pp. 127-140, ISSN 1097-0177; 1058-8388

Thored, P., Arvidsson, A., Cacci, E., Ahlenius, H., Kallur, T., Darsalia, V., Ekdahl, C.T., Kokaia, Z. & Lindvall, O. (2006). Persistent Production of Neurons from Adult Brain Stem Cells during Recovery After Stroke. *Stem Cells (Dayton, Ohio),* Vol.24, No.3, pp. 739-747, ISSN 1066-5099

Vana, A.C., Flint, N.C., Harwood, N.E., Le, T.Q., Fruttiger, M. & Armstrong, R.C. (2007). Platelet-Derived Growth Factor Promotes Repair of Chronically Demyelinated White Matter. *Journal of Neuropathology and Experimental Neurology,* Vol.66, No.11, pp. 975-988, ISSN 0022-3069

Vasse, M., Pourtau, J., Trochon, V., Muraine, M., Vannier, J.P., Lu, H., Soria, J. & Soria, C. (1999). Oncostatin M Induces Angiogenesis in Vitro and in Vivo. *Arteriosclerosis, Thrombosis, and Vascular Biology,* Vol.19, No.8, pp. 1835-1842, ISSN 1079-5642

Villoslada, P. & Genain, C.P. (2004). Role of Nerve Growth Factor and Other Trophic Factors in Brain Inflammation. *Progress in Brain Research,* Vol.146, pp. 403-414, ISSN 0079-6123

Vincent, V.A., Robinson, C.C., Simsek, D. & Murphy, G.M. (2002). Macrophage Colony Stimulating Factor Prevents NMDA-Induced Neuronal Death in Hippocampal Organotypic Cultures. *Journal of Neurochemistry,* Vol.82, No.6, pp. 1388-1397, ISSN 0022-3042

Wang, L., Li, Y., Chen, X., Chen, J., Gautam, S.C., Xu, Y. & Chopp, M. (2002). MCP-1, MIP-1, IL-8 and Ischemic Cerebral Tissue Enhance Human Bone Marrow Stromal Cell Migration in Interface Culture. *Hematology,* Vol.7, No.2, pp. 113-117, ISSN 1024-5332

Wang, M., Crisostomo, P.R., Herring, C., Meldrum, K.K. & Meldrum, D.R. (2006). Human Progenitor Cells from Bone Marrow Or Adipose Tissue Produce VEGF, HGF, and IGF-I in Response to TNF by a p38 MAPK-Dependent Mechanism. *American Journal of Physiology.Regulatory, Integrative and Comparative Physiology,* Vol.291, No.4, pp. R880-4, ISSN 0363-6119

Wang, Y., Jin, K., Mao, X.O., Xie, L., Banwait, S., Marti, H.H. & Greenberg, D.A. (2007a). VEGF-Overexpressing Transgenic Mice show Enhanced Post-Ischemic Neurogenesis and Neuromigration. *Journal of Neuroscience Research,* Vol.85, No.4, pp. 740-747, ISSN 0360-4012

Wang, Y.Q., Guo, X., Qiu, M.H., Feng, X.Y. & Sun, F.Y. (2007b). VEGF Overexpression Enhances Striatal Neurogenesis in Brain of Adult Rat After a Transient Middle Cerebral Artery Occlusion. *Journal of Neuroscience Research,* Vol.85, No.1, pp. 73-82, ISSN 0360-4012

Weiss, T.W., Samson, A.L., Niego, B., Daniel, P.B. & Medcalf, R.L. (2006). Oncostatin M is a Neuroprotective Cytokine that Inhibits Excitotoxic Injury in Vitro and in Vivo. *The FASEB Journal,* Vol.20, No.13, pp. 2369-2371, ISSN 1530-6860; 0892-6638

Wells, W.A. (2002). Is Transdifferentiation in Trouble? *The Journal of Cell Biology,* Vol.157, No.1, pp. 15-18, ISSN 0021-9525

Widera, D., Holtkamp, W., Entschladen, F., Niggemann, B., Zanker, K., Kaltschmidt, B. & Kaltschmidt, C. (2004). MCP-1 Induces Migration of Adult Neural Stem Cells. *European Journal of Cell Biology,* Vol.83, No.8, pp. 381-387, ISSN 0171-9335

Wilkins, A., Chandran, S. & Compston, A. (2001). A Role for Oligodendrocyte-Derived IGF-1 in Trophic Support of Cortical Neurons. *Glia,* Vol.36, No.1, pp. 48-57, ISSN 0894-1491

Woodbury, D., Schwarz, E.J., Prockop, D.J. & Black, I.B. (2000). Adult Rat and Human Bone Marrow Stromal Cells Differentiate into Neurons. *Journal of Neuroscience Research,* Vol.61, No.4, pp. 364-370, ISSN 0360-4012

Wright, D.W., Kellermann, A.L., Hertzberg, V.S., Clark, P.L., Frankel, M., Goldstein, F.C., Salomone, J.P., Dent, L.L., Harris, O.A., Ander, D.S., Lowery, D.W., Patel, M.M., Denson, D.D., Gordon, A.B., Wald, M.M., Gupta, S., Hoffman, S.W. & Stein, D.G. (2007). ProTECT: A Randomized Clinical Trial of Progesterone for Acute Traumatic Brain Injury. *Annals of Emergency Medicine,* Vol.49, No.4, pp. 391-402, 402.e1-2, ISSN 1097-6760

Xin, H., Li, Y., Shen, L.H., Liu, X., Wang, X., Zhang, J., Pourabdollah-Nejad, D.S., Zhang, C., Zhang, L., Jiang, H., Zhang, Z.G. & Chopp, M. (2010). Increasing tPA Activity in Astrocytes Induced by Multipotent Mesenchymal Stromal Cells Facilitate Neurite Outgrowth After Stroke in the Mouse. *PloS One,* Vol.5, No.2, pp. e9027, ISSN 1932-6203

Xiong, Y., Qu, C., Mahmood, A., Liu, Z., Ning, R., Li, Y., Kaplan, D.L., Schallert, T. & Chopp, M. (2009). Delayed Transplantation of Human Marrow Stromal Cell-Seeded Scaffolds Increases Transcallosal Neural Fiber Length, Angiogenesis, and Hippocampal Neuronal Survival and Improves Functional Outcome After Traumatic Brain Injury in Rats. *Brain Research,* Vol.1263, pp. 183-191, ISSN 1872-6240; 0006-8993

Yabe, T., Samuels, I. & Schwartz, J.P. (2002). Bone Morphogenetic Proteins BMP-6 and BMP-7 have Differential Effects on Survival and Neurite Outgrowth of Cerebellar Granule Cell Neurons. *Journal of Neuroscience Research,* Vol.68, No.2, pp. 161-168, ISSN 0360-4012

Yamada, M., Tanabe, K., Wada, K., Shimoke, K., Ishikawa, Y., Ikeuchi, T., Koizumi, S. & Hatanaka, H. (2001). Differences in Survival-Promoting Effects and Intracellular Signaling Properties of BDNF and IGF-1 in Cultured Cerebral Cortical Neurons. *Journal of Neurochemistry,* Vol.78, No.5, pp. 940-951, ISSN 0022-3042

Yan, Y.P., Sailor, K.A., Lang, B.T., Park, S.W., Vemuganti, R. & Dempsey, R.J. (2007). Monocyte Chemoattractant Protein-1 Plays a Critical Role in Neuroblast Migration After Focal Cerebral Ischemia. *Journal of Cerebral Blood Flow and Metabolism,* Vol.27, No.6, pp. 1213-1224, ISSN 0271-678X

Yi, J.J., Barnes, A.P., Hand, R., Polleux, F. & Ehlers, M.D. (2010). TGF-Beta Signaling Specifies Axons during Brain Development. *Cell,* Vol.142, No.1, pp. 144-157, ISSN 1097-4172; 0092-8674

Yoo, S.W., Kim, S.S., Lee, S.Y., Lee, H.S., Kim, H.S., Lee, Y.D. & Suh-Kim, H. (2008). Mesenchymal Stem Cells Promote Proliferation of Endogenous Neural Stem Cells and Survival of Newborn Cells in a Rat Stroke Model. *Experimental & Molecular Medicine,* Vol.40, No.4, pp. 387-397, ISSN 1226-3613

Yung, H.S., Lai, K.H., Chow, K.B., Ip, N.Y., Tsim, K.W., Wong, Y.H., Wu, Z. & Wise, H. (2010). Nerve Growth Factor-Induced Differentiation of PC12 Cells is Accompanied by Elevated Adenylyl Cyclase Activity. *Neuro-Signals,* Vol.18, No.1, pp. 32-42, ISSN 1424-8638; 1424-862X

Zanier, E.R., Montinaro, M., Vigano, M., Villa, P., Fumagalli, S., Pischiutta, F., Longhi, L., Leoni, M.L., Rebulla, P., Stocchetti, N., Lazzari, L. & Simoni, M.G. (2011). Human Umbilical Cord Blood Mesenchymal Stem Cells Protect Mice Brain After Trauma. *Critical Care Medicine,* ISSN 1530-0293; 0090-3493

Zechel, S., Werner, S., Unsicker, K. & von Bohlen und Halbach, O. (2010). Expression and Functions of Fibroblast Growth Factor 2 (FGF-2) in Hippocampal Formation. *The Neuroscientist,* Vol.16, No.4, pp. 357-373, ISSN 1089-4098; 1073-8584

Zhang, Z.X., Guan, L.X., Zhang, K., Zhang, Q. & Dai, L.J. (2008). A Combined Procedure to Deliver Autologous Mesenchymal Stromal Cells to Patients with Traumatic Brain Injury. *Cytotherapy,* Vol.10, No.2, pp. 134-139, ISSN 1477-2566; 1465-3249

Zhao, L.R., Singhal, S., Duan, W.M., Mehta, J. & Kessler, J.A. (2007). Brain Repair by Hematopoietic Growth Factors in a Rat Model of Stroke. *Stroke,* Vol.38, No.9, pp. 2584-2591, 1524-4628; 0039-2499

Zhong, C., Qin, Z., Zhong, C.J., Wang, Y. & Shen, X.Y. (2003). Neuroprotective Effects of Bone Marrow Stromal Cells on Rat Organotypic Hippocampal Slice Culture Model of Cerebral Ischemia. *Neuroscience Letters,* Vol.342, No.1-2, pp. 93-96, ISSN 0304-3940

Zhu, W., Cheng, S., Xu, G., Ma, M., Zhou, Z., Liu, D. & Liu, X. (2011). Intranasal Nerve Growth Factor Enhances Striatal Neurogenesis in Adult Rats with Focal Cerebral Ischemia. *Drug Delivery,* Vol.18, No.5, pp. 338-343, ISSN 1521-0464; 1071-7544

4

Development of Foamy Virus Vectors for Gene Therapy for Neurological Disorders and Other Diseases

Yingying Zhang[1**], Guoguo Zhu[1**], Yu Huang[1**],
Xiaohua He[1,2*] and Wanhong Liu[1,2*]
[1]*School of Basic Medical Sciences, Wuhan University, Wuhan*
[2]*Centre for Medical Research, Wuhan University, Wuhan*
China

1. Introduction

The complexities of neurological diseases make it difficult to develop effective methods to treat them. In addition, it is difficult for the drugs used in neurological diseases to reach target cells at a sufficient concentration due to the blood-brain barrier, which may lead to side-effects in other organs, even though newly developed drugs are targeted directly to the origin of the diseases. Nevertheless, as the field of gene delivery gradually matures, new ways to deliver therapies for diseases become possible, and there are reasons to believe that gene therapy would be an optional treatment for neurological diseases.

There are two main classes of vectors used for gene delivery: nonviral vectors and viral vectors (Gardlik et al., 2005). As viral vectors display a higher efficiency and specificity than nonviral vectors, they have been developed as therapeutic gene transfer carriers for various organ systems throughout the body in which the nervous system is involved (Glorioso et al., 2003). The four major viral vector systems used for neurological diseases are recombinant lentivirus (LV), adenovirus (Ad), herpes-simplex virus (HSV), and recombinant adeno-associated virus (rAAV) (Manfredsson et al., 2010). However, the utilization of these vectors is limited by safety concerns because of their pathogenicity (Zhang et al., 2010).

Foamy viruses (FVs), widespread, complex retroviruses with a large genome approximately 12-13 kb, are syncytial viruses containing two different promoters termed IP (internal promoter) and P (promoter) (Löchelt et al., 1995). Due to the specific structure of the viruses and their innocuousness in both human and primate infections, FV vectors have potential as a safe and capable vehicle with a larger capacity for transgenes (Williams, 2008). It has been reported that FV are potentially safer than gammaretroviruses and lentiviral vectors (Trobridge et al., 2009). In this review, we discuss the use of FV vectors as a safe and efficient carrier to deliver therapeutic genes for neurological disorders and other diseases.

---

*Corresponding author
**Equal contribution to this work

2. Characteristics of foamy virus (Figure 1)

2.1 Construction

FVs were first described 50 years ago and are widely distributed in the natural world (Loh et al., 1992). They have been isolated from several mammals, including nonhuman primates, cattle, cats, and horses.

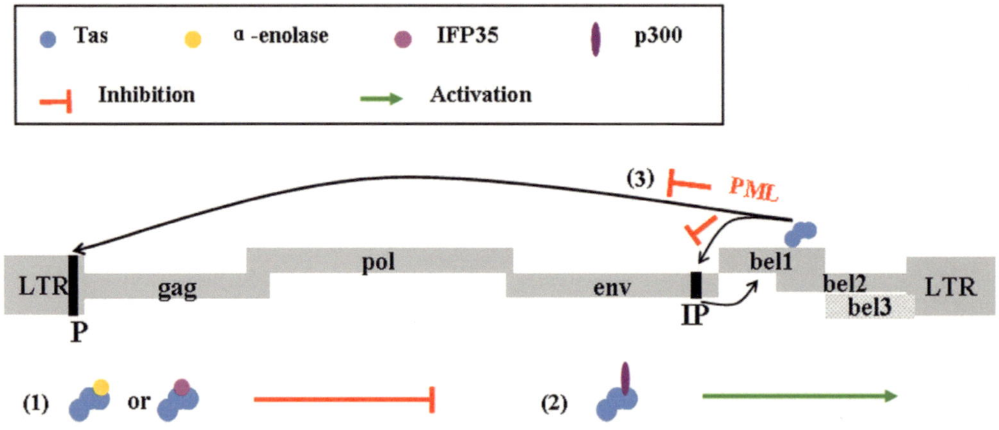

(1) IFP35 can interact with the bovine Tas (BTas) and arrest the replication of BFV; and Bel-1 interacts with α-enolase, then represses the activation of LTR and IP ; (2) Tas can be acetylated by p300, and activate the virus replication ; (3) PML inhibits the binding of Tas to IP and LTR.

Fig. 1. The genomic organization of FVs and Tas of FVs interacted with other proteins in cells

Once infected by FVs, life-long latency of the infected cell is obtained (Maxine et al., 2000). FVs contain the largest genome and possess the most complex gene structure of all the retroviruses. For example, the human foamy virus (HFV, also called primate foamy virus (PFV)) contains LTR (long terminal repeat) sequences at the 5′and 3′ ends of its genome, and there are three structural genes between these two LTRs that are found in all viral genomes: *gag*, *pol*, and *env* (Saïb et al., 1995). Several ORFs (open reading frames), often two or three, are located between the *env* and the LTR at the 3′end of all sequenced FVs, which encode autologous transactivators, including Tas, an important transactivator (Linial, 2000). The Tas protein is required by both the promoter (P) in the U3 region of the 5′ LTR and another unique internal promoter (IP) at the end of the *env* gene for high-level expression (Linial, 2000).

2.1.1 Promoters

2.1.1.1 LTR

Long terminal repeats (LTRs), located at the 5' and 3' end of the viral genome, are noncoding regions that exist in all types of retroviruses. The LTR is required for the integration of the viral genome into the host genome and is related to the replication, kinetics, tissue tropism, and pathogenicity of the virus. A U3-R-U5 (unique 3' subregion-repeat subregion-unique 5' subregion) structure forms the LTR. The LTR promoter, containing a component of the U3-R-U5 region, is a traditional retroviral promoter. The prototypical HFV U3 region is approximately 777 nt and includes a TATA box, transcription regulatory signals and several BREs (Bel1 transactivator response elements) that are located at ~89-116 nt, ~284-327 nt, ~348-360 nt, ~418-454 nt and ~506-559 nt, respectively (Lee et al., 1993; Verdin et al., 1995). As there are a number of BRE regions, Choy, Kerr et al. suggested that the Bel1 regions regulate gene expression by integrating with intracellular transcription factors and transcription initiation complexes without binding directly to BREs and act as enhancers that work together to make a change (Lee et al., 1993; Choy et al., 1993; Kerr et al., 1993; Yang et al., 1997; Löchelt et al., 1994)). The negative control region in the RU5 inhibits the gene expression of HFV, and the viral mRNA R-U5 forms a stable secondary structure (Nabel et al., 1987). There is a splice donor site (SD) 51 nt downstream of the transcription site of the R region, where the posttranscriptional splicing of the *gag*, *pol*, *env*, and *bel* genes is initiated by the 5′ LTR promoter start site (Li et al., 1999).

2.1.1.2 IP

All FVs possess a promoter in the U3 region of the LTR. In addition to the LTR promoter P, they also contain another unique internal promoter, termed IP (Löchelt et al., 1993). The internal promoter is located at the end of *env* gene. These two promoters require Tas for high-level expression (Löchelt et al., 1994). Compared with the LTR promoter, Tas has a higher affinity for the IP (Kang et al., 1998). In the early stage of viral infection, the IP initially regulates the expression of Tas transcription through an LTR cis-acting effect and the participation of as yet unknown cytokines. Next, Tas affects the IP through its self-activating mechanism to elevate its synthesis level; when the Tas protein reaches a certain level, the activated LTR initiates the transcription and expression of the structural gene and performs transformation of gene transcription and expression from the early non-structural gene to the late structural gene.

2.1.2 Structural genes

Following the 5' LTR of FVs, there are three structural genes (*gag*, *pol*, *env*). The newly synthesized 74/78 kDa precursor protein encoded by the *gag* gene is located in the nuclei of the infected cells (Schliephake et al., 1994), and it is cleaved into the matrix, capsid, and nucleocapsid structural protein by the viral protease (Saïb et al., 1995). The nucleocapsid (NC) domain of Gag protein lacks Cys-His boxes found in all other retroviral Gag proteins, but its C terminus possesses three glycine-arginine motifs (GR boxes) that are required for RNA packaging (Stenbak et al., 2004; Yu et al., 1996; Maurer et al., 1998). The *pol* gene overlaps the *gag* gene, and its product does not contain any Gag protein determinant; however, unlike other conventional retroviruses, there is no Gag-Pol fusion protein synthesized in the course of viral transcription, but the underlying mechanism remains unknown (Stenbak et al., 2004; Yu et al., 1996). The precursor protein encoded by the *env* gene, which is approximately 130 kDa, is cleaved into the SU and TM subunits during the process of maturation (Saïb et al., 1995; Aguzzi, 1993). Linial et al. found that the extracellular virions of HFV require the Env protein for further production but that the formation of intracellular particles seems to be independent of the Env protein (Baldwin et al., 1993). Unfortunately, the role of Gag, Pol, and Env in the assembly of the FVs remains uncertain.

2.1.3 Regulatory genes

There are several ORFs encoding accessory genes or regulatory genes that are located between the *env* and the LTR and are therefore named *bel* genes. These ORFs encode autologous transactivators, including *bel-1*, *bel-2*, *bel-3* and *bet*.

2.1.3.1 Tas

The regulatory gene *bel-1*, which is approximately 902 bp in length, is located in the nucleus of expressing cells and is essential for HFV replication. FVs transactivators of different genera have been named differently; the simian FVs transactivator, for example, was termed *taf*. However the First International Foamy Virus Meeting determined that these transactivators, including Taf and Bel1, should be designated Tas (Zou et al., 1996). The activity of the functional IP and P of FVs depends on this transactivator. Transcription starts from the integration of Tas and the IP, leading to transactivation of the IP. However, the LTR promoter will not be activated until the level of Tas reaches a certain level (Linial, 2000). In view of the fact that the Tas protein plays an important role in the transcription and replication of FVs, it has received increasing attention and interest among virologists.

The interactions between Tas and other cellular molecules are complex. For example, Tas can be acetylated by p300 and PCAF (Bodem et al., 2007). Recently, an interaction between Tas and transcriptional coactivators, such as HATs, was reported. Studies show that only acetylated Tas enhances viral transcription (Bodem et al., 2007). Interferon-induced proteins (IFPs) complete multiple functions through various interferon signals. IFP35, which is approximately 35 kDa, is a member of the IFP family. It interacts with the bovine foamy virus Tas regulatory protein, and its overexpression disturbs viral gene transcription and replication of the bovine foamy virus Tas protein. Furthermore, IFP35 plays a crucial role in the interferon-induced anti-foamy virus host response (Tan et al., 2008). First discovered by Lohman and Mayerhof in 1934 (Lohman et al., 1934), α-enolase was later shown to be a highly conserved enzyme that catalyses the transformation of 2-phosphoglyceric acid to enolphosphopyruvate in the Embden-Meyerhof-Parnas pathway (Wold, 1971). α-Enolase interrupts the transactivation of Tas with the promoters during viral transcription (Wu et al., 2009). The promyelocytic leukemia protein (PML) is a cell growth and tumor suppressor gene, which is expressed in the nucleus and whose expression is increased significantly in the response to interferon (IFN) (Wang et al., 1998). Regad et al. found that PML inhibits the binding of Tas to the IP and LTR by direct interaction with Tas (Regad et al., 2001).

2.1.3.2 Bet

Bet is a second IP regulating protein. Generated by the combination of the spliced mRNA of the Tas region and the Bel2 ORF (Linial, 2000), overexpression of Bet prevents the virus from infecting the host and inhibits viral integration at the initial stage of viral infection (Bock et al., 1998). A variant RNA can be generated by the LTR promoter, which has the ability to generate Bet protein fragments that, after reverse transcription, could induce the expression of a ΔTas provirus (Saïb et al., 1993). Because of the deficiency of Tas in the provirus, ΔTas plays a significant role in the preservation and latency of FVs, which clarifies that the LTR does not initiate the synthesis of viral protein, whereas the expression of Bet is induced by IP (Linial, 2000). Transcription may be different in diverse cell types. Additionally, the combination site of Tas for the internal promoter IP is different from that for the LTR promoter, and the required cytokines are different. High expression of the virus would be suppressed under conditions in which the IP promoter was active in various cell types, yet cytokines, which the LTR promoter requires, exist in a select few cells. The transcription of integral provirus is mainly initiated by IP and will express Tas and Bet but virus will not.

2.2 Replication and transcription

As mentioned previously, FVs are a member of the spumavirus genus of the retroviridae family. It is believed that the replication and transcription mechanisms of various family members are similar (Coffin, 1990). However, Yu et al. found that although HFV possesses a replication pathway with features of both retroviruses and hepadnaviruses, there are also unique features contained in the assembly and reverse transcription pathway (Yu et al., 1996).

At an early stage of viral infection, Tas is expressed due to the high level of transcription of IP, which in turn transactivates the expression of IP and LTR, leading to the expression of accessory and structural genes, respectively, inducing late stage viral infection (Löchelt et al., 1994). The Gag-Pol fusion protein is synthesized during the transcription of other retroviruses. However, as discussed above, the *pol* gene product in foamy viruses does not contain any Gag protein determinant, which means there is no Gag-Pol fusion protein synthesized in the course of viral transcription. Therefore, unknown mechanisms exist in the synthesis of *pol* gene products. As there are two promoters present in the genome of foamy virus, it is presumed that IP functionally replaces the post-transcriptional regulatory protein of other retroviruses and thus provides a temporal pattern with stage-specific promoters (Mergia, 1994).

Although FVs infection can result in a unique foam-like cytopathic effect and syncytia in cell cultures, they are nonpathogenic in naturally or experimentally infected animals, and the pathogenicity to their hosts remains unknown. However, more and more research groups are attracted to FVs due to the lack of pathogenicity; thus, increased attention has been given to the development of FVs as vectors of target gene delivery.

3. The development of human foamy virus (HFV) (Figure 2)

3.1 Replication-competent HFV

The first described FVs vectors (pFOV-1, pFOV-3 and pFOV-7) were replication-competent. Noncoding sequences in *bel-2* and *bel-3* were deleted, and two termination codons and a *bel-1* splice donor site mutation were introduced into these vectors (Schmidt et al., 1995). The vector pFOV-7, containing the herpes virus type 1 (HSV-1) thymidine kinase (tk), the *E.coli* cytosine deaminase (cd) and the polynucleotide phosphorylase (*pnp*) genes, was introduced into tumor cells and promoted their death (Nestler et al., 1997).

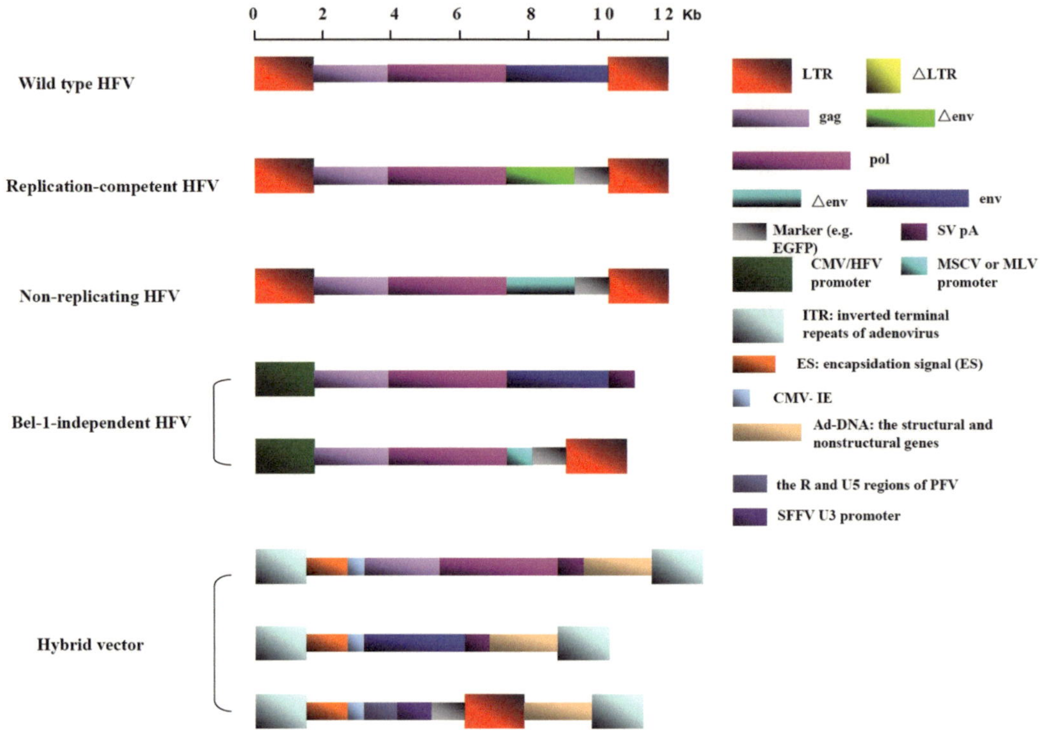

Fig. 2. The development of HFV vectors. The replication-competent FV vectors were deleted noncoding sequences in *bel-2* and *bel-3*. The non-replicating FV vectors were constructed by the portion of the *env* gene replaced by marker gene. The bel-1-independent FV vector system contains relevant packaging plasmid and the vector plasmid carrying exogenous gene. The adenovirus and human foamy virus hybrid vector system express separately the HFV structural genes *gag* and *pol*, the HFV structural gene *env*, and the transgene.

3.2 Non-replicating HFV

The second generation FV vectors were non-replicating HFV, lacking portions of the structure gene. The recombinant foamy virus vectors (pFGPSN and pFGPMAP) were constructed by replacing a portion of the *env* gene with the neomycin phosphotransferase gene under the control of the SV40 early promoter and the human placental alkaline phosphatase gene under the control of the MLV LTR promoter, respectively (David & Russell, 1996). These vectors were capable of transducing diverse cells (David & Russell, 1996), including human fibroblasts, COS-7 cells, Vero cells, Cf2Th cells, etc. Furthermore, these vectors transduced cells from different species, including steer, sheep, dog, cat, rat and hamster and at different stages of the cell cycle, thus suggesting that HFV could transduce dividing and non-dividing cells.

3.3 Bel-1-independent HFV

The third generation FV vectors were Bel-1-independent HFV. This foamy virus vector system contained relevant packaging plasmid (pCGPES) and vector plasmids (pCGPMAPDBel and pCGPMscvF) (Vassilopoulos et al., 2001). In this vector, a constitutive CMV/HFV fusion promoter derived from the cytomegalovirus (CMV) promoter replaced the HFV LTR U3 region sequences (Trobridge & Russell, 1998). The *gag*, *pol*, and *env* were placed under control of an SV40 polyadenylation site (SV pA) in the packaging plasmid pCPGES, and the reporter gene, AP or GFP, was expressed respectively by internal MLV LTR or murine stem cell virus (MSCV) promoters (Vassilopoulos et al., 2001). Thus, the *gag* and *pol* genes were not expressed in transduced cells after reverse transcription. Researchers demonstrated that the 5′ portion of gag and 3′ portion of *pol* were critical for viral product (Heinkelein et al., 1998; Erlwein et al., 1998). Thus, it may be possible for foamy virus vectors to contain fewer viral sequences in the future.

3.4 Human foamy virus hybrid vector

To improve the viral titer, adenovirus and human foamy virus hybrid vector systems (pFAD-2 and pFAD-7) were developed (Picard-Maureau et al., 2004). An infectious extracellular particle could be produced by pFAD-2 containing the PFV gene. The pFAD-7 lacked the PFV *env* gene required for viral capsid export and could therefore only undergo an intracellular replication cycle. Both of these FV vectors were controlled by the tetracycline-regulatable system. The other adenoviral/PFV hybrid vector was generated from three different adenoviruses and achieved gene transfer in vitro (Russell et al., 2004). These vectors separately expressed the PFV structural genes *gag* and *pol* (Ad-GagPolDPacI), the PFV structural gene *env* (Ad-Env), and the transgene (Ad-MD9). After co-transduction by the three adenoviruses, release of recombinant PFV was generated, and a titer of up to 10^3 vector particles/ml was achieved.

It has been shown that these hybrid vectors can effectively improve the titer and integrate into host genome. Additional foamy virus hybrid vectors have been developed, and more research needs to be undertaken to verify their effectiveness and safety.

3.5 FVs derived from other species

In addition to the prototypic PFV (Trobridge et al., 1998; Heinkelein et al., 1998; Trobridge et al., 2002; Schmidt et al., 1995; Nestler et al., 1997; Heinkelein et al., 2002), a variety of FV vectors have been developed, including simian foamy virus type 1 (SFV-1, macaque) (Wu et al., 1998; Park et al., 2002) and feline foamy virus (FFV) (Bastone et al., 2006; Bastone et al., 2007). A series of vectors and helper plasmids derived from SFV-1 have been constructed, and the minimum vector sequence required for efficient gene transduction has been established. This minimum vector contained the 5′ untranslated region to the first 637 nucleotides of the *gag*, 596 nucleotides of *pol*, while the 3′ LTR removed 1131 nucleotides. Therefore, with different packaging plasmids and helper plasmids, this vector can carry an 8930 base-size heterologous DNA fragment.

4. The advantages of FV

Research groups have designed a novel type of vehicle based on FVs for use as gene delivery vectors. FVs are classified in the subfamily Spumaretroviridae (Khan et al., 2009). FVs have been reported to be prepotent in relation to other retroviral subfamilies, such as HIV and HTLV, in terms of safety and efficiency. FVs have many advantages that allow them to transduce target cells for treating nervous system disorders. The advantages of functional gene transfer vectors derived from foamy viruses are as follows.

a. FVs have a wide range of hosts and can infect a variety of tissues and cells (Heneine et al., 1998; Russell & Miller, 1996). They were first found in mammalian species, while humans can be infected through occupational and non-occupational exposure to infected animals and their tissues, blood or body fluids (Khan et al., 2009). The feature of a broad host tropism makes FVs suitable for wide use in gene therapy.
b. Most retroviral vectors derived from FVs are nonpathogenic to humans (Caprariello et al., 2009). There is not enough evidence indicating the ability of foamy viruses to be transmitted between populations (Liu et al., 2005; Mergia et al., 2001). Furthermore, long-term studies of animal care workers and experimental researchers infected by foamy viruses have failed to show negative consequences (Mergia et al., 2001; Saib et al., 1997). Thus, there is little or no risk of developing malignancies in patients treated with gene therapy by FV vectors.
c. The size of the foamy virus genome is the largest amongst all retroviruses (Flugel et al., 1991; Trobridge et al., 2002). Thus, it is able to transport large fragments of foreign genetic material into cells. As therapeutic genes can be too large to be delivered by common retroviral vectors, the ability of FV vectors to package foreign genes is significant. FVs can be used as gene therapy vectors for the diseases that are caused by the loss of large fragments of functional genes.
d. FVs possess a dual-promoter, which makes them unique. Whereas all retroviruses have a promoter in their U3 region of the long terminal repeat sequence, FVs have an internal promoter that is located at the end of the env (Liu et al., 2005; Lochelt et al., 1993). The two promoters co-regulate the expression of therapeutic genes at both temporal and spatial levels in target cells.
e. FVs have a distinct integration pattern compared with other retroviral vectors. Bauer et al. have studied these patterns, and unlike gammaretroviral and lentiviral vectors, there seems to be an inverse correlation between gene density and integration frequency. Furthermore, FV vectors integrated significantly fewer times near oncogenes, as demonstrated using integration-site and statistical analysis (Bauer et al., 2008). The unique integration pattern indicates that FVs prefer inserting into non-transcribed areas of the chromosome, which promotes the development of FV vectors in gene therapy.
f. Recently, researchers have found that the number of integration sites in a cell gradually increased over several weeks following viral infection. Most of the additional integration sites appeared in regions of low gene density (Bauer et al., 2008). This may be, to some extent, why FV vectors are safer and have a higher expression as well as long-term efficacy.
g. FVs particles are simple and convenient to obtain for basic medical research and clinical trials. FVs are stable enough to be concentrated by ultracentrifugation and maintain the ability to introduce and express genes in target cells (Josephson et al., 2004).

These unique characteristics of FVs make them suitable to be used as foreign gene delivery systems in treating genetic diseases, especially nervous disorders. However, low viral titer limits the application of FV vectors to clinical treatments. Furthermore, it is uncertain whether a mutation could occur after integration, which would be a serious threat to the health and survival of individuals undergoing gene therapy treatment.

5. Transduction of neural and other cells by FV vectors

5.1 Transduction of a variety of cells derived from diverse species

FV vectors can transduce diverse human cells (David & Russell, 1996), including human fibroblasts, 293 cells and COS-7 cells. FV vectors can also transduce cells derived from other species, such as, Vero and Cf2Th cells. These cells can be transduced by FV vectors at different stages (M phase or stationary phase) of the cell cycle (Figure 3).

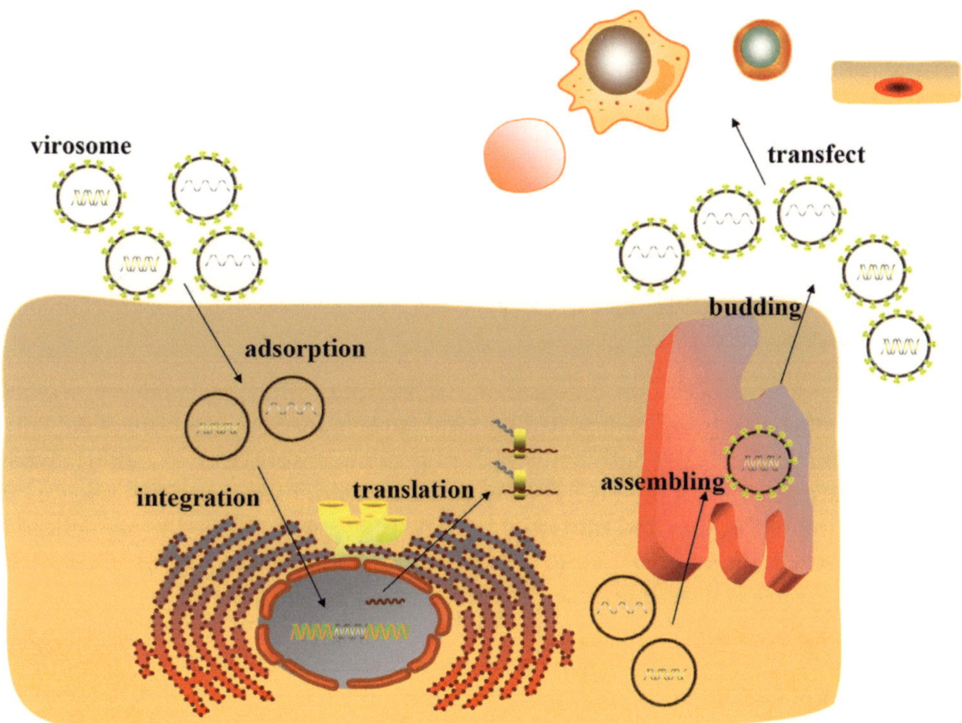

Fig. 3. The cell model transduced by FVs. Infectious viral particles enter cells and concentrate around the centrosomes. Under the help of centrosomes, the PIC enter the nucleus. After integration, the viral genes are expressed, and the viral proteins are synthesized. The viral particles are assembled in internal membranes, and released by budding.

5.2 Transduction of growth-arrested cells

Research has demonstrated that FV vectors can transduce MRC5 cells and human fibroblasts that have been arrested using aphidicolin (G1/S phase) (Saib et al., 1997; Trobridge et al., 2004), although the integration pattern (integration or non-integration) remains unclear.

5.3 Transduction of neural cells and brain tissues

NT2.N neurons, a postmitotic human neuronal cell line, can be transduced by simian foamy virus-1 (SFV-1) vectors (Mergia et al., 2001). Neural cells, cultured astrocytes, cultured rat hippocampal and dorsal root ganglia neurons are also transducible by FV vectors (Liu et al., 2005; Liu et al., 2007; Liu et al., 2008). Brain tissues can be transduced by FV vectors in a rat model (Caprariello et al., 2009).

6. Possible mechanisms for the transduction of neural cells and other growth-arrested cells

Although the underlying mechanism of foamy viral transduction in neural and nondividing cell is unclear, some clues can be acquired from the unique life cycle of FVs (Figure 3).

The viral structure of foamy viruses is special. FVs possess two coordinated promoters (Liu et al., 2005; Lochelt et al., 1993): one is located in the U3 region of the LTR, while the other, termed IP, is located at the end of the *env* gene. With the largest genome among all retroviruses (11,021 bp), FV vectors can carry a large transgene cassette (9.2 kb) (Flugel et al., 1991; Trobridge et al., 2002.)

Foamy viral reverse transcription, integration, transcription and packaging processes are also distinct. The reverse transcription during viral particle formation produces 20% of viral particles containing the full-length viral cDNA genome (Mergia et al., 2001), which is conducive to the formation of the PIC. The Tas (transactivator of spumavirus) plays a critical role in foamy viral replication and transcription. The *pol* gene of FVs is directly spliced from the mRNA, which is unique to FVs (Yu et al., 1996; Enssle et al., 1996). Therefore, the protease reverse-transcriptase-integrase proteins, derived from the Pol, are activated early and may facilitate the formation of the preintegration complex (PIC). As an element of the PIC, the Gag protein is cleaved into a mature product near the C-terminus. The entrance of the PIC into the nucleus utilizes the centrioles. The frequency of foamy viral integration is inversely correlated with gene density, with foamy virus preferring to integrate into regions of low gene density (Bauer et al., 2008).

7. Application of FV vectors in neurological disorders and other diseases

It has been reported that 2 of 11 children who received gene therapy developed leukemia due to the use of retroviral vectors, which may lead to the insertional activation of nearby oncogenes (Marshall, 2002; Marshall, 2003). In contrast, foamy virus is a safe and promising vector system for gene transfer into various cell types, including neurocytes. The potential applications of FV vectors for gene therapy are summarized below and in Table 1.

Virus	Diseases	Transgenes	References
HFV	Parkinson's disease	GAD gene	Liu et al. 2007
HFV	Neuropathic pain	GAD gene	Liu et al. 2008
FV	Lukocyte adhesion deficiency	MSCV- CD18	Bauer et al. 2008
FV	Lukocyte adhesion deficiency	PGK-CD18	Bauer et al. 2011
PFV	Gioblastoma xenograft model	FOV-7/pnp, FOV-7/ntr, FOV-7/tk suicide gene	Heinkelein et al. 2005
HFV	Cancer	Interleukin-24	Chen et al. 2010
HFV	HIV infection	Interferon-tau	Fujii et al.2004
SFV-1	SIV infection	R2 siRNA	Park et al. 2005
FV	HIV infection	RevM10, Sh1 and maC46	Taylor et al.2008
HFV	Hpatitis B	siRNA	Sun et al. 2007
FV	Cronic granulomatous disease	gp91^{phox}	Chatziandreou et al. 2011

Table 1. Foamy Virus Vectors used in Neurological Disorders and other diseases

7.1 Parkinson's disease

Parkinson's disease (PD) is the second most common age-related progressive neurodegenerative disorder (Feng et al., 2010). Currently, the treatment of PD is focused on the amelioration of symptoms and does not have a satisfactory therapeutic effect. Caprariello and colleagues demonstrated that high-titer FV, which is able to efficiently transduce brain parenchyma, had the potential for gene therapy of disorders of the central nervous system (CNS) (Caprariello et al., 2009). FV-vector-mediated gene transfer to neural progenitor cells that are potential vehicles for delivery of therapeutic agents into the brain can achieve differentiation-dependent gene expression (Rothenaigner et al., 2009). In a rat model of PD, replication-defective HFV vectors were used to transduce astrocytes, which were then injected into the subthalamic nucleus (STN) region of PD animal models. The HFV vector-derived glutamic acid decarboxylase (GAD) expression in the astrocytes resulted in behavioral recovery of the rats. The transduction of the GAD vector achieved isoform-specific expression of GAD, synthesis of a significant amount of gamma-aminobutyric acid (GABA) and the release of tonically active GABA (Liu et al., 2007). GABA is primarily synthesized from glutamate (glutamic acid) by the pyridoxal-5-phosphate-dependent glutamic acid decarboxylase. GAD65 and GAD67 are two isoforms of GAD in the brain, which provide a dual system for the control of neuronal GABA (Figure 4). GAD65 is mainly present as an inactive apoenzyme and can be induced by nerve activity, whereas GAD67 is a pyridoxal phosphate-bound permanently active holoenzyme (Lindefors, 1993). In this study, replication-defective vector (rdv) GAD67 or rdvGAD65 were injected into the rat STN. There was a significant decrease in the rotation rates of the rdvGAD65 rats while the rdvGAD67 rats did not. This study demonstrates that HFV vector-derived GAD expression in astrocytes provides a potential approach to repair GABA transmission in neurological disorders (Liu et al., 2007).

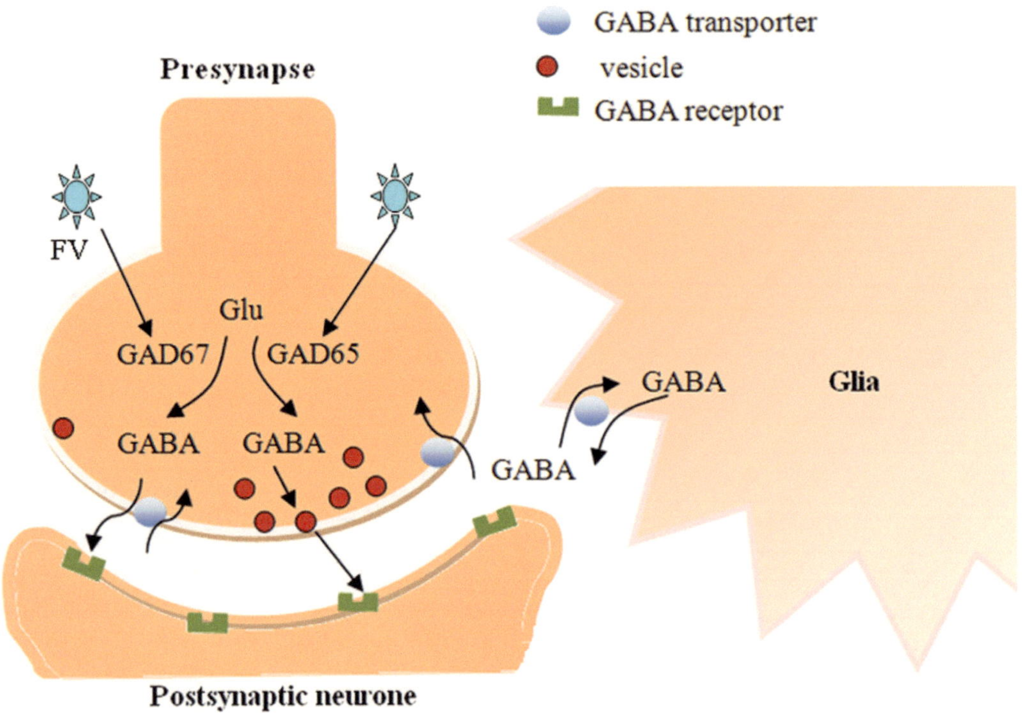

Fig. 4. GABA is primarily synthesized from glutamate (glutamic acid) by GAD67 and GAD65. GAD67, which might preferentially synthesize cytoplasmic GABA, appears to be distributed more uniformly in neurons. GAD65, which might preferentially synthesize GABA for vesicular release, tends to be concentrated in nerve terminals. In most physiological circumstances, GABA-uptake transporters rapidly remove GABA that is released from the synapse into the extracellular space. However, the GABA transporter can reverse its action and release GABA from neurons or glial cells under certain conditions. FV vectors encoding GAD65 or GAD67 can achieve significant synthesis and release of GABA, which may ameliorate neurological disorders associated with hyperexcitable or diminished inhibitory activity.

7.2 Neuropathic pain

Neuropathic pain is an important health concern that is often refractory to medical management. Further studies of neuropathic pain have made the development of gene therapy a possibility. Subcutaneous inoculation of a replication-defective HFV vector expressing GAD67 attenuated below-injury level central neuropathic pain after spinal cord injury (SCI). To achieve the release of GABA, the GAD67 gene was transferred into dorsal root ganglion (DRG) cells for 7 days after T13 spinal cord hemisection. The result suggests that HFV-mediated gene transfer to DRG could be applied to treat below-injury level central neuropathic pain after incomplete SCI (Liu et al., 2008). The inhibitory effect of GABA, which is the major inhibitory neurotransmitter in the mammalian central nervous system, is mediated by $GABA_A$, $GABA_B$ and $GABA_C/GABA_{A\text{-}\rho}$ receptors (Rissman et al., 2011). GABA-mediated depolarization influences the excitability of sensory neurons both in cell bodies and nerve terminals by inactivating other voltage-sensitive channels, such as Ca^{2+} and Na^{+}. It is also possible that the GABA-activated a Cl^{-} current directly that inhibits an ATP-evoked excitatory current in DRG neurons (Naik et al., 2008).

7.3 Leukocyte adhesion deficiency

Gene transfer into hematopoietic stem cells (HSCs) is a promising treatment approach for many hematologic and genetic diseases. FV vectors can overcome safety concerns and the low HSC transduction rates found with oncoretroviral vectors. Recombinant FV vectors efficiently transduced human umbilical cord blood $CD34^{+}$ cells that were injected into nonobese diabetic/severe combined immunodeficiency (NOD/SCID) mice (Leurs et al., 2003; Josephson et al., 2002; Josephson et al., 2004; Zucali et al., 2002). The transduced human cells expressed high levels of the transgene in lymphoid, myeloid, and progenitor cells (Leurs et al., 2003; Vassilopoulos et al., 2001; Josephson et al., 2002). Additionally, there was no transgene silencing (Vassilopoulos et al., 2001; Josephson et al., 2002). Compared with FV, human immunodeficiency virus type 1 (HIV-1)-based lentiviral vectors pseudotyped with gibbon ape leukemia virus envelope (GALV Env) and murine leukemia virus (MLV)-based oncoretroviral vectors were inefficient in transducing NOD/SCID repopulating cells (Leurs et al., 2003). Bauer et al. demonstrated that FV vectors expressing the canine CD18 gene from an internal murine stem cell virus (MSCV) promoter could correct the lymphocyte proliferation and neutrophil adhesion defects characteristic of canine leukocyte adhesion deficiency (LAD). This work was the first successful use of FV vectors to treat a genetic immunodeficient disease. In addition, genotoxic complications were not observed, and compared with gammaretroviral vectors, integration site analysis revealed a polyclonality of transduced cells and a decreased risk of integration near oncogenes (Bauer et al., 2008). In another study, an FV vector expressing canine CD18 from a phosphoglycerate kinase (PGK) gene promoter, without an enhancer that would activate neighboring genes, expressed CD18 efficiently in canine neutrophils and $CD34^{+}$ cells. However, dogs continued to suffer from LAD after treatment of hematopoietic stem cells transduced with the PGK-CD18 vector. This suggests that the PGK promoter cannot effectively replace the MSCV promoter in CD18-expressing FV vectors and that a strong promoter-enhancer may be necessary in FV vectors for the treatment of human LAD (Bauer et al., 2011).

7.4 Cancer

Selective introduction of a foreign gene into tumor cells to produce an enzyme is the basis of suicide gene therapy as an anticancer strategy. The gene product activates an inert prodrug to its cytotoxic form, which results in tumor cell death (Bhaumik, 2011). To evaluate the effect of tumor growth suppression utilizing suicide gene therapy, FV vectors expressing the purine nucleoside phosphorylase (FOV-7/pnp), the nitroreductase (FOV-7/ntr), or the thymidine kinase (FOV-7/tk) suicide genes were injected into the nude-mouse/human subcutaneous U87 glioblastoma xenograft model. Mice with vector virus-injected tumors were treated with the respective prodrug, resulting in a significant inhibition of tumor growth. Without prodrug treatment, a similar suppression of tumor growth was also observed both in mice with vector virus-injected U87 tumor cells and in the G59 glioma model that received the FOV-7/pnp virus vector. Furthermore, wild-type FV, instead of the suicide gene-transducing vectors, was able to inhibit tumor growth, suggesting an oncolytic activity of foamy virus replication in a nude-mouse glioblastoma xenograft tumor model. However, the vector is not restricted to the tumor and persists in various mouse tissues. This persistence limits its potential use in clinical trials (Heinkelein et al., 2005). Replication-defective HFV vectors expressing interleukin-24 also exhibited an inhibitory effect on cancer cells (Chen et al., 2010).

7.5 Acquired immunodeficiency syndrome

FV vectors have the potential for gene therapy of acquired immunodeficiency syndrome in patients who are resistant to traditional antiviral therapy. The nonpathogenic HFV mediated intracellular expression of ovine interferon-tau permitted cells to be resistant to HIV infection (Fujii et al., 2004). Vectors developed from SFV expressing anti-rev/env (R2) short-interfering RNA (siRNA) effectively inhibited simian immunodeficiency virus (SIV) replication. This result shows that R2 siRNA reduces the rev and env gene expression and is a potent inhibitor of SIV replication (Park et al., 2005). Taylor and co-workers used three anti-HIV transgenes, including a dominant negative version of the viral rev protein (RevM10), a short hairpin RNA directed against a conserved overlapping sequence of the *tat* and *rev* genes (Sh1), and a membrane-attached peptide blocking HIV cell entry (maC46). These transgenes, expressed by foamy virus vectors both individually and collectively, were used to determine if they were able to effectively block HIV replication in macrophages. HIV replication was specifically blocked by maC46 or sh1 transgene expression. Entry inhibition by the maC46 transgene was the most effective method of blocking HIV replication among these three individual transgenes. In addition, the three anti-HIV transgenes expressed by FV vectors together effectively blocked HIV infection in primary macrophages derived from transduced, peripheral blood CD34-selected cells and in a cell line used for propagating HIV (Taylor et al., 2008).

7.6 Hepatitis B Virus (HBV)

Double-stranded RNA initiates and directs sequence-specific, post-transcriptional silencing of homologous genes. The use of RNA interference (RNAi), which is mediated by double-stranded small interfering RNA (siRNA), has received attention for the treatment of infectious diseases caused by viral or parasitic infection (Arenz et al., 2003). To successfully apply RNAi in the treatment of HBV infection, it was necessary to screen specific RNAi targeting sequences that could effectively knock down HBV transcripts. In a cell-based HBV infection model, two effective siRNA sequences designated S2 and X1 were cloned into HFV-based vectors to produce single siRNA expression vectors (HFVU6-siS2, HFVU6-siX1) and a dual siRNA expression vector (HFVU6-siSX). These siRNA vectors achieved long-term inhibition of HBV gene expression and viral DNA replication. HFVU6-siSX simultaneously expressing the two siRNAs that targeted the S and X genes of HBV was the most potent inhibitor of HBV replication, suggesting HFVU6-siS2 and HFVU6-siX1 may cooperate to inhibit HBV mRNA expression (Sun et al., 2007).

7.7 Chronic granulomatous disease

Chronic granulomatous disease (CGD) is a fatal genetic defect in leukocyte function caused by mutations in any of the four genes encoding the subunits ($p22^{phox}$, $gp91^{phox}$, $p47^{phox}$ and p67^{phox}) of phagocyte NADPH oxidase (Kume et al., 2000; Chatziandreou et al., 2011). The majority of CGD cases are due to sex-linked recessive inheritance resulting from mutations in the CYBB gene encoding gp91^{phox}. Chatziandreou et al. evaluated the gene transfer potential of FV vectors in an X-linked form of chronic granulomatous disease (X-CGD). FV vectors expressing the human codon-optimized gp91^{phox} reconstituted NADPH activity in vitro in the X-CGD cell line, ex vivo in primary murine HSCs and in vivo in the X-CGD mouse model of the disease. Sustained long-term expression of the gp91^{phox} transgene and a high percentage of superoxide-producing cells in the peripheral blood of transplanted X-CGD mice was achieved by FV vectors, suggesting that FV-based vectors were effective therapeutic vehicles for the genetic correction of X-CGD (Chatziandreou et al., 2011).

8. Perspectives

Because foamy virus infections are nonpathogenic, FVs have been considered potential vectors for the advancement of gene therapy. Moreover, the discovery of the internal promoter, IP, and the transactivator, Tas, have greatly promoted the research on foamy viruses. However, new issues have arisen in the course of foamy virus research; for example, studies have mainly focused on the primate foamy virus, which limits the field. Additionally, the products and functions of the structural and regulatory genes are not completely understood. Furthermore, although FVs are widespread, the host cell receptors are not yet known. These unknown features make the development of foamy virus gene therapy vectors difficult, yet there is still an interest in their development.

The use of viral mediated gene transfer is challenged by serious defects, yet they remain a potential tool of gene therapy for various diseases (Bastone et al., 2007). Therefore, it is critical to find a refined vector that is efficient and safe for treatment of the diseases, especially for nervous system therapy. To date, it is believed that FVs are nonpathogenic to the host, and their regulation of gene expression has been widely studied. Foamy virus is a widespread retrovirus with a unique structure that is innocuous in both human and primate infections. Thus, compared with the four major viral vector systems, the FV vectors appear to be a harmless and capable vehicle. With the increased understanding of neurological diseases and the improvement of gene therapy, the potential future of FV-based vectors carrying therapeutic genes for nervous systems and other organic systems is bright.

9. Acknowledgments

This work was supported by the National Natural Sciences Foundation of China (No. 30870856, 30970145 and 81171577), the Scientific Research Foundation for the Returned Overseas Scholars by the Ministry of Education of China, the Research Fund for the Doctoral Program of Higher Education of China (No. 20090141110010), and the Fundamental Research Funds for the Central Universities of China (No.3081002).

10. References

Aguzzi A. (1993). The foamy virus family: molecular biology, epidemiology and neuropathology. Biochim Biophys Acta., Vol. 271, No. 5255, (May 1993) pp.1-24, ISSN

Arenz, C. & Schepers, U. (2003). RNA interference: from an ancient mechanism to a state of the art therapeutic application? Naturwissenschaften., Vol.90, No.8, (Aug 2003) pp.345-359. ISSN

Baldwin, D.N.; Linial, M.L. (2003). The roles of Pol and Env in the assembly pathway of human foamy virus. J Virol., Vol. 72, No. 5. (May 1998) pp. 3658-3665, ISSN

Bastone, P.; Bravo, I.G. (2006). Lochelt M. Feline foamy virus-mediated marker gene transfer: identification of essential genetic elements and influence of truncated and chimeric proteins. Virology., Vol. 348, No. 1 (Apr 2006) pp. 190-9, ISSN

Bastone, P.; Romen, F.; Liu, W.; Wirtz, R.; Koch, U.; Josephson, N.; Langbein, S.; Löchelt, M. (2007). Construction and characterization of efficient, stable and safe replication-deficient foamy virus vectors, Gene Ther., Vol. 14, No. 7, (Apr 2007) pp. 613-620, ISSN

Bauer, TR. Jr.; Allen, J.M.; Hai, M.; Tuschong, L.M.; Khan, I.F.; Olson, E.M.; Adler, R.L.; Burkholder, T.H.; Gu, Y.C.; Russell, D.W. & Hickstein, D.D. (2008). Successful treatment of canine leukocyte adhesion deficiency by foamy virus vectors. Nat Med., Vol.14, No.1, (Jan 2008) pp. 93-97, ISSN

Bauer, TR. Jr.;Olson, E.M.; Huo, Y.; Tuschong, L.M.; Allen, J.M.; Li, Y.; Burkholder, T.H.; & Russell, D.W. (2011). Treatment of canine leukocyte adhesion deficiency by foamy virus vectors expressing CD18 from a PGK promoter. Gene Ther., Vol.18, No.6, (Jun 2011) pp.553-559, ISSN

Bhaumik, S. (2011). Advances in imaging gene-directed enzyme prodrug therapy. Curr Pharm Biotechnol., Vol.12, No.4, (Apr 2011) pp.497-507, ISSN

Bock, M.; Heinkelein, M.; Lindemann, D.; Rethwilm, A. (1998). Cells expressing the human foamy virus (HFV) accessory Bet protein are resistant to productive HFV superinfection. Virology., Vol. 250, No. 1 (Oct 1998) pp. 194-204, ISSN

Bodem, J.; Kräusslich, H.G.; Rethwilm, A. (2007). Acetylation of the foamy virus transactivator Tas by PCAF augments promoter-binding affinity and virus transcription. J Gen Virol., Vol. 88, No.1 (Jan 2007) pp. 259-263, ISSN

Caprariello, A.V.; Miller R.H. & Selkirk S.M. (2009). Foamy virus as a gene transfer vector to the central nervous system. Gene Ther., Vol. 16, No. 3, (Mar 2009) pp. 448-452, ISSN

Chatziandreou, I.; Siapati, E.K. & Vassilopoulos, G. (2011). Genetic correction of X-linked chronic granulomatous disease with novel foamy virus vectors. Exp Hematol., Vol. 39, No. 6, (Jun 2011) pp. 643-652, ISSN

Chen, S.C.; Yao, C.; Chen, F.; Liu, W.H.; Tao, W.P. & Li, W.X. (2010). Inhibitive effect of human foamy virus induced IL-24 on cancer cells. Xi Bao Yu Fen Zi Mian Yi Xue Za Zhi., Vol. 26, No. 2, (Feb 2010) pp. 121-124, ISSN

Choy, B.; Green, M.R. (1993). Eukaryotie activators function during multiple steps of preintiation complex assembly. Nature., Vol. 366, No. 6455, (Dec 1993) pp. 531-536, ISSN

Enssle, J.; Jordan, I. ; Mauer, B. ; Rethwilm, A. (1996). Foamy virus reverse transcriptase is expressed independently from the Gag protein. Proc Natl Acad Sci U S A., Vol. 93, No. 9, (Apr 1996) pp. 4137-41, ISSN

Erlwein, O.; Bieniasz, P.D.; McClure, M.O. (1998). Sequences in pol are required for transfer of human foamy virus-based vectors. J Virol., Vol. 72, No. 7, (Jul 1998) pp.5510-6, ISSN

Feng, L.R. & Maguire-Zeiss, K.A. (2010). Gene therapy in Parkinson's disease: rationale and current status. CNS Drugs., Vol. 24, No. 3, (Mar 2010) pp.177-192, ISSN

Flugel R.M. (1991). Spumaviruses: A group of complex retrovirus. J Acquir Immune Defic Syndr., Vol. 4, No. 8, (1991) pp.739-50, ISSN

Fujii, Y.; Murase, Y.; Otake, K.; Yokot, Y.; Omoto, S.; Hayashi, H.; Okada, H.;, Okada, N.; Kawai, M.; Okuyama, H. & Imakawa, K. (2004). A potential live vector, foamy virus, directed intra-cellular expression of ovine interferon-tau exhibited the resistance to HIV infection. J Vet Med Sci., Vol. 66, No. 2, (Feb 2004) pp. 115-121, ISSN

Gardlík, R.; Pálffy, R.; Hodosy, J.; Lukács, J.; Turna, J.; Celec P. (2005). Vectors and delivery systems in gene therapy. Med Sci Monit., Vol. 11, No. 4, (Apr 2005) 110-121, ISSN

Glorioso, J.C.; Mata, M.; Fink, D.J. Therapeutic gene transfer to the nervous system using viral vectors. J NeuroVirol., (2003). Vol. 9, No. 2, (Apr 2003) pp. 165-172, ISSN

Heinkelein, M.; Dressler, M.; Jármy, G.; Rammling, M.; Imrich, H.; Thurow, J.; Lindemann, D.; Rethwilm, A. (2002). Improved primate foamy virus vectors and packaging constructs. J Virol., Vol. 76, No. 8, (2002 Apr) pp. 3774-83, ISSN

Heinkelein, M.; Hoffmann, U.; Lücke, M.; Imrich, H.; Müller, J.G.; Meixensberger, J.; Westphahl, M.; Kretschmer, A. & Rethwilm, A. (2005). Experimental therapy of allogeneic solid tumors induced in athymic mice with suicide gene-transducing replication-competent foamy virus vectors. Cancer Gene Ther., Vol. 12, No. 12, (Dec 2005) pp. 947-953, ISSN

Heinkelein, M.; Schmidt, M.; Fischer, N.; Moebes, A.; Lindemann, D.; Enssle.; J.; Rethwilm, A. (1998). Characterization of a cis-acting sequence in the Pol region required to transfer human foamy virus vectors. J Virol., Vol. 72, No. 8 (Aug 1998) pp. 6307-14, ISSN

Heneine, W.; Switzer, W.M.; Sandstrom, P.; Brown, J.; Vedapuri, S.; Schable, C.A.; Khan, A.S.; Lerche, N.W.; Schweizer, M.; Neumann-Haefelin, D.; Chapman, L.E.; Folks, T.M. (1998). Identifcation of a human population infected with simian foamy viruses. Nat Med., Vol. 4, No. 4, (Apr 1998) pp. 403-7, ISSN

Josephson, N.C.; Trobridge, G.; Russell, D.W. (2004). Transduction of long-term and mobilized peripheral blood-derived NOD/SCID repopulating cells by foamy virus vectors. Hum Gene Ther., Vol. 15, No. 1, (Jan 2004) pp. 87-92, ISSN

Josephson, N.C.; Vassilopoulos, G.; Trobridge, G.D,; Priestley, G,V.; Wood, B.L.; Papayannopoulou, T. & Russell, D.W. (2002). Transduction of human NOD/SCID-repopulating cells with both lymphoid and myeloid potential by foamy virus vectors. Pnas., Vol. 99, No. 12, (Jun 2002) pp. 8295-300, ISSN

Kang, Y.; Blair, W.S.; Cullen, B.R. (1998). Identification and functional characterization of a high-affinity Bel1 DNA-binding site located in the human foamy virus internal promoter. J Virol., Vol. 72, No. 1 (Jan 1998) pp.504-11, ISSN

Kerr, L.D.; Ransone, L.J.; Wamsley, P.; Schmitt, M.J.; Boyer, T.G.; Zhou, Q.; Berk, A.J.; Verma, I.M. (1993). Association between proto-oncoprotein Rel and TATA-binding proteins mediates transcriptional activation by NF-KB. Nature., Vol. 364, No. 6445, (Sep 1993) pp. 412-419, ISSN

Khan, A.S. (2009). Simian foamy virus infection in humans:prevalence and anagement. Expert Rev Anti Infect Ther., Vol. 7, No. 5, (Jun 2009) pp. 569-80, ISSN

Kume, A. & Dinauer, M.C. (2000). Gene therapy for chronic granulomatous disease. J Lab Clin Med., Vol. 135, No. 2, (Feb 2000) pp.122-128, ISSN

Lee, K.J.; Lee, A.H.; Sung. Y.C. (1993). Multiple Positive and Negative cis-Acting Elements That Mediate Transactivation by bell in the Long Terminal Repeat of Human Foamy Virus. Journal of Virology., Vol. 67, No. 4, (Apr 1993) pp. 2317-2326, ISSN

Leurs, C.; Jansen, M.; Pollok, K.E.; Heinkelein, M.; Schmidt, M.; Wissler, M.; Lindemann, D.; Von Kalle, C.; Rethwilm, A.; Williams, D.A. & Hanenberg, H. (2003). Comparison of three retroviral vector systems for transduction of nonobese diabetic/severe combined immunodeficiency mice repopulating human CD34+ cord blood cells. Hum Gene Ther., Vol. 14, No. 6, (Apr 2003) pp. 509-519, ISSN

Li, Z.; Yang, P.; Li W. (1999). Research Advances on Human Spuma Retrovirus. J. Wuhan Univ., Vol. 45, No. 6, (Dec. 1999) pp. 901-904, ISSN

Lindefors, N. (1993). Dopaminergic regulation of glutamic acid decarboxylase mRNA expression and GABA release in the striatum: A review. Prog Neuropsychopharmacol Biol Psychiatry., Vol. 17, No. 6, (Nov 1993) pp.887-903, ISSN

Linial, M. (2000). Why aren't foamy viruses pathogenic? Trends In Microbiology., Vol. 8, No. 6, (Jun 2000) pp. 284-289, ISSN

Liu, W.; He, X.; Cao, Z.; Sheng, J.; Liu, H.; Li, Z.; Li, W. (2005). Efficient therapeutic gene expression in cultured rat hippocampal neurons mediated by human foamy virus vectors: a potential for the treatment of neurological diseases. Intervirology., Vol. 48, No. 5, (2005) pp. 329-35, ISSN

Liu, W.; Liu, Z.; Cao, X.; Cao, Z.; Xue, L.; Zhu, F.; He, X. & Li, W. (2007). Recombinant human foamy virus, a novel vector for neurological disorders gene therapy, drives production of GAD in cultured astrocytes. Mol Ther., Vol. 15, No. 10, (Oct 2007) pp. 1834-1841, ISSN

Liu, W.; Liu, Z.; L. Liu.; Xiao, Z.; Cao, X.; Cao, Z.; Xue, L.; Miao, L.; He, X. & Li, W. (2008). A novel human foamy virus mediated gene transfer of GAD67 reduces neuropathic pain following spinal cord injury. Neurosci Lett., Vol. 432, No. 1, (Feb 2008) pp. 13-18, ISSN

Löchelt, M.; Flügel, R.M.; Aboud, M. (1994). The Human Foamy Virus Internal Promoter Directs the Expression of the Functional Bel 1 Transactivator and Bet Protein Early after Infection. J Virol., Vol. 68, No. 4, (Feb 1994) pp. 638-645, ISSN

Löchelt, M.; Muranyi, W.; Flügel, R.M. (1993). Human foamy virus genome possesses an internal Bel-1-dependent and functional promoter. Proc Natl Acad Sci U S A., Vol. 90, No. 15, (Aug 1993) pp. 7317-21, ISSN

Löchelt, M.; Yu, S.F.; Linial, M.L.; Flügel, R.M. (1995). The human foamy virus internal promoter is required for efficient gene expression and infectivity. Virology., Vol. 206, No. 1, (Jan 1995) pp. 601-610, ISSN

Lohman, K.; Uber, E.O. (1934). Enzymatic transformation of phosphoglyceric acid into pyruvic and phosphoric acid. Biochem Z., Vol. 273, No. 1. pp. 60-72, ISSN

Manfredsson, F.P.; Mandel, R.J. (2010). Development of Gene Therapy for Neurological Disorders. Discov Med., Vol. 9, No. 46, (Mar 2010) pp. 204-11, ISSN

Marshall, E. (2002). Gene therapy a suspect in leukemia-like disease. Science., Vol. 4, No. 298, (Oct 2002) pp. 34-35, ISSN

Marshall, E. (2003). Gene therapy. Second child in French trial is found to have leukemia. Science., Vol.17, No.299, (Jan 2003) pp. 320, ISSN

Maurer, B.; Bannert, H.; Darai, G.; Flügel, R.M. (1998). Analysis of the Primary Structure of the Long Terminal Repeat and the gag and pol Genes of the Human Spumaretrovirus, J Virol., Vol. 62, No. 5. (May 1988) pp.1590-1597, ISSN

Mergia, A. (1994). Simian foamy virus type 1 contains a second promoter located at the 3' end of the env gene. Virology., Vol. 1999, No. 1 (Feb 1994) pp. 219-222, ISSN

Mergia, A.; Chari, S.; Kolson, D.L.; Goodenow, M.M.; Ciccarone, T. (2001). The efficiency of simian foamy virus vector type-1 (SFV-1) in nondividing cells and in human PBLs. Virology., Vol. 280, No. 2, (Feb 2001) pp. 243-52, ISSN

Nabel, G.; Baltimore, D. (1987). An inducible transcription factor activates expression of human immunodeficiency virus in T cells. Nature., Vol. 326, No. 6114. (Apr 1987) pp. 711-713, ISSN

Naik, A.K.; Pathirathna, S. & Jevtovic-Todorovic, V. (2008). GABAA receptor modulation in dorsal root ganglia in vivo affects chronic pain after nerve injury. Neuroscience., Vol. 154, No. 4, (Jul 2008) pp. 1539-1553, ISSN

Nestler, U.; Heinkelein, M.; Lücke, M.; Meixensberger, J.; Scheurlen, W.; Kretschmer, A.; Rethwilm, A. (1997). Foamy virus ectors for suicide gene therapy. Gene Ther., Vol. 4, No. 11, (Nov 1997) pp. 1270-7, ISSN

Park, J.; Nadeau, P.; Zucali, J.R.; Johnson, C.M. & Mergia, A. (2005). Inhibition of simian immunodeficiency virus by foamy virus vectors expressing siRNAs. Virology., Vol. 343, No. 2, (Dec 2005) pp. 275-282, ISSN

Park, J.; Nadeau, P.E.; Mergia, A. (2002). A minimal genome simian foamy virus type 1 vector system with efficient gene transfer. Virology., Vol. 302, No. 2, (Oct 2002) pp. 236-44, ISSN

Picard-Maureau, M.; Kreppel, F.; Lindemann, D.; Juretzek, T.; Herchenröder, O.; Rethwilm, A.; Kochanek, S.; Heinkelein, M. (2004). Foamy virus--adenovirus hybrid vectors. Gene Ther., Vol. 11, No. 8, (Apr 2004) pp. 722-8, ISSN

Regad, T.; Saib, A.; Lallemand-Breitenbach, V.; Pandolfi, P.P.; de Thé, H.; Chelbi-Alix, M.K. (2001). PML mediates the interferon-induced antiviral state against a complex retovirus via its association with the viral transactivator. EMBO J., Vol. 20, No. 13. (Jul 2001) pp. 3495-3505, ISSN

Rissman, R.A. & Mobley, W.C. (2011). Implications for treatment: GABAA receptors in aging, Down syndrome and Alzheimer's disease. J Neurochem., Vol. 117, No. 4, (May 2011) pp. 613-622, ISSN

Rothenaigner, I.; Kramer, S.; Meggendorfer, M.; Rethwilm, A. & Brack-Werner, R. (2009). Transduction of human neural progenitor cells with foamy virus vectors for differentiation-dependent gene expression. Gene Ther., Vol. 16, No. 3, (Mar 2009) pp. 349-358, ISSN

Russell, D.W.; Miller, A.D. (1996). Foamy virus vectors. J Virol., Vol. 70, No. 1, (Jan 1996) pp. 217-22, ISSN

Russell, R.A.; Vassaux, G.; Martin-Duque, P. ; McClure, M.O. (2004). Transient foamy virus vector production by adenovirus. Gene Ther., Vol. 11, No. 3, (Feb 2004) pp. 310-6, ISSN

Saïb, A. ; Puvion-Dutilleul, F. ; Schmid, M. ; Périès, J. ; de Thé, H. (1997). Nuclear Targeting of Incoming Human Foamy Virus Gag Proteins Involves a Centriolar Step. J Virol., Vol. 71, No. 2, (Feb 1997) pp. 1155-61, ISSN

Saïb, A.; Périès, J.; de Thé H. (1995). Recent insight into the biology of human foamy virus. Trends In Microbiology., Vol. 3, No. 5, (May 1995) pp. 173-178, ISSN

Saïb, A.; Périès, J.; de Thé, H. (1993). A defective human foamy provirus generated by pregenome splicing. EMBO J., Vol. 12, No. 11. (Nov 1993) pp. 4439-4444, ISSN

Schliephake, A.W.; Rethwilm, A. (1994). Nuclear Localization of Foamy Virus Gag Precursor Protein. J Virolog., Vol. 68, No. 8. (Aug 1994) pp. 4946-4954, ISSN

Schmidt, M. & Rethwilm, A. (1995). Replicating foamy virus-based vectors directing high level expression of foreign genes. Virology., Vol. 210, No. 1, (Jun 1995) pp. 167-78, ISSN

Stenbak, C.R.; Linial, M.L. (2004). Role of the C Terminus of Foamy Virus Gag in RNA Packaging and Pol Expression. J Virol., Vol. 78, No. 17. (Sept 2004) pp. 9423-9430, ISSN

Sun, Y.; Li, Z.; Li, L.; Li, J.; Liu, X. & Li, W. (2007). Effective inhibition of hepatitis B virus replication by small interfering RNAs expressed from human foamy virus vectors. Int J Mol Med., Vol. 19, No. 4, (Apr 2007) pp.705-711, ISSN

Tan, J.;Qiao, W.; Wang, J.; Xu, F.; Li, Y.; Zhou, J.; Chen, Q.; Geng, Y. (2008). IFP35 is involved in the antiviral function of interferon by association with the viral tas transactivator of bovine foamy virus. J Virol., Vol. 82, No. 9. (May 2008) pp. 4275-4283, ISSN

Taylor, J.A.; Vojtech, L.; Bahner, I.; Kohn, D.B.; Laer, D.V.; Russell, D.W. & Richard, R.E. (2008). Foamy virus vectors expressing anti-HIV transgenes efficiently block HIV-1 replication. Mol Ther., Vol. 16. No. 1, (Jan 2008) pp. 46-51, ISSN

Trobridge G, Russell DW (2004). Cell cycle requirements for transduction by foamy virus vectors compared to those of oncovirus and lentivirus vectors. J Virol., Vol. 78, No. 5, (2004 Mar) pp. 2327-35, ISSN

Trobridge, G.; Josephson, N.; Vassilopoulos, G.; Mac, J.; Russell, D.W. (2002). Improved foamy virus vectors with minimal viral sequences. Mol Ther., Vol. 6, No. 3, (Sep 2002) pp. 321-8, ISSN

Trobridge, G.D. (2009). Foamy virus vectors for gene transfer. Expert Opin Biol Ther., Vol. 9, No. 11, (Nov 2009) pp. 1427-1436, ISSN

Trobridge, G.D.; Russell, D.W. (1998). Helper-free foamy virus vectors. Hum Gene Ther., Vol.9, No. 17, (Nov 1998) pp. 2517-25, ISSN

Vassilopoulos, G.; Trobridge, G.; Josephson, N.C. & Russell, D.W. (2001). Gene transfer into murine hematopoietic stem cells with helper-free foamy virus vectors. Blood., Vol. 98, No. 3, (Aug 2001) pp. 604-609, ISSN

Wang, Z.G.; Ruggero, D.; Ronchetti, S.; Zhong, S.; Gaboli, M.; Rivi, R.; Pandolfi, P.P. (1998). PML is essential for multiple apoptotic pathways, Nat Genet., Vol. 20, No. 3. (Nov 1998) pp. 266-272, ISSN

Williams, D.A. (2008). Foamy Virus Vectors Come of Age. Molecular Therapy., Vol. 16, No. 4 (Apr 2008) pp. 635-636, ISSN

Wu, M.; Chari, S.; Yanchis, T.; Mergia, A. (1998). cis-Acting sequences required for simian foamy virus type 1 vectors. J Virol., Vol. 72, No. 4, (1998 Apr) pp. 3451-4, ISSN

Wu, Y.; Zhang, Q.; Li, Z.; Tang, S.; Xu, F.; Chen, Q. (2009).α-Enolase Repress Bell-mediated Transcriptional Activation of LTR and IP. Acta Scientiarum Naturallum., Vol. 42, No. 5. ISSN

Yang, P.; Zemba, M.; Aboud M. (1997). Deletion analysis of both the long terminal repeat and the internal promoter of the human foamy virus. Virus Genes., Vol. 15, No. 1, (1997) pp. 17-23, ISSN

Yu, S.F.; Baldwin, D.N.; Gwynn, S.R.; Yendapalli, S.; Linial, M.L. (1996). Human foamy virus replication: a pathway distinct from that of retroviruses and hepadnaviruses. Science., Vol. 271, No. 5255. (Mar 1996) pp. 1579-1582, ISSN

Yu, S.F.; Edelmann, K.; Strong, R.K.; Moebes, A.; Rethwilm, A.; Linial, M.L. (1996). The Carboxyl Terminus of the Human Foamy Virus Gag Protein Contains Separable Nucleic Acid Binding and Nuclear Transport Domains, J Virol., Vol. 70, No. 12. (Dec 1996), pp. 8255-8262, ISSN

Zhang, Y.; Liu Y.; Zhu, G.; Qiu, Y.; Peng, B.; Yin, J.; Liu, W.; and He, X. (2010). Foamy virus: an available vector for gene transfer in neural cells and other nondividing cells. Journal of NeuroVirology., Vol. 16, No. 6, (Nov 2010) pp. 419-426, ISSN

Zou, J.X.; Luciw, P.A. (1996). The transcriptional transactivator of simian foamy virus 1 binds to a DNA target element in the viral internal promoter(J). Proc. Natl. Acad. Sci., Vol. 93, No. 1. (Jan 1996) pp. 326-330, ISSN

Zucali, J.R.; Ciccarone, T.; Kelley, V.; Park, J.; Johnson, C.M. & Mergia, A. (2002). Transduction of umbilical cord blood CD34+ NOD/SCID-repopulating cells by simian foamy virus type 1 (SFV-1) vector. Virology., Vol. 302, No. 2, (Oct 2002) pp.229-235, ISSN

5

Real-Time Analysis of Intracranial Pressure Waveform Morphology

Fabien Scalzo, Robert Hamilton and Xiao Hu
Neural Systems and Dynamics Laboratory (NSDL), UCLA
USA

1. Introduction

The cranial vault is composed of four fundamental components: arterial blood, venous blood, cerebrospinal fluid (CSF), and brain parenchyma. Intracranial pressure (ICP) represents the pressure within the brain parenchyma and cerebrospinal fluid (CSF). The environment within the cranial vault is unique compared to other organ systems; it is enclosed within a rigid skull and thus small volumetric changes in any of the four elements lead to significant changes in ICP. One example of this, is the periodic influx of arterial blood over the cardiac cycle; this change causes the ICP pulse pressure waveform. The pulse pressure waveform has three characteristic peaks hypothesized to correspond to different physiologic components. Early work [1] demonstrated the relationship between pulsations in the choroid plexus and the pulse pressure waveform. Moreover, other studies [2] compared the right atrium (venous) and the aortic (arterial) pressures to the intracranial waveform in the cistern magna and showed that although the cranial pulse pressure is related to arterial pulsations, there is also a venous component. The results of these studies support the current theories for the etiology of the characteristic peaks in the ICP pulse pressure waveform. The majority of the literature indicates that P1, the percussion wave, corresponds with the pulsation of the choroid plexus and/or large intracranial conductive vessels [3-5]. The rebound of the percussion wave is thought to contribute to P2, which has also been related to cerebral compliance [5]. Finally, the dicrotic wave, or P3, is thought to be venous in origin [2, 4, 6].

ICP monitoring is fundamental to the management of numerous intracranial pathologies, including the management of traumatic brain injury (TBI), subarachnoid hemorrhage (SAH), hydrocephalous, and any other conditions where pathological changes in intracranial volume (ICV) may occur. Maintaining an ICP within normal limits is vital for adequate perfusion of the brain. An increase in ICP (intracranial hypertension) reduces arterial blood flow into the cranial vault, while decreased ICP (intracranial hypotension) results in severe headaches. Although the importance of monitoring ICP is well established, only recently has ICP pulse pressure waveform morphology yielded promising results due to advancing technology. However, the importance of ICP pulse pressure waveform morphology has been known for years; special interest should be focused not only on the height of mean ICP, but also on the pressure pulse curve, because the configuration and pulse amplitude of the CSF pulsations can be regarded to a certain extent as an index of the state of intracranial elastance or cerebral bulk compliance [6].

Methods for monitoring ICP include: epidural, subarachnoid, intraventricular, and intraparenchymal pressure probes. For the investigation of ICP morphology, a continuous measurement of ICP must be achieved. There have been several recent advances by various groups to analyze continuous ICP waveform morphology. An analysis method [7] that utilizes 6-sec time windows to extract average amplitude and latency information for the given window was developed. Our group has recently developed a time-domain analysis toolbox for intracranial waveform morphology known as Morphological Clustering and Analysis of Continuous Intracranial Pulse (MOCAIP)[8]. The details of this algorithm will be presented in the subsequent chapter. Several groups have successfully utilized pulse pressure waveform morphology analysis in the diagnosis and management of various conditions. For example, pulse pressure amplitude has been linked to several conditions with promising results in normal pressure hydrocephalus (NPH) for predicting shunt responsiveness [9, 10]. Work has also been done in chronic headaches; again, showing the usefulness of pulse pressure amplitude. Furthermore, our group has investigated several conditions using ICP morphological metrics including: detection of cerebral hyoperfusion [11], prediction of ICP hypertension [12], segmentation of ICP slow waves [13], changes in vasoreactivity (vasodilatation) [14]. ICP monitoring has been fundamental for the diagnosis and management of several conditions for decades. In this chapter, we present a few of the recent advances in the analysis of ICP pulse pressure waveforms and its applications as described above.

2. Automatic analysis of ICP morphology

As previously described, the ICP pulse pressure signal contains three characteristic peaks [5]. From those peaks, it is possible to describe in a parametric way the amplitude and timing information of the pulse for further examination. While several studies have focused on the offline analysis of the ICP waveform [15-17] and the extraction of its morphological features, processing ICP signals to extract the three peaks in a continuous way is challenging because the signal is commonly affected by various types of noise and artifacts. MOCAIP algorithm [18, 19] was developed by our group to address these issues. MOCAIP is capable of extracting morphological features of ICP pulses in real-time by recognizing legitimate ICP pulses, and by detecting the three peaks from average waveforms computed from segments of ICP.

Recently, two main extensions have been developed from the original framework. MOCAIP++ (Section 2.1) is a generalization of MOCAIP that allows different peak recognition techniques to be used and uses intermediate features to make the peak detection more robust to the variations observed in the clinical conditions. The latest extension of MOCAIP is presented in Section 2.2 and poses the peak detection problem in terms of Bayesian inference.

2.1 MOCAIP++

MOCAIP++ [20] generalizes MOCAIP in two ways. First, it proposes a unifying framework where different peak recognition techniques can be integrated. Second, it allows the algorithm to take advantage of additional ICP features to improve the peak recognition. A summary of the algorithm is described in the following subsections.

ICP Segmentation: The continuous raw ICP signal is segmented into a series of individual ICP pulses using a pulse extraction technique [21] combined with the ECG QRS detection [17, 22] that locates each ECG beat. Because ICP recordings are subject to various noise and artifacts during the acquisition process, an average pulse is extracted from a series of consecutive ICP pulses using hierarchical clustering [23].

Peak Candidates: Peak candidates, each being a potential match to one of the three peaks, are detected at curve inflections of the average ICP pulse using the second derivative of the signal.

Second-order ICP Features: We have shown in a recent study [20] that the first derivative of the ICP signal is very useful to discriminate between ICP peaks and therefore preoviding improve recognition. In our previous work, the first L_x demonstrated the best improvements in comparison with the second derivative and the curvature within MOCAIP++ framework. The derivative L_x is computed according to the smoothed version L of the ICP,

$$L_x = L(x,\sigma) - L(x+1,\sigma). \tag{1}$$

where the ICP signal $I(x)$ is first convolved with a Gaussian smoothing filter $G(x;\sigma)$ with the standard deviation σ to generate $L(x,\sigma)$,

$$L(x,\sigma) = G(x;\sigma) * I(x). \tag{2}$$

Peak Recognition: The peak recognition tasks consists in recognizing the three peaks (p_1, p_2, p_3) among the set of candidate peaks detected within the pulse. Several techniques have been developed and can be used such as independent Gaussian models [18], Gaussian Mixture Models (GMM), and spectral regression (SR) analysis [19]. Depending on the technique, it can exploit the latency of the peak candidates, the raw ICP pulse, or different features extracted from the pulse.

Morphological metrics: Once the peaks have been detected in an ICP pulse, a set of metrics (Fig. 1) is used to describe the shape morphology in a parametric way. This allows to obtain a better understanding about the type of variations that take place.

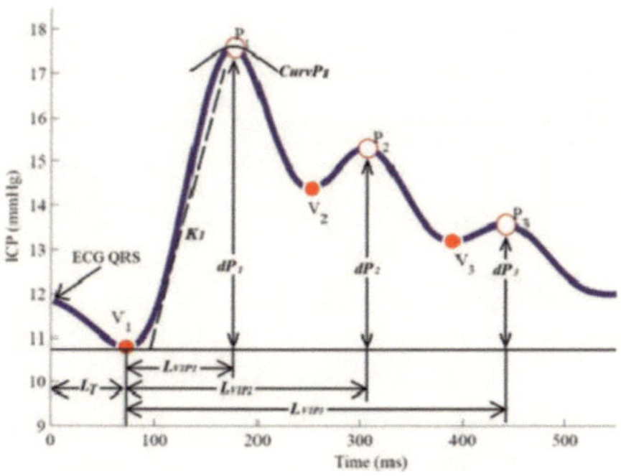

28 Basic metrics extracted from individual landmarks or over all characteristics	
dV1, dV2, dV3, dP1, dP2, dP3	Amplitude of landmark relative to the minimum point prior to initial rise
L_{V1P1}, L_{V1P2}, L_{V1P3}, L_{V2P2}, L_{V3P3}	Time delay among landmarks
$Curv_{v1}$, $Curv_{v2}$, $Curv_{v3}$, $Curv_{p1}$, $Curv_{p2}$, $Curv_{p3}$	Absolute curvature of each landmark
K1, K2, K3, RC1, RC2, RC3	K1, K2, K3 are slope of each rising edge and RC1, RC2, RC3 are time-constants of each descending edge
mICP, diasICP	Mean ICP and diastolic ICP
L_T	Time delay of V_1 to ECG QRS peak
mCurv	Mean absolute curvature of the pulse
WaveAmp	Maximum among dP1–dP3
100 extended metrics calculated as ratios among metrics within each group	
$dP_{p1p2,...}$	Ratio among landmark amplitudes
$L_{V1P1}/L_{T,...}$	Ratio among time delays
$Curv_{v1}/Curv_{v2,...}$	Ratio among curvatures
$K_1/RC_{1,...}$	Ratio among slopes/RCs

Fig. 1. Illustration of morphological metrics extracted From ICP peaks (reproduced with permission from [14] and [66]).

2.2 Bayesian tracking of ICP morphology

In this section, we present a probabilistic framework [24] to track ICP peaks in real time. The tracking is posed as inference in a graphical model that associates a continuous random variable to the position of each of the three peaks, in terms of their latency within the pulse and pressure level. The model (Section 2.3) represents the dependencies between the peaks using a Kernel Density Estimation (KDE) from evidence collected from manually annotated pulses, while Nonparametric Belief Propagation (NBP) [25] is used during the detection process (Section 2.4).

We assume that the tracking framework is presented with a series of raw pulses extracted from the ICP signal. The model consists of three distinct states $[x_{t,1}, x_{t,2}, x_{t,3}]$ at time t, one for the position of each peak. A state $x_{t,i} = \{\mu_{t,i}, v_{t,i}\}$ is two-dimensional that defines the latency $\mu_{t,i} \in R$, and the ICP elevation $v_{t,i} \in R$ of the peak. To each state $x_{t,i}$ is associated an observation $y_{t,i}$ directly extracted from the position of the peak within the current pulse.

2.3 Probabilistic tracking framework

The graphical model used in our tracking framework defines relations between pairs of nodes. States $x_{t,i} \in x$ and observations $y_{t,i} \in y$ are represented in the graphical model and illustrated in Fig. 2 by white, and shaded nodes, respectively. Edges represent dependencies between states, and possibly observations, by two types of functions: observation potentials $\phi(x_{t,i}, y_{t,i})$ that are the equivalent of the likelihood part $p(y_{t,i} | x_{t,i})$, and compatibility potentials $\psi_{ij}(x_{t,i}, x_{t,j})$ that embed the conditional parts $p(x_{t,i} | x_{t,j})$, $p(x_{t,j} | x_{t,i})$ of the Bayesian formulation and can be used by conditioning them in either directions during inference. By introducing compatibility potentials between states of the same peak at successive times $\psi(x_{t,i}, x_{t-1,i})$, that we name temporal potentials, the model becomes a dynamic Markov model.

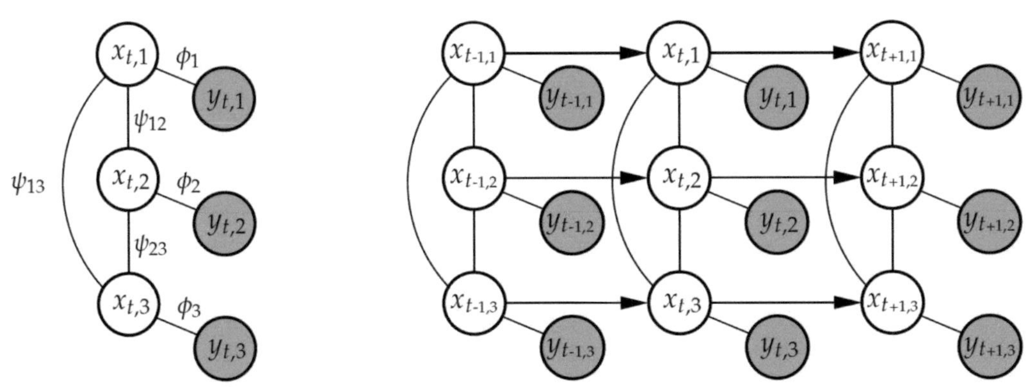

Fig. 2. The graphical model represents the dependence through pairwise potentials ($\psi_{12}, \psi_{13}, \psi_{23}$) between hidden nodes ($x_1, x_2, x_3$), and likelihood functions (ϕ_1, ϕ_2, ϕ_3) between hidden and observable nodes (y_1, y_2, y_3) (a). By introducing temporal potentials between successive nodes (b), the graphical model becomes dynamic and allows for tracking ICP peaks in real time (reproduced from permission from [24]).

2.3.1 Observation model

An observation $y_{t,i} \in \{R^2 \cup \varnothing\}$ corresponds to the position of the ith peak, in terms of latency and ICP elevation, that was produced by a peak detector at time t. Our framework uses MOCAIP as peak detector but any other peak detection technique can be used within our model. Observations $y_{t,i}$ are linked to their state $x_{t,i}$ through an observation potential $\phi(x_{t,i}, y_{t,i})$. Equation (3) formalizes the integration of the observation using a Gaussian model,

$$\phi(x_{t,i}, y_{t,i}) = \begin{cases} exp(-\alpha^{-1} \mid y_{t,i} - x_{t,i} \mid^2), if(y_{t,i} \neq \varnothing) \\ \lambda_i, if(y_{t,i} = \varnothing) \end{cases} \tag{3}$$

where α is a smoothing parameter, and λ_i is a constant factor that accounts for missing peaks by the detector.

2.3.2 Compatibility and Temporal potentials

Temporal potentials $\psi(x_{t-1,i}, x_{t,i})$ define the relationship between two successive states of a peak. They are defined as a Gaussian difference between their arguments,

$$\psi(x_{t-1,i}, x_{t,i}) = exp(-\mid x_{t-1,i} - x_{t,i} \mid^2 / \sigma_t^2) \tag{4}$$

where the standard deviation σ_t of the model was previously estimated using maximum likelihood (ML) on training data. Compatibility potentials $\psi_{i,j}(x_{t,i}, x_{t,j})$, however, are not expected to follow a Gaussian distribution. Each potential is represented by a KDE [26] $\psi_{i,j}(x_{t,i}, x_{t,j}) = \hat{f}(x_{ij}; \Theta)$ that is constructed by collecting co-occurring ICP peak positions across the training set.

2.4 Tracking ICP peaks using nonparametric bayesian inference

Detecting peaks in an ICP pulse at time t amounts to estimating $p(x_t \mid y_{\{1...t\}})$, the posterior belief associated with the states $x_t = \{x_{t,1}, x_{t,2}, x_{t,3}\}$ given all observations $y_{\{1...t\}} = \{y_{\{1...t\},1}, y_{\{1...t\},2}, y_{\{1...t\},3}\}$ accumulated so far. Thus, peak detection is achieved through inference in our graphical model. One way to do this efficiently is to use Nonparametric Belief Propagation [25]. It is a message passing algorithm for graphical models that generalizes particle filtering and Belief Propagation (BP). Messages are repeatedly exchanged between nodes to perform inference. Following the notation of BP, a message m_{ij} sent from node i to j is written [1],

$$m_{i,j}(x_j) \leftarrow \int \psi_{i,j}(x_i, x_j)\, \phi_i(x_i, y_i) \prod_{k \in N_i \setminus j} m_{k,i}(x_i) dx_i \tag{5}$$

---

[1]To simplify the notation, we discard the temporal subscript t of each node which is not necessary to explain the inference.

where $N_{i\setminus j}$ is the set of neighbors of state i where j is excluded, $\psi_{i,j}(x_i,x_j)$ is the pairwise potential between nodes i,j, and $\phi_i(x_i,y_i)$ is the observation potential. Each message $m_{i,j}(x_j)$ as well as each node $x_i \in x$ distribution is represented through a multivariate KDE.

To compute an outgoing message $m_{i,j}(x_j)$, NBP requires the pairwise potential $\psi_{i,j}(x_i,x_j)$, which represents the joint distribution between the nodes, to be conditioned on the source state x_i. This task is achieved by sampling N_a particles $s_j^k \leftarrow \psi_{i,j}(x_i = s_i^k, x_j)$ from the potential.

After any iteration of message exchanges, each state can compute an approximation $\hat{p}(x_i \mid y_{\{1...t\}})$, called belief, to the marginal distribution $p(x_i \mid y_{\{1...t\}})$ by combining the incoming messages with the local observation:

$$\hat{p}(x_i \mid y_{\{1...t\}}) \leftarrow \phi_i(x_i,y_i) \prod_{k \in R_i} m_{k,i}(x_i) \tag{6}$$

An example of inference is provided in Fig. 3 where the latency and the elevation of the three peaks is tracked simultaneously and in real-time on a pulse-by-pusle fashion.

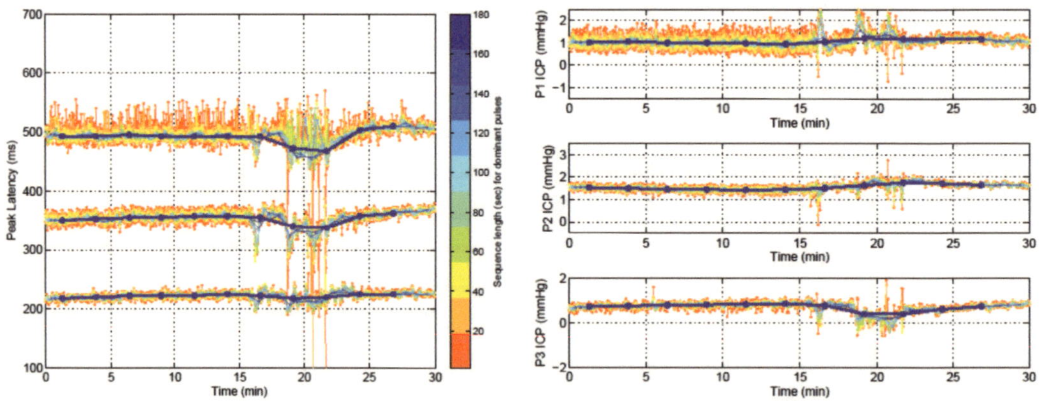

Fig. 3. Peak latency (left) and ICP elevation (right) estimated on ICP sequences by NBP tracking algorithm. The predictions of the tracking are obtained in real-time and are robust to transient perturbations that frequently occur during the ICP signal recording.

3. Detection of decreased cerebral blood flow (CBF)

The measure of cerebral blood flow (CBF) is an indicator of perfusion and is therefore very useful in neurocritical care. While imaging techniques provide a snapshot in time and invasive monitors offer continuous readings of the CBF, they usually carry additional risks and require additional equipments and increased cost. Furthermore, non-invasive techniques for CBF monitoring only provide intermittent measures of CBF. There is therefore a need to create a continuous, low cost technique that would not increase risk and could be easily integrated to bedside monitors.

Drawing from the fact that a physiological relation exists between ICP and CBF, we recently investigated if the ICP signal holds predictive information about CBF. Such a complex relationship has only been partially explored such that mean ICP (mICP) is used in the following equation to derive the driving pressure of blood flow through the cerebral vasculature:

$$CPP = ABP - mICP \tag{7}$$

where CPP stands for cerebral perfusion pressure, and ABP for systemic arterial blood pressure (ABP). To date, the influence of cerebral vascular changes on both ICP and CBF remain poorly understood. Subtle changes in the morphology of ICP pulses may reflect cerebral vascular changes. Because an ICP waveform can be thought as arising from an incidental arterial pressure pulse influenced by different intracranial compartments, we hypothesize that the ICP waveform carries information composed of changes in cerebral vasculature and hence CBF. In this section, we report our study [11] investigating the ability of ICP morphoology metrics to detect low CBF. A multi-modal dataset originating from brain injured patients with ICP monitoring, global average CBF, and Transcranial Doppler (TCD) assessment was analyzed. Detection of low CBF was posed as a classification problem and implemented using a regularized linear discriminant analysis (LDA). To further improve the performance of the framework, an optimization algorithm was used to find the subset of morphological metrics that maximizes a measure based on the combination of positive predictivity and sensitivity.

3.1 Data

The dataset used in our study originates from 63 patients among which 31 were admitted for SAH from aneurysm rupture and 26 had a TBI. The remaining patients were admitted either with arteriovenous malformation, brain tumor, and Intraparenchyma hemorrhage.

The mean global CBF was measured using the intravenous ^{133}Xenon clearance technique [27] for 11 minutes. TCD [28] was used to insonate the extracranial internal carotid artery (ICA) and the basilar artery (BA). Blood samples were taken immediately before or after CBF measurement. In addition to ECG, ICP was monitored using ventriculostomy and waveforms were recorded from bedside monitors at a sampling rate of 240 Hz. The ICP signal (selected as a one hour segment closest to the CBF measurement) was processed by MOCAIP to extract 24 morphological metrics for each three minute segment of data. A total number of 199 CBF-TCD-ICP segments were extracted from the 63 patients. In addition to the 24 morphological metrics extracted from ICP, the eight following variables weren also extracted: 1) average flow velocities of the right and the left internal carotid artery (ICA); 2) average diastolic flow velocities of the right and the left ICA; 3) average pulsatility indices (PI) of the right and the left ICA; 4) partial carbon dioxide pressure (CO_2); 5) total amount of hemoglobin (Hgb); 6) fraction of the blood composed of red blood cells (Hct); 7) mean arterial blood pressure (MAP); 8) amount of CSF drainage in the hour of CBF measurement.

3.2 Experiments

A classification experiment was designed to evaluate the power of ICP morphology to discriminate between low and normal CBF value (averaged globally, threshold of 20 ml/min/100g). Four combinations of all 32 available metrics were considered, within which an optimal subset was obtained using the classifier training algorithm described below; with (a) all 32 metrics, (b) only includes MOCAIP, CSF drainage and TCD metrics, (c) only morphological ICP and CSF drainage metrics, and (d) only seven TCD and blood analysis metrics. Using those features, a regularized version [29] of the Gaussian quadratic classifier (QDC) was chosen, and differential evolution (DE) [30] used to optimize the model using feature selection. The objective function for the optimization algorithm is the average of the sensitivity and the positive predictivity (PPV). Each evaluation of the objective function involves a leave-one-patient-out cross-validation.

3.3 Results

A sensitivity of $81.8 \pm 0.9\%$ and specificity of $50.1 \pm 0.2\%$ were obtained using the optimal combination (d) of conventional TCD and blood analysis metrics as input. Using the optimal combination of the morphological metrics alone (c) was able to achieve a sensitivity of $92.5 \pm 0.7\%$ and specificity of $84.8 \pm 0.8\%$. Searching for the optimal combination of all available metrics (a) achieved the best result that was marginally better than those from using morphological metrics alone (c). To visually assess how ICP pulse morphology is associated with different perfusion states, we present one typical case in Fig. 4 from a traumatic brain injury patient who had ICP recordings both in the normal and in the low CBF states. In each plot, we overlap the average ICP pulses extracted from every three minutes of data. In addition, we display the CBF value associated with the ICP recording. We observe that the elevation of the third peak within the pulse is associated with low CBF value. This pattern of elevated third peak was observed in six out of the eight patients with positive cases.

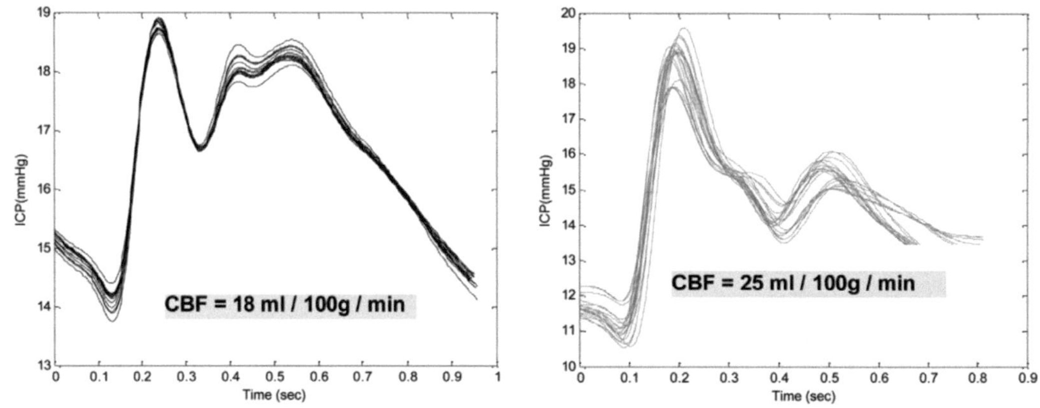

Fig. 4. Illustration of average ICP pulse with low (left) and normal (right) CBF (reproduced with permission from [11]).

Table 1 lists the mean and standard deviation of sensitivity, specificity, and positive predictivity value of the three after the leave-one-out (LOO) cross-validation and the bootstrapping (BS) cross-validation. Based on the bootstrapping results, it is observed that combining morphological ICP metrics, TCD, and blood analysis achieves the best performance. The biggest gain of the performance is caused by the incorporation of the morphological ICP metrics. The number of times each metrics was selected over the experiment was accumulated and analyzed. The following metrics were always selected; dP_{13}, dP_3, diasP, mICP, L_t, L_3, and ICAEd. There are 10 more metrics, including ICAPI and Hct, were selected for majority of the runs. Also, there are 10 metrics that were never selected as part of classifier features including PCO_2, Hgb, and ICAMean. The complete list of the metrics can be found in the original paper.

Exp.	Val.	SE	SPE	PPV
MOCAIP+TCD+BA	LOO	0.933 ± 0.000	0.862 ± 0.003	0.356 ± 0.005
	BS	0.941 ± 0.014	0.852 ± 0.013	0.341 ± 0.024
MOCAIP + TCD	LOO	0.933 ± 0.000	0.853 ± 0.005	0.342 ± 0.008
	BS	0.920 ± 0.014	0.846 ± 0.011	0.316 ± 0.018
MOCAIP	LOO	0.933 ± 0.000	0.851 ± 0.003	0.339 ± 0.005
	BS	0.925 ± 0.007	0.848 ± 0.008	0.320 ± 0.020
BA	LOO	0.867 ± 0.000	0.516 ± 0.000	0.127 ± 0.000
	BS	0.818 ± 0.009	0.501 ± 0.002	0115 ± 0.001

Se: sensitivity; Spe: specificity; PPV: positive predictivity value; LOO: leave-one out; BS: bootstrapping.

Table 1. Illustration of the CBF classification results.

Besides the metrics that reflect P_3 elevation were selected as classifier features, the metrics including L_t, L_1, L_2, and L_x were also frequently selected. The engagement of L_t in the classification process can be probably explained by the fact that it measures the timing difference between ECG QRS peak and the onset of ICP pulse, which is significantly influenced by systemic arterial blood pressure. Therefore, L_t is a relevant measure as it contains information about the driving pressure of the cerebral blood flow.

3.4 Discussion

We tested the hypothesis that low global CBF may be detected using morphological metrics extracted from the ICP waveforms through a trained classifier. The main finding was that the incorporation of morphological metrics of ICP was able to significantly improve the performance as compared to only using conventional TCD and blood analysis measurements. Although the study was retrospective and data-driven, we believe that it should motivate further studies to investigate the implications and the underlying mechanisms of the association between ICP pulse morphology and cerebral blood perfusion.

One of the findings from the classification experiment is that the elevation of the third peak of an ICP pulse may indicate low global cerebral perfusion. Some questions can be raised regarding whether controlling ICP can also lead to the control of cerebral venous pressure. This is important because the true perfusion pressure is actually determined by the difference between arterial and venous pressure. Even when the mean ICP is well within the prescribed limit, the true perfusion pressure may be still low in situation of cerebral venous hypertension.

4. Predicting intracranial hypertension

Intracranial hypertension (IH) poses a constant threat to head injured patients because it may lead to secondary injuries due to decreased cerebral perfusion pressure and cerebral ischemia. Because bedside monitors are usually designed to report only a short-term history of the ICP, large scale patterns and trends on average ICP that might help to prevent IH are not available to the bedside clinician. Therefore, the constant attention of the nursing staff and their prompt reaction following detecting of an IH episode are critical aspects during the management of patients with IH issues. There is a clear need for a computerized monitoring support that would be accurate in predicting ICP hypertension several minutes ahead, offering enough time to attract the full attention of the bedside clinician.

The main hypothesis is that precursor features can be detected in the ICP signal prior to the elevation. Several studies have verified this hypothesis and offer various insights into which form the predictive features might take. Amplitude of ICP [31, 32], variance of changes [33-35], and rounding of pulse waveform [36] have been shown to correlate with changes of the mean ICP. Decreases in ABP were observed at the beginning of plateau waves [37], and A waves [38]. Moreover, system analysis [39] suggested that a change in the transfer function that relates ABP to ICP may precede elevations. Several other investigators have also attempted to make predictions using wavelet decomposition of the ICP signal [40-42]. More recently, two studies [12, 43] demonstrated that morphological features extracted from the ICP waveform at various times before the elevation onset contains predictive information for IH. Despite more than 30 years [44, 45] of investigation, the automatic, real-time prediction of ICP hypertension is still beyond current methods. Drawing from the studies [12, 36, 43] indicating that ICP morphology contains relevant predictors of IH, we present in this section a framework [65] to predict IH based on morphological features of ICP. A key contribution of this study is to test the effectiveness of ensemble classifiers (AdaBoost, Extremely Randomized Decision Trees) to make temporal prediction. The proposed framework is evaluated on a representative database of 30 neurosurgical patients admitted for various intracranial pressure related conditions.

4.1 Methods

4.1.1 Data source and pre-processing

The dataset of ICP signals originates from the University of California, Los Angeles (UCLA) Medical Center. The ICP and ECG signals were acquired continuously at a rate of 240 Hz or 400 Hz using intraparenchymal sensors from a total of 30 patients treated for various intracranial pressure related conditions. These patients were monitored because of headache symptoms (idiopathic intracranial hypertension, Chiari syndrome, and slit ventricle patients with clamped shunts) with known risks of ICP elevation.

Intracranial hypertension episodes, defined as an elevated ICP greater than 20 mmHg for a period longer than five minutes, were manually delineated by retrospective analysis. The elevation onset was marked at the beginning of the plateau. From this analysis, 13 patients were identified with at least one IH episode, leading to a total of 70 episodes. Based on the expert review of the ICP signal and the manual annotation of the elevation onset, ICP and ECG segments were extracted to cover the period from 20 minutes before to one minute after the onset.

Control segments were constructed by randomly extracting ten-minute ICP segments from the 17 control patients who did not present a single episode of ICP elevation, and from the IH patients no less than an hour before or after an ICP elevation episode. There were a total of 70 control segments which are evenly distributed among all patients. The 140 IH and NON-IH ICP segments were then processed by MOCAIP so that morphological waveform features were extracted to describe each one minute segments of ICP.

4.2 Experimental setup

The prediction of ICP elevation is posed as a classification problem where each input example $x_i \in X$ is a set of N_s MOCAIP vectors $x_i = \{\alpha_0,\ldots,\alpha_{N_s-1}\}$ calculated over a series of successive one-minute ICP segments. The corresponding output $y_i \in Y$ is a binary variable which equals 1 if the ICP segment led to a treated IH episode. The performance in terms of Area Under the Curve (AUC) is reported for input segments x_i extracted at various time-to-onset for the predictive model. The impact of the number N_s of successive ICP segments used to construct the input vectors $x_i = \{\alpha_0,\ldots,\alpha_{N_s-1}\}$ is evaluated for different prediction techniques. The main purpose of the experiment is to test the hypothesis that the use of ensemble classifiers improves the prediction of IH because it can exploit more efficiently the morphological information contained in longer ICP segments located prior to the elevation onset.

4.2.1 Performance Evaluation by Time-To-Onset Variation

For evaluation, a ten-fold cross-validation at the patient level is performed and three different prediction techniques are compared; Multiple Linear Regression (MLR) [46], Adaptive Boosting (AdaBoost) [47], and Extremely Randomized Decision Trees (Extra Trees) [48]. The models are trained on each fold such that each positive example $x_i = \{\alpha_0,\ldots,\alpha_{N_s-1}\}$ corresponds to the $N_s - 1$ vectors of morphological metrics $\alpha_i \in R^{N_f}$, where $Nf = 24$ is the number of MOCAIP metrics used in this study. The negative examples are randomly sampled from the pulses of the control set such that the training dataset is balanced and contains an equal number of positive and negative examples. For testing, the models are evaluated on the excluded fold by varying the time-to-onset ρ at which the ICP segments $x_i = \{\alpha_{0+\rho},\ldots,\alpha_{N_s-1+\rho}\}$ are extracted.

4.2.2 Number of morphological ICP segments

This experiment aims at evaluating if the use of additional morphological vectors extracted up to ten minutes ($N_s = 10$) prior to the tested time-to-onset can improve the prediction performance of the models. To do so, the classifiers are trained such that the input x_i of the positive examples are the N_s morphological vectors $\{\alpha_0, \alpha_1, \ldots, \alpha_{N_s-1}\}$ extracted from the segments prior to the onset plus the segment concurrent to the IH onset. Training of the models is performed for ten different lengths $N_s = \{1, \ldots, 10\}$, from one to ten minutes. Controls of corresponding lengths are randomly extracted from the current fold but remain the same across the different time-to-onset. Each model is evaluated using the average AUC results computed from a ten-fold cross-validation, and ten different time-to-onset $\rho = \{0, \ldots, 9\}$.

4.3 Results

The best results of each method are reported in Fig. 5 in terms of AUC. While the linear classifiers obtain an AUC of [0.87,0.78,0.71] for the time-to-onset corresponding to [1,3,6] minutes prior to the elevation respectively, the use of ensemble classifiers significantly improves the AUC. AdaBoost reaches an AUC [0.93,0.84,0.80], and Extra-Trees performs even better with an AUC of [0.96,0.91,0.87].

The Extra-Trees method shows significant improvement in terms of average AUC when the length of the input is increased. For [1,5,10] minute(s)-long segments, the AUC is respectively [0.77,0.88,0.9]. AdaBoost also shows significant increases in AUC, from [0.75,0.83,0.84] for segments of [1,5,10] minute(s) length, respectively. The linear models are unable to efficiency exploit the larger segments of morphological ICP data. AUC results are [0.76,0.65,0.73] for segments of [1,5,10] minute(s) length, respectively. The best average AUC for the linear model was observed using a single ICP segment $N_s = 1$. In contrast, the best performance for AdaBoost and Extra-Trees models is obtained with $N_s = 10$ ICP segments, corresponding to ten minutes of ICP data extracted prior to the tested time-to-onset.

Although the previous experiments demonstrate that the ensemble classifier models trained over ten minutes of ICP data perform better than the one trained over shorter segments, it is not clear if each additional one minute ICP segment contribute independently to the improvements, or if they are complementary; in which case the dynamic of change of ICP morphology over time would appear to be useful. To test these hypothesis, three different learning strategy of the Extra-Trees models are compared. The first model (a), which is used as baseline, is trained on a single ($N_s = 1$) one-minute long segment $x_i = \{\alpha_1\}$. The second strategy (b) consists in learning independently ten different models on each one-minute long segment and then fuse their output using an arithemic mean. Finally, (c) is to build a single model trained on a series of ten ($N_s = 10$) one-minute long segments concatenated to a single input vector $x_i = \{\alpha_1, \ldots, \alpha_{10}\}$. Although, the use of ten independent classifiers (b) improves the overall performance versus the use of only one classifier (a), there is an additional increase in AUC by using all ten vectors at the same time (c). This results indicates that the relative values of successive morphological vectors contain relevant precursors of IH. It is an important finding because it means that the dynamic of ICP changes holds critical predictive information.

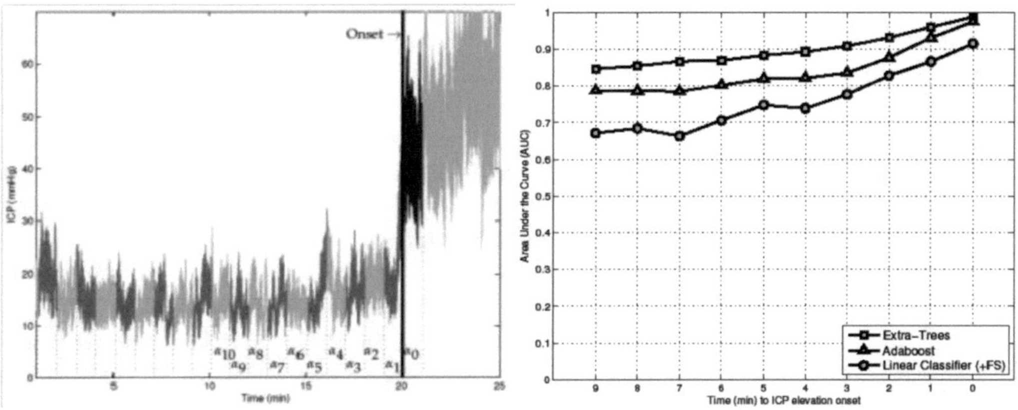

Fig. 5. Illustration of an IH ICP episode (left). Elevated episodes are divided into 21 segments of one minute. For each segment, MOCAIP is applied to extract morphological vectors. On the right, the AUC is reported after a leave-one-out crossvalidation for each technique. Extra-trees ranks first and is followed by the AdaBoost and Multi-linear classifiers (reproduced with permission from [65]).

4.4 Discussion

Thanks to the use of a series of successive one minute ICP segments as input to classifier ensemble techniques, the proposed study has demonstrated that ensemble classifiers can exploit more efficiently the morphological information contained in the pulse. The performance improvement observed in our experiments can be attributed to the following reasons:

- First, as it has been shown in other applications, the two ensemble classifiers perform better than the multiple linear classifier because they can better capture the nonlinearity between the morphological vectors and the outcome.
- Second, the use of a larger segment of ICP segment prior to the onset improves the accuracy.
- Finally, the use of a full sequence of successive morphological vectors at once leads to better models than the one based on individual vectors which indicates that the relative values and the order between successive morphological vectors contain additional precursors.

Although the ICP of brain injured patients is continuously managed by the bedside clinicians, changes in ICP prior to elevation are reflected by complex variations in the morphology of the signal that are difficult to be recognized in real-time. Decision support tools that would alert the bedside clinicians of future ICP elevation would add a new proactive dimension to the current treatment of ICP elevations, which largely remains a reactive procedure. Further improvement of the technical methodology and a better understanding of the physiological meaning of these morphological variations should be possible. Ideally, we would like to translate the rules learned by ensemble classifiers into a physiological model in an attempt to represent ICP dynamics explicitly.

5. Acute hypercapnic cerebral vasodilatation

The influence of changes within the cerebral vasculature and there impact on ICP remain poorly understood in humans. Studies [49] have shown that in head injured patients, the cerebral perfusion pressure is inversely proportional to the amplitude of pulsatile inflow and, consequently, the exponential shape of the pressure-volume relationship is not the only factor influencing the magnitude of ICP pulse wave [50]. This section presents a recent study [14] conducted by our group to test the hypothesis that acute hypercapnic cerebral vasodilatation induces consistent changes in ICP waveform morphology. This hypothesis is tested on a dataset of ICP signals of uninjured patients undergoing a CO_2 inhalation challenge in which hypercapnia induced acute cerebral vasodilatation. For each morphological metrics extracted from the ICP waveforms using MOCAIP, the consistency and rate of change were analyzed.

5.1 Materials and methods

The hypercapnic dataset consists of the ICP and ECG recordings of four patients, who were admitted at UCLA medical center for the evaluation of their chronic headaches. During their hospitalization, the patients received continuous ICP monitoring using intraparenchymal microsensors situated in the right frontal lobe. They also underwent a CO_2 challenge test by inhaling a 5% CO_2 mixture for less than three minutes. During the test, ICP and ECG signals were recorded at a sampling rate of 400 Hz at the bedside with a dedicated acquisition system.

To quantify the rate of change of each metric over a specific time segment, a line was first fitted to the segment of interest and then the slope of this line was used to calculate the rate of the metric change. The sign of the obtained hourly rate of change (negative vs. positive) was used to determine the trend of change (decreasing vs. increasing).

5.2 Experimental protocol

The average duration of the selected data segment was (5.1 ± 0.7 minutes) which included (1.5 ± 0.5 minutes) of baseline, (2.5 ± 0.5 minutes) of CO_2 challenge test and (1.1 ± 0.2 minutes) of post-test data. The slope of the lines fitted to each of the extracted metrics over the rising edge of ICP signal during CO_2 challenge test and the falling edge of ICP signal during the post-test normal breathing, were used to define the hourly rate of change during the test and post-test normal breathing, respectively. For the purpose of comparing the hourly rate of change between different metrics, each metric rate was normalized by the average value of the corresponding metric over either the last ten beats of the baseline or the first ten beats of the stabilized part of the post-test data.

To evaluate the results from baseline, test, and post-test, we report 1) the consistency of changes of individual metrics; 2) differences in rate of metric changes; and 3) which of the peak regions (P1, P2 and P3) has a more dramatic change during the cerebral vasodilation; the specifics of how the region assignments were defined are in the publication [14]. In addition, we calculated the region-weighted relative hourly rate of change averaged over the subset of consistent metrics.

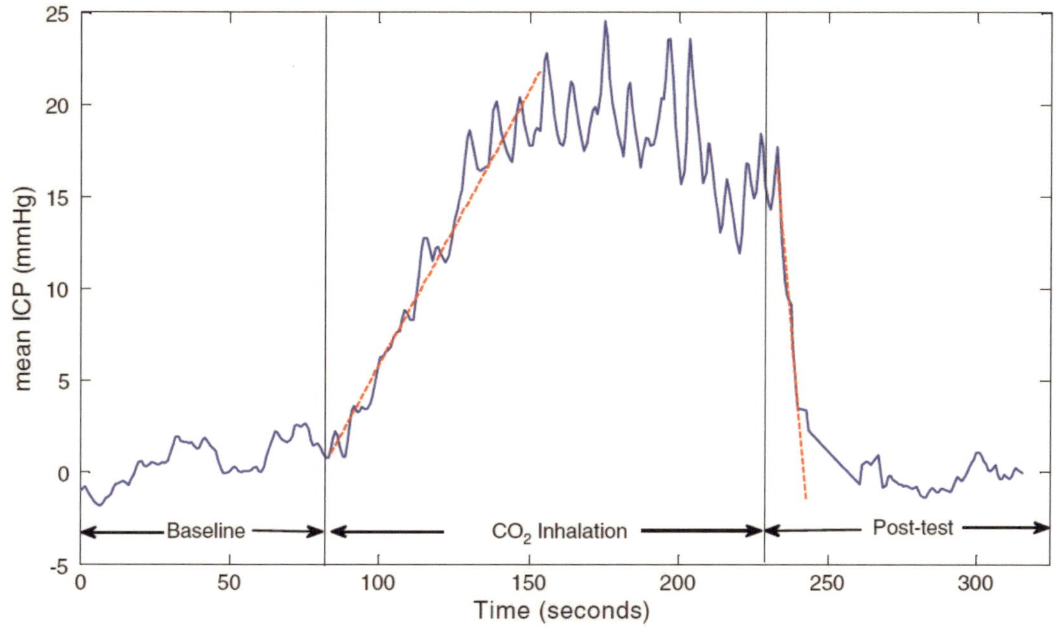

Fig. 6. Illustration of induced hypercapnia for a headache patient. There are three segments (Baseline, CO_2 Inhalation, and Post-test) with the linear fits shown by dotted lines (reproduced with permission from [14]).

5.3 Results

Fig. 6 depicts the mean ICP value for one of the headache patients during the baseline, the CO_2 challenge test, and the post-test normal breathing. When the patient inhales the 5% mixture of CO_2, mean ICP increases over time, reaches a saturation level, and then stabilizes. When the patient returns to breathing normal concentrations of CO_2, the mean ICP returned to baseline in less than one minute.

Investigating the hourly rate of change for all 128 ICP metrics during the hypercapnic and normal breathing post-test data, reveal that; out of 128 ICP metrics, 72 metrics had consistent changes in association with CO_2 changes for all four subjects. We observe that no metrics had the same trend during both the hypercapnic and normal breathing post-test data. This observation is consistent with our expectation that, if a variable has a specific trend of change in one condition, the change would be in the opposite direction as the condition is reversed. We also observe that for all subjects, 50 metrics consistently increased ("+" metrics) during hypercapnia and decreased when patients switched back to room air and 22 metrics consistently decreased ("-" metrics) during CO_2 inhalation phase and increased during post-test normal breathing.

The region-weighted (P1, P2, P3) relative hourly rate of change of the 50 "+" metrics were (0.518, 1.076, and 0.976), respectively. Conversely, for the 22 "-" metrics, the region-weighted relative hourly rate of change averaged over 22 "-" metrics were (0.20, 0.32 and 0.27), respectively.

5.4 Discussion

Acute vasodilatation caused consistent changes in a total of 72 ICP pulse morphological metrics. In addition, it appears that the P_2 sub-region responded to cerebral vascular changes in the most consistent way with the greatest changes as compared to P_1 and P_3 sub-regions. Information with regard to how ICP pulse morphology responds to vasodilatation and vasoconstriction may allow surrogate, continuous monitoring of the cerebral vasculature.

In summary, the present work provides positive preliminary results related to the hypothesis that the dilation/constriction of the cerebral vasculature results in detectable consistent changes in ICP morphological metrics. Acute vasodilatation caused consistent changes in a total of 72 ICP pulse morphological metrics. In addition, it appears that the P_2 sub-region responded to cerebral vascular changes in the most consistent way with the greatest changes as compared to P_1 and P_3 sub-regions.

6. Morphological ICP waveform characteristics during slow waves

The diagnosis and management of NPH remain challenging mostly due to a lack of reliable methods of selecting candidates for shunt implantation and third ventriculostomy. There exists positive [51, 52] and negative [53-55] evidence that frequent presence of ICP slow waves predicts a positive outcome after shunt implant. ICP slow waves, also known as Lundberg's B-waves, are defined as oscillations with a frequency of 2-0.5/minute and large amplitude [56]. There exists indirect evidence that certain characteristics of ICP slow waves may contain useful information for correctly diagnosing NPH and predicting shunt response. It was recently found that increased ICP pulse pressure amplitude has a predictive value for shunt response [9, 57]. In this section, we describe our recent attempt [13] to detect and separate periods of ICP slow waves (BW, "B-wave") from those of flat or nearly flat ICP (NW, "no wave") in an overnight ICP recording. We hypothesized that mean values and variations of ICP pulse morphological metrics extracted by the MOCAIP algorithm can be effectively used as input feature vectors to a classification algorithm to distinguish between periods of flat ICP (NW) and those with slow waves (BW). Such a classifier can then be used to construct an automated ICP slow wave recognition algorithm.

6.1 Materials and methods

Pre operative (shunt) overnight ICP recordings performed in 44 patients hospitalized at the UCLA Adult Hydrocephalus Center. Hydrocephalus was diagnosed for all patients. An intraparenchymal ICP sensor was inserted in the right frontal lobe and simultaneous recordings of ICP and ECG signals were performed at a sampling rate of either 400 Hz or 240 Hz. The signal recordings were visually screened by three independent experts to select both BW and NW patterns. Fig. 7 presents an example of ICP overnight monitoring where initially fairly stable ICP recording transforms into clearly distinguishable slow waves with relatively high amplitude and asymmetrical shape. In our study, small ICP slow waves with amplitude less than six mmHg were classified as NW pattern. As both patterns of ICP (BW and NW) might occur multiple times during overnight monitoring in the same patient, we included several selections from the same study. The total number of selected patterns was 276 (NW-131 and BW- 145).

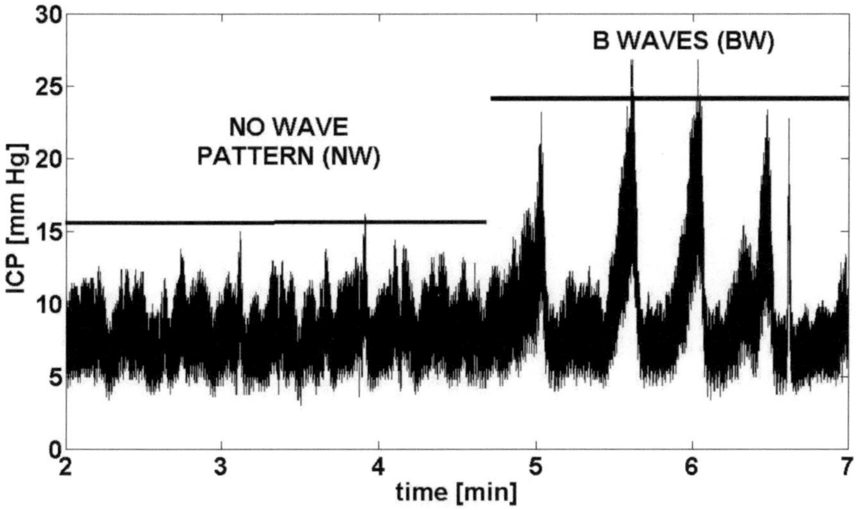

Fig. 7. Illustration of B wave segment (reproduced with permission from [13]).

6.1.1 Feature selection and classification

A total of 48 metrics (comprising 24 morphological metrics plus their standard deviation) were used to described the morphology of each ICP pulse.

To optimize the classification performance, three feature selection techniques (differential evolution (DE), discriminant analysis (DA) and analysis of variance based on Anova (V)) were applied to find an optimal set of MOCAIP metrics under different criteria. In addition, we selected three sets of metrics common to those found by combination of two selection methods, to be used as classification features (differential evolution and analysis of variance, discriminant analysis and analysis of variance, and combination of differential evolution and discriminant analysis).

A regularized linear quadratic classifier was used discriminate between BW from NW based on morphological ICP features. We repeated classification experiment seven times: first time for the set of optimal ICP metrics chosen by DE algorithm, second time for the set of ICP metrics selected based on analysis of variance (V), the third time for these metrics picked by step-wise DA approach, the next three runs were repeated for the metrics overlapped two sets: DE+V, DA+V and DE+DA, and finally we used only one parameter -- S.D. of mean ICP to confirm possible advantage of using combination of metrics over single metric (SM). To compare the performance of classification for different sets of metrics, we ran the bootstrapping procedure 25 times to calculate average and S.D. of performance metrics including Se, Spe, PPV and Ac.

6.1.2 Results and discussion

Results indicate that the changes in six morphological metrics (S.D. of: dP_2, dP_{12},dP_{13}, $Curv_T$, dICP, mICP) were sufficient to distinguish between BW from NW with high specificity 96.2% and acceptable accuracy 88.9%.

Based on our experiments, using DE in conjunction with Anova to derive the final set of metrics leads to the best classification results. The combination of methods: DA+V as well as DE+DA did not improve the classification performance. Combining DE and V methods appeared to be complementary in our study. Since accuracy of classification experiment for Anova+DE is the highest (88.9%) and the number of input metrics is reasonable small (six metrics), we ranked this method as the best for separating BW from NW.

The final list of six metrics selected by DE+V (S.D. of: dP_2, dP_{12}, dP_{13}, $Curv_T$, dICP, mICP) reflects the most salient changes associated with ICP increase due to slow waves. We found that amplitude of P_2 component notably increases during ICP slow wave occurrence (hence S.D. of dP_2), which is also associated with increase in total curvature of the pulse (hence S.D. of $Curv_T$). Amplitude of P_1, most likely related to systole of arterial pressure [58], shows a moderate increase during BW in comparison with both dP_2 and dP_3 (hence S.D. of dP_{12}, S.D. of dP_{13}).

7. Predicting lumbar drain outcome from ICP morphology

Due to the complication rate and malfuction assoicated with existing shunt technologies, differentiating patient with NPH that will benefit from shunt implantation is significant. Extended lumbar drain (LD) for 72 hours has become a popular pre-shunt workup in many neurosurgical centers [59-61]. Its popularity stems from the findings of an excellent study which demonstrated the high specificity and sensitivity of predicting shunt response based on LD test outcome [60, 62]. However, the mechanistic relationship between positive LD outcome and shunt response remains to be elucidated. Therefore, many centers also employ additional tests to assess patients for predicting their shunt response. Overnight ICP monitoring is one of such tests. It has been reported in many studies that overnight ICP monitoring is able to reveal many phenomena that a short-term ICP monitoring or lumbar puncture cannot reveal, e.g., large but slow oscillations of ICP that are termed B-waves. However, the capability of overnight ICP monitoring to predict shunt response remains controversial. [51, 53-55].

Given these existing contradicting results, elucidating the potential prognostic value of overnight ICP monitoring is significant. Overnight ICP monitoring could be an important economic alternative to LD because it requires a shorter hospital stay for patients if its prognostic value can be fully explored. Unfortunately, many existing analysis methods applied to overnight ICP recordings are very subjective and usually extract limited amounts of information from overnight ICP recordings. On the other hand, a few studies utilizing more advanced ICP signal analysis methods [7, 10] have demonstrated that the amplitude of ICP pulse has excellent predictive value for shunt response. In addition to lack of complex analysis methods of overnight ICP, a potential limit to the existing studies that use shunt response as an end-point is that such outcome is also determined by many other post-implantation factors not necessarily associated with overnight ICP characteristics.

Therefore, this work aims to develop an automated method of feature extraction and decision rule construction from overnight ICP recording. This method is used to assess the predictive accuracy of LD outcome instead of shunt outcome.

Specifically, we used the MOCAIP algorithm to analyze the overnight ICP recordings. MOCAIP was applied to consecutive short segments of an ICP recording resulting in 128 metrics per each segment. Then various feature functions were designed to summarize the distribution of the 128 metrics from all the segments per each ICP recording. The predictive value of each feature-metric pair was then assessed using the area under curve [60] of the receiver operator characteristic (ROC) curve. Based on the ROC curve, a simple decision rule involving one metric can be derived for predicting LD outcome. To further improve the performance, we proposed an automated way to combine two such rules.

7.1 Materials and methods

The present retrospective study involved 54 patients undergoing pre-shunt workup that included overnight ICP monitoring and extended lumbar drain (three-day) while hospitalized at the UCLA Adult Hydrocephalus Center. An intraparenchymal ICP microsensor (Codman and Schurtleff, Raynaud, MA) was inserted in the right frontal lobe and monitoring started at least one night before the placement of the LD. Continuous waveform data including ECG and ICP was captured using the BedMaster system with a sampling rate of 240 Hz. Patients were assessed both pre-LD and post-LD before discharge from the hospital by ten meter walking exam, and an NPH routine assessment which includes the Mini-mental state examination (MMSE). The LD outcome used in the present work was retrospectively collected as indicated from the clinical report of the follow-up visit after the LD procedure and predominantly focused on the improvement in gait. The average age and standard deviation of the 54 patients is 72.05 ± 9.63 years respectively, with a gender distribution of 35 males and 19 females. Among the patient cohort, 12 patients (seven males and five females) showed no improvement in gait following the procedure.

7.2 Feature functions

Once the metrics for each dominant pulse have been computed an additional processing step is used to summarize each of the 128 MOCAIP metrics for one overnight ICP recording via five feature functions. For example, if a patient has ten hours of continuous ICP data there will be approximately 1200 dominant pulses, for each dominant pulse there is 128 MOCAIP metrics, each of the MOCAIP metrics can be summarized with the five feature functions (below). There is no prior knowledge with regard to the best way of summarizing an overnight ICP recording. Therefore, it is necessary to allow for an automated process to identify the best candidates. We have evaluated the following feature functions:

Average feature: This feature function simply calculates the average of each individual metric across one overnight ICP recording.

Standard deviation feature: This function calculates the standard deviation of each individual metric across one overnight ICP recording.

Percentage feature: This function calculates the percentage of time when a metric is greater than a threshold. This threshold is determined by pooling data from all patients and then determined as the average of the corresponding MOCAIP metric.

Percentage of standard deviation feature: This function calculates the percentage of time of the standard deviation of MOCAIP metrics greater than a threshold calculated from a five-minute ICP. The threshold was determined as the standard deviation of pooled MOCAIP metrics from all patients.

Range feature: This function calculates the difference between the 95 percentile and the 5 percentile of each individual metric of an overnight ICP recording.

7.3 Optimal single-metric rule

After applying a feature function, an overnight ICP recording is reduced to a vector of 128 metric-feature pairs. We next seek for a single-metric rule to predict LD outcome in the following form: if a metric-feature of an overnight recording is greater (or smaller) than a threshold, then LD outcome will be positive. Note, rules published in several existing studies [10, 63] can be considered as specific instances of the above form. For each metric-feature, we generate a sequence of threshold values by pooling all the data. This sequence of threshold values can be used to generate two ROC curves for each metric-feature, one of which corresponds to the greater than situation and another of which corresponds to the less than situation. Then we retain the ROC that has an AUC greater than 0.5 and discard the other for each metric. Next, for each feature the optimal metric is defined as the one with the greatest AUC. The impact of the optimal metric selection (as a function of AUC) is explained in the results section. Following the optimal metric determination for each feature, one natural step further is to determine if one can combine two such rules to obtain a better performance (a combination of two of the five features described above). Considering the combination of two features (A and B) with the corresponding set of false positive, true positive, false negative, and true negative cases represented (from rule A) as FPA, TPA, FNA, TNA, respectively, the notation is analogous for rule B. Furthermore, we shall consider two possible combination operations: AND and OR. If the OR operator is used for combination, then the resultant sets of false positive, true positive, false negative, and true negative are FPA ∪ FPB, TPA ∪ TPB, FNA ∩ FNB, and TNA ∩ TNB. On the other hand, if the AND operator is used for combination, then the corresponding sets are FPA ∩ FPB, TPA ∩ TPB, FNA ∪ FNB, and TNA ∪ TNB. Based on this analysis, the accuracy of the combined predictive rules can be calculated using their respective true positive and true negative values along with the total number of patients. Therefore, one can choose the combinations with the maximal accuracy.

7.4 Data analysis protocol

In this section, we summarize the data analysis protocol used in the present work to determine the best rule combination and its accuracy. The following steps were taken to analyze the 54 overnight ICP recordings:

1. Each recording is analyzed using the MOCAIP algorithm on consecutive 30-second segments.
2. Resultant MOCAIP metrics are then manually checked for any errors in recognizing legitimate dominant pulse and placement of the landmarks. This step is facilitated by using software developed in house.
3. Generate the threshold sequence for each metric that will be used to generate ROC curve. The i-th value of the sequence of thresholds is calculated for each metric-feature by the following equations: (i-1) where L is the mean plus the ten standard deviation of the metric-feature divided by the number of steps, which is 100 in the present work.
4. Each value of the threshold sequence is used to form two simple rules (greater than and less than), which are then used to assess the 54 cases. The corresponding false positive rate (FPR) and true positive rate (TPR) are obtained. After sweeping through the sequence, two ROC curves are obtained but only the one with AUC greater 0.5 is retained.
5. Determine the optimal metric-feature. This is achieved by selecting one metric-feature that has the largest AUC per each feature function evaluated. In other words, for each feature defined above, the metric (out of the 128 calculated by MOCAIP) with the greatest AUC is defined as the optimal metric-feature (five total, one for each feature).
6. Determine the rule. For the optimal metric-feature, the optimal point on the ROC curve is selected as the operating point, which gives a false positive rate less than 0.35.
7. Then the accuracy of the ten pairs (two combination rules and five feature) are calculated.
8. The best rule combination is then determined as the one with the greatest accuracy.

7.5 Results

Panel F of Fig. 8 displays ROC curves of each of the 128 metric-features (average feature function is used here as an example). The ROC curve shown in bold represents the metric with the greatest AUC; which was selected as the optimal metric-feature for rule construction. The ROC curves of optimal metric-pair corresponding to each of the five feature functions (A: Average feature function; B: Standard deviation feature function; C: Percentage of average feature function; D: Percentage of five-minute standard deviation feature function; E: Inter 5-95 percentile feature function) are shown in Panels A through E of Fig. 8 where the selected MOCAIP metric is also spelled out. On each curve, the operating point is circled, which corresponds to the particular threshold value selected for rule construction.

In summary, the individual metric-feature rules found in the present work are: 1.If standard deviation of RLv2p2Lp1p2 of overnight ICP recording is > 0.0547, then patient will respond to LD. 2.If average RCurvp3Curvv2 of overnight ICP recording is > 0.9808, then patient will respond to LD. 3.If percentage of RC1 of overnight ICP recording greater than 8.76 is < 41.48%, then patient will respond to LD. 4.If percentage of five minute segments of ICP having a standard deviation of RRC3k2 greater than 57.68 is > 0.49%, then patient will respond to LD drain. 5.If the inter 95-5 quartile range of RCurvp2Curvp3 of overnight ICP recording is < 64.25, then patient will respond to LD. The accuracy for the corresponding features is: 70.4%, 72.2%, 74.1%, 72.2%, and 79.6% respectively. Finally, the OR combination of rules 4 and 5 achieves the best accuracy of 88.9%.

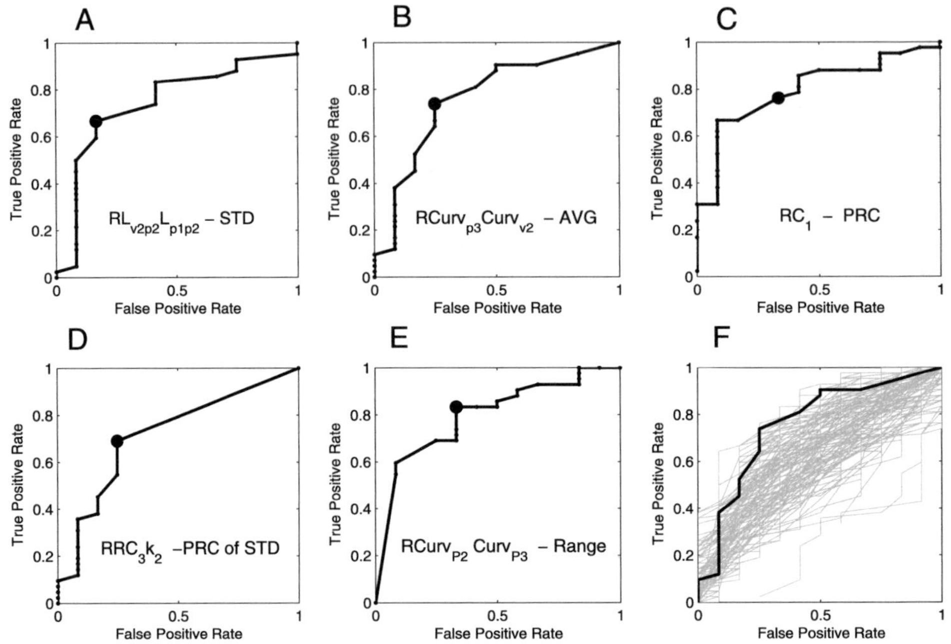

Fig. 8. Illustration of LD ROCs (reproduced with permission from [67]).

7.6 Discussion

We have demonstrated a systemic way of deriving two-rule combination of simple decision rules from overnight ICP recording to predict the corresponding outcome of three-day LD for patients with NPH clinical triad undergoing pre-shunt evaluation. Using a cohort of 54 patients, we are able to find optimal two-rule combination that reaches an accuracy of 88.9%. This rule can be explained in plain English such that it can be readily communicated to non-technical clinicians and patients. Although further validation with large patient cohort is needed, technically, the rules found in the present work in combination with an automated analysis of overnight ICP using the existing MOCAIP algorithm can readily be built into a decision support system of NPH diagnosis and evaluation that has the potential to reduce the time and cost associated with the existing three-day LD procedure.

A systemic way of discovering predictive rules is needed if a large number of ICP pulse morphological metrics are involved to construct rules. Compared to the existing studies that focus on either mICP or ICP pulse amplitude, the increased number of ICP metrics demands an objective way of discovering rules to guarantee optimality and avoid bias. Indeed, the five individual optimal metrics found in the present work do not include either mean ICP or ICP wave amplitude demonstrating the potential power of adopting a more comprehensive ICP pulse morphology characterization.

The proposed rule discovery framework can be easily extended in several aspects. We have proposed five simple feature functions to summarize an overnight ICP recording. More complex feature function can certainly be implemented in future work. In particular, we believe that feature functions characterizing the relationship among MOCAIP metrics could potentially offer better predictive power as compared to single-metric feature functions used here. Furthermore, we have only studied the combination of two rules, one could readily derive the equations to calculate the accuracy of combining multiple rules and check if the predictive accuracy can be further improved.

One fundamental limitation of the present work is the lack of cases to conduct independent evaluation of the discovered rules. It therefore remains to be demonstrated whether the same level of predictive accuracy can be retained when applying the rules discovered using our dataset to process data from other centers and how the data from multi-centers can be utilized to refine the rules. The present work has clearly demonstrated the technical feasibility of such future studies and hopefully more precise and robust predictive rules can be discovered through multi-center collaboration and the adoption of advanced ICP signal analysis and data mining methods.

8. Conclusions

Pulse pressure amplitude has been linked to several conditions with promising results in NPH for predicting shunt responsiveness [9, 10]. Work has also been done in chronic headaches; again, showing the usefulness of pulse pressure amplitude. Recent, detailed pulse pressure morphology analysis by our group has shown promise as a possible indicator of low global cerebral blood perfusion [11]. The resistance from many clinicians and researchers is the unknown relationship between these pulse pressure metrics (MOCAIP) and their physiologic meaning. Therefore, the additional information provided by knowing the origins of these pulse pressure features would help bridge the gap between a strictly data mining approach and physiologic meaning. Finally, the importance of this work was confirmed in a recent review article by Wagshul et al.:

"Given the success of invasive pulsatility measurements in clinical prognosis, studies which can provide a link between changes in pulse pressure and changes in non-invasive TCD- or MRI-based measures of pulsatility will be particularly valuable." [64]

9. Acknowledgements

The work presented in this chapter was supported in part by the National Institute of Neurological Disorders and Stroke (NINDS) and grants R21-NS055998, R21-NS055045, R21-NS059797, R01-NS054881, R01-NS066008, along with a research fund for international young scientists NSFC-31050110122.

10. References

[1] E. A. Bering, Jr., "Choroid plexus and arterial pulsation of cerebrospinal fluid; demonstration of the choroid plexuses as a cerebrospinal fluid pump," *AMA Arch Neurol Psychiatry,* vol. 73, pp. 165-72, Feb 1955.

[2] R. J. Adolph, H. Fukusumi, and N. O. Fowler, "Origin of cerebrospinal fluid pulsations," *Am J Physiol,* vol. 212, pp. 840-6, Apr 1967.

[3] J. Y. Fan, C. Kirkness, P. Vicini, R. Burr, and P. Mitchell, "Intracranial pressure waveform morphology and intracranial adaptive capacity," *Am J Crit Care,* vol. 17, pp. 545-54, Nov 2008.

[4] O. Hirai, H. Handa, M. Ishikawa, and S. H. Kim, "Epidural pulse waveform as an indicator of intracranial pressure dynamics," *Surg Neurol,* vol. 21, pp. 67-74, Jan 1984.

[5] E. R. Cardoso, J. O. Rowan, and S. Galbraith, "Analysis of the cerebrospinal fluid pulse wave in intracranial pressure," *J Neurosurg,* vol. 59, pp. 817-21, Nov 1983.

[6] J. Hamer, E. Alberti, S. Hoyer, and K. Wiedemann, "Influence of systemic and cerebral vascular factors on the cerebrospinal fluid pulse waves," *J Neurosurg,* vol. 46, pp. 36-45, Jan 1977.

[7] P. K. Eide, "A new method for processing of continuous intracranial pressure signals," *Med Eng Phys,* vol. 28, pp. 579-87, Jul 2006.

[8] X. Hu, P. Xu, D. J. Lee, V. Paul, and M. Bergsneider, "Morphological changes of intracranial pressure pulses are correlated with acute dilatation of ventricles," *Acta Neurochir Suppl,* vol. 102, pp. 131-6, 2008.

[9] P. K. Eide and A. Brean, "Intracranial pulse pressure amplitude levels determined during preoperative assessment of subjects with possible idiopathic normal pressure hydrocephalus," *Acta Neurochir (Wien),* vol. 148, pp. 1151-6; discussion 1156, Nov 2006.

[10] P. K. Eide and W. Sorteberg, "Diagnostic intracranial pressure monitoring and surgical management in idiopathic normal pressure hydrocephalus: a 6-year review of 214 patients," *Neurosurgery,* vol. 66, pp. 80-91, Jan 2006.

[11] X. Hu, T. Glenn, F. Scalzo, M. Bergsneider, C. Sarkiss, N. Martin, and P. Vespa, "Intracranial pressure pulse morphological features improved detection of decreased cerebral blood flow," *Physiol Meas,* vol. 31, pp. 679-95, May 2010.

[12] R. Hamilton, P. Xu, S. Asgari, M. Kasprowicz, P. Vespa, M. Bergsneider, and X. Hu, "Forecasting intracranial pressure elevation using pulse waveform morphology," *Conf Proc IEEE Eng Med Biol Soc,* vol. 2009, pp. 4331-4, 2009.

[13] M. Kasprowicz, S. Asgari, M. Bergsneider, M. Czosnyka, R. Hamilton, and X. Hu, "Pattern recognition of overnight intracranial pressure slow waves using morphological features of intracranial pressure pulse," *J Neurosci Methods,* vol. 190, pp. 310-8, Jul 15 2010.

[14] S. Asgari, M. Bergsneider, R. Hamilton, P. Vespa, and X. Hu, "Consistent changes in intracranial pressure waveform morphology induced by acute hypercapnic cerebral vasodilatation," *Neurocrit Care,* vol. 15, pp. 55-62, Aug.

[15] T. Ellis, J. McNames, and M. Aboy, "Pulse morphology visualization and analysis with applications in cardiovascular pressure signals," *IEEE Trans Biomed Eng,* vol. 54, pp. 1552-9, Sep 2007.

[16] H. Takizawa, T. Gabra-Sanders, and J. D. Miller, "Changes in the cerebrospinal fluid pulse wave spectrum associated with raised intracranial pressure," *Neurosurgery,* vol. 20, pp. 355-61, Mar 1987.

[17] M. Aboy, J. McNames, T. Thong, D. Tsunami, M. S. Ellenby, and B. Goldstein, "An automatic beat detection algorithm for pressure signals," *IEEE Trans Biomed Eng,* vol. 52, pp. 1662-70, Oct 2005.

[18] X. Hu, P. Xu, F. Scalzo, P. Vespa, and M. Bergsneider, "Morphological clustering and analysis of continuous intracranial pressure," *IEEE Trans Biomed Eng,* vol. 56, pp. 696-705, Mar 2009.

[19] F. Scalzo, P. Xu, S. Asgari, M. Bergsneider, and X. Hu, "Regression analysis for peak designation in pulsatile pressure signals," *Med Biol Eng Comput,* vol. 47, pp. 967-77, Sep 2009.

[20] F. Scalzo, S. Asgari, S. Kim, M. Bergsneider, and X. Hu, "Robust peak recognition in intracranial pressure signals," *Biomed Eng Online,* vol. 9, p. 61, 2010.

[21] X. Hu, P. Xu, D. J. Lee, P. Vespa, K. Baldwin, and M. Bergsneider, "An algorithm for extracting intracranial pressure latency relative to electrocardiogram R wave," *Physiol Meas,* vol. 29, pp. 459-71, Apr 2008.

[22] V. X. Afonso, W. J. Tompkins, T. Q. Nguyen, and S. Luo, "ECG beat detection using filter banks," *IEEE Trans Biomed Eng,* vol. 46, pp. 192-202, Feb 1999.

[23] Kaufman, Leonard, Rousseeuw, and J. Peter, *Finding groups in data : an introduction to cluster analysis of Wiley series in probability and mathematical statistics*. Hoboken, N.J: Wiley, 2005.

[24] F. Scalzo, S. Asgari, S. Kim, M. Bergsneider, and X. Hu, "Bayesian tracking of intracranial pressure signal morphology," *Artif Intell Med,* Oct 2 2011.

[25] E. Sudderth, A. Ihler, W. T. Freeman, and A. S. Willsky, "Nonparametric Belief Propagation," in *IEEE Computer Society Conference on Computer Vision and Pattern Recognition (CVPR)*, 2003, pp. 605-612

[26] E. Parzen, " On Estimation of a Probability Density Function and Mode," *The Annals of Mathematical Statistics,* vol. 33, pp. 1065-1076, 1962.

[27] W. Obrist and D. Marion, "Xenon techniques for CBF measurement in clinical head injury," *Neurotrauma,* 1995.

[28] R. Aaslid, T. M. Markwalder, and H. Nornes, "Noninvasive transcranial Doppler ultrasound recording of flow velocity in basal cerebral arteries," *J Neurosurg,* vol. 57, pp. 769-74, Dec 1982.

[29] J. Friedman, " Regularized Discriminant-Analysis," *J Am Stat Assoc,* 1989.

[30] R. Storn and K. Price, "Differential evolution - a simple and efficient heuristic for global optimization over continuous spaces," *J Global Optim,* 1997.

[31] J. McNames, C. Crespo, J. Bassale, M. Aboy, M. Ellenby, S. Lai, and B. Goldstein, "Sensitive Precursors to Acute Episodes of Intracranial Hypertension," in *4th International Workshop Biosignal Interpretation*, 2002.

[32] J. Szewczykowski, P. Dytko, A. Kunicki, J. Korsak-Sliwka, S. Sliwka, J. Dziduszko, and B. Augustyniak, "Determination of critical ICP levels in neurosurgical patients: A statistical approach," *Intracranial Pressure II,* pp. 392-393, 1975.

[33] R. Hornero, M. Aboy, D. Abasolo, J. McNames, and B. Goldstein, "Interpretation of approximate entropy: analysis of intracranial pressure approximate entropy during acute intracranial hypertension," *IEEE Trans Biomed Eng,* vol. 52, pp. 1671-80, Oct 2005.

[34] X. Hu, C. Miller, P. Vespa, and M. Bergsneider, "Adaptive computation of approximate entropy and its application in integrative analysis of irregularity of heart rate

variability and intracranial pressure signals," *Med Eng Phys,* vol. 30, pp. 631-9, Jun 2008.

[35] J. Turner, D. McDowall, R. Gibson, and H. Khaili, "Computer analysis of intracranial pressure measurements: Clinical value and nursing response," *Intracranial Pressure III,* pp. 283-287, 1976.

[36] H. D. Portnoy and M. Chopp, "Cerebrospinal fluid pulse wave form analysis during hypercapnia and hypoxia," *Neurosurgery,* vol. 9, pp. 14-27, Jul 1981.

[37] M. Czosnyka, P. Smielewski, S. Piechnik, E. A. Schmidt, P. G. Al-Rawi, P. J. Kirkpatrick, and J. D. Pickard, "Hemodynamic characterization of intracranial pressure plateau waves in head-injury patients," *J Neurosurg,* vol. 91, pp. 11-9, Jul 1999.

[38] M. Rosner, "Pathophysiology and management of increased intracranial pressure," *Neurosurgical Intensive Care,* pp. 57-112, 1993.

[39] I. R. Piper, J. D. Miller, N. M. Dearden, J. R. Leggate, and I. Robertson, "Systems analysis of cerebrovascular pressure transmission: an observational study in head-injured patients," *J Neurosurg,* vol. 73, pp. 871-80, Dec 1990.

[40] M. Swiercz, Z. Mariak, J. Krejza, J. Lewko, and P. Szydlik, "Intracranial pressure processing with artificial neural networks: prediction of ICP trends," *Acta Neurochir (Wien),* vol. 142, pp. 401-6, 2000.

[41] B. Azzerboni, G. Finocchio, M. Ipsale, F. La Forestal, and F. C. Morabito, "Intracranial Pressure Signals FOrecasting with Wavelet Transform and Neuro-Fuzzy Network," in *EMBS-BMES conference* Houston, TX, USA, 2002.

[42] F. Tsui, M. Sun, C. Li, and R. Sclabasi, "A Waveelet Based Neural Network For Prediction of ICP Signal," in *IEEE EMBC,* 1995, pp. 1045-1046.

[43] X. Hu, P. Xu, S. Asgari, P. Vespa, and M. Bergsneider, "Forecasting ICP elevation based on prescient changes of intracranial pressure waveform morphology," *IEEE Trans Biomed Eng,* vol. 57, pp. 1070-8, May 2010.

[44] R. Allen, "Time series methods in the monitoring of intracranial pressure. Part 1: Problems, suggestions for a monitoring scheme and review of appropriate techniques," *J Biomed Eng,* vol. 5, pp. 5-18, Jan 1983.

[45] D. Price, R. Dugdale, and J. Mason, "The control of ICP using three asynchronous closed loop," *Intracranial Pressure IV,* pp. 395-399, 1980.

[46] S. Chatterjee and A. S. and Hadi, "Influential observations, high leverage points and outliers in linear regression," *Statistical Science,* vol. 1, pp. 379-393, 1986.

[47] R. Schapire, "The Strength of Weak Learnability," *Mach. Learn,* vol. 5, pp. 197--227, 1990.

[48] P. Geurts, D. Ernst, and L. Wehenkel, "Extremely randomized trees," *Mach Learn,* vol. 63, pp. 3-42, 2006.

[49] K. H. Chan, J. D. Miller, N. M. Dearden, P. J. Andrews, and S. Midgley, "The effect of changes in cerebral perfusion pressure upon middle cerebral artery blood flow velocity and jugular bulb venous oxygen saturation after severe brain injury," *J Neurosurg,* vol. 77, pp. 55-61, Jul 1992.

[50] M. Czosnyka, E. Guazzo, M. Whitehouse, P. Smielewski, Z. Czosnyka, P. Kirkpatrick, S. Piechnik, and J. D. Pickard, "Significance of intracranial pressure waveform

analysis after head injury," *Acta Neurochir (Wien),* vol. 138, pp. 531-41; discussion 541-2, 1996.

[51] C. Raftopoulos, C. Chaskis, F. Delecluse, F. Cantraine, L. Bidaut, and J. Brotchi, "Morphological quantitative analysis of intracranial pressure waves in normal pressure hydrocephalus," *Neurol Res,* vol. 14, pp. 389-96, Dec 1992.

[52] L. Symon and N. W. Dorsch, "Use of long-term intracranial pressure measurement to assess hydrocephalic patients prior to shunt surgery," *J Neurosurg,* vol. 42, pp. 258-73, Mar 1975.

[53] H. Stephensen, N. Andersson, A. Eklund, J. Malm, M. Tisell, and C. Wikkelso, "Objective B wave analysis in 55 patients with non-communicating and communicating hydrocephalus," *J Neurol Neurosurg Psychiatry,* vol. 76, pp. 965-70, Jul 2005.

[54] M. A. Williams, A. Y. Razumovsky, and D. F. Hanley, "Comparison of Pcsf monitoring and controlled CSF drainage diagnose normal pressure hydrocephalus," *Acta Neurochir Suppl,* vol. 71, pp. 328-30, 1998.

[55] G. F. Woodworth, M. J. McGirt, M. A. Williams, and D. Rigamonti, "Cerebrospinal fluid drainage and dynamics in the diagnosis of normal pressure hydrocephalus," *Neurosurgery,* vol. 64, pp. 919-25; discussion 925-6, May 2009.

[56] N. Lundberg, "Continuous recording and control of ventricular fluid pressure in neurosurgical practice," *Acta Psychiatr Scand Suppl,* vol. 36, pp. 1-193, 1960.

[57] M. Czosnyka, Z. Czosnyka, N. Keong, A. Lavinio, P. Smielewski, S. Momjian, E. A. Schmidt, G. Petrella, B. Owler, and J. D. Pickard, "Pulse pressure waveform in hydrocephalus: what it is and what it isn't," *Neurosurg Focus,* vol. 22, p. E2, 2007.

[58] E. Carrera, D. J. Kim, G. Castellani, C. Zweifel, Z. Czosnyka, M. Kasparowicz, P. Smielewski, J. D. Pickard, and M. Czosnyka, "What shapes pulse amplitude of intracranial pressure?," *J Neurotrauma,* vol. 27, pp. 317-24, Feb 2010.

[59] L. S. Governale, N. Fein, J. Logsdon, and P. M. Black, "Techniques and complications of external lumbar drainage for normal pressure hydrocephalus," *Neurosurgery,* vol. 63, pp. 379-84; discussion 384, Oct 2008.

[60] A. Marmarou, H. F. Young, G. A. Aygok, S. Sawauchi, O. Tsuji, T. Yamamoto, and J. Dunbar, "Diagnosis and management of idiopathic normal-pressure hydrocephalus: a prospective study in 151 patients," *J Neurosurg,* vol. 102, pp. 987-97, Jun 2005.

[61] R. Walchenbach, E. Geiger, R. T. Thomeer, and J. A. Vanneste, "The value of temporary external lumbar CSF drainage in predicting the outcome of shunting on normal pressure hydrocephalus," *J Neurol Neurosurg Psychiatry,* vol. 72, pp. 503-6, Apr 2002.

[62] A. Marmarou, M. Bergsneider, P. Klinge, N. Relkin, and P. M. Black, "The value of supplemental prognostic tests for the preoperative assessment of idiopathic normal-pressure hydrocephalus," *Neurosurgery,* vol. 57, pp. S17-28; discussion ii-v, Sep 2005.

[63] P. K. Eide and A. Brean, "Cerebrospinal fluid pulse pressure amplitude during lumbar infusion in idiopathic normal pressure hydrocephalus can predict response to shunting," *Cerebrospinal Fluid Res*, vol. 7, p. 5, 2010.

[64] M. E. Wagshul, P. K. Eide, and J. R. Madsen, "The pulsating brain: A review of experimental and clinical studies of intracranial pulsatility," *Fluids Barriers CNS*, vol. 8, p. 5, 2011.

[65] F. Scalzo, R. Hamilton, S. Asgari, S. Kim, and X. Hu. Intracranial Hypertension Prediction using Extremely Randomized Decision Trees. *Med Eng Phys*. In press, 2011.

[66] S. Kim, X. Hu, D. McArthur, R. Hamilton, M. Bergsneider, T. Glenn, N. Martin, and P. Vespa, "Inter-Subject Correlation Exists Between Morphological Metrics of Cerebral Blood Flow Velocity and Intracranial Pressure Pulses," *Neurocrit Care*, Dec 7 2010.

[67] X. Hu, R. Hamilton, K. Baldwin, P. Vespa, and M. Bergsneider, "Automated Extraction of Decision Rules for Predicting Lumbar Drain Outcome by Analyzing Overnight Intracranial Pressure," *Acta Neurochir Suppl*, vol. 114, In press, 2011.

Part 2

Proteomic Analysis in Neurological Disorders

6

Developing Novel Methods for Protein Analysis and Their Potential Implementation in Diagnosing Neurological Diseases

Olgica Trenchevska[1*], Vasko Aleksovski[2], Dobrin Nedelkov[1,3] and Kiro Stojanoski[1]

[1]Institute of Chemistry, Faculty of Natural Sciences and Mathematics, Sts.Cyril and Methodius University, Skopje,
[2]Clinic of Neurology, Medical Faculty, Sts.Cyril and Methodius Univerisity, Skopje
[3]Intrinsic Bioprobes Inc., Tempe, AZ,
[1,2]Macedonia
[3]USA

1. Introduction

The objective of this paper is to introduce a new chapter in protein analyses and profiling in general, and to discuss on the potential practical implementation in detecting neurological diseases. A need for such a research occurs due to the arguable fact that new techniques and methods for protein analyses have been developing, and only a few have actually been implemented in routine clinical practice. This study is a part of a larger effort to develop methods in order to understand protein diversity and specificity of a human proteome in health and disease. Primarily, we will introduce and discuss some standard and already implemented techniques in clinical practice, and further we will focus on the new methods for cerebrospinal fluid (CSF) analysis as a primary biological media for study of neurological diseases.

1.1 Proteins in neurological diseases

Neurological conditions in patients occur as a result of a structural or biochemical abnormality in the brain, spinal cord or in the nerves leading to and from them. After the onset of symptoms, additional parameters are analyzed in order to distinguish between different, so called, patterns and contribute to the diagnosis of a disease. Protein profiling has been introduced in clinical practice 100 years ago (W. Bruno 1956; Vesterberg 1989). Cerebrospinal fluid is the media used for such investigations, due to its close proximity to the brain; therefore being a biological fluid that can potentially obtain first-hand information about the potential causes of the induced change. Changes usually occur either in the CSF physical appearance, or can be manifested through the intrinsic characteristics – mainly the protein content and composition. Protein profiling in neurological diseases, therefore,

* Corresponding author

contributes to the overall clinical diagnosis. However, in order to acquire the complete clinical state in a patient one must include comparative protein analysis in the other biological fluids (serum, plasma or urine). Since proteins in CSF are derived from the plasma, changes in the composition or concentration in either of these media will result in changes in the other (Andersson, Alvarez-Cermeno et al. 1994). Total protein concentration reveals only little about the function of blood-brain barrier and exploits changes only after the onset of symptoms related to a neurological disorder. Also, there are neurological disorders, among others multiple sclerosis, which are characterized with normal or moderately increased total protein concentration (although changes in the individual protein concentration occurs) (Link and Muller 1971). This serious neurological disorder, and many others, mostly related to demyelization processes in the CNS; do not exhibit changes in total protein concentration (Hein Nee Maier, Kohler et al. 2008). Other neurodegenerative disorders such as Alzheimer disease (AD), Parkinson disease (PD), or amyotrophic lateral sclerosis (ALS) have different causes and affect different regions of the nervous system, and are characterized by abnormal accumulation of protein aggregates and organelles along the axon due to disruption of axonal transport. As a consequence, an early pathogenic event leading to the demise of neurons occurs (Chevalier-Larsen and Holzbaur 2006; De Vos, Grierson et al. 2008). This remark only contributes to the importance of analyzing proteins and protein profiles in such diseases.

In order to achieve our goal and to be able to correlate proteins to certain disease, we must first address to understanding the origin of the complexity of the proteome in human cells and body fluids. The importance of studying cells at the proteome level is underscored by the difficulty in predicting protein characteristics from genomic sequence data alone. These characteristics include post-translational modifications, subcellular distribution, stability, biomolecular interactions, and function. In contrast to DNA and RNA, proteins can be modified by phosphorylation, glycosylation, acetylation, nitrosation, poly(ADP ribosylation), ubiquitination, farnesylation, sulfation, linkage to glycosyl-phosphatidylinositol anchors, and SUMOylation. In total, there are about 300 different posttranslational modifications that have been reported. These modifications can profoundly affect protein conformation, stability, localization, binding interactions, and function (Aebersold and Goodlett 2001). Separate media further complicate the application of protein analyses. Cerebrospinal fluid is a hurdle media for protein analyses for one basic reason - limited amount of starting material that is often insufficient to carry out all the analysis required. Additional reasons for the difficult analysis of body fluid proteome is their large dynamic range reflected by the presence of very abundant proteins like albumin, and in the case of CSF, minute quantities of brain-derived proteins (Anderson and Anderson 1998). Further complicating the analysis of CSF is the possible infiltration of serum proteins that is caused by a leaky blood-brain barrier that is especially pronounced in patients with brain disorders. As a consequence, it is often impossible to know if a protein that is found in CSF is derived from the brain or serum. And not only proteins fitting in a specific family, but the separate protein fractions, and moreover, the individual proteins and even protein variants, produce useful information about the presence of all types of disorders. Considerable fact is that additional modifications in proteins occur after translation of the information written in the genes. Having this remark in mind, it is obvious that the proteome is practically more related to the phenotype of an individual, and hence, protein profiling will result in the most precise understanding of disease mechanisms as well as the molecular effects of drugs (Turck, Maccarrone et al. 2005). The ultimate goal of proteomics in medicine, and its sub disciplines is therefore, to provide quantitative and qualitative data of sample proteins that reflect a certain phenotype, disease state or a response to disease treatment.

1.2 Methods for protein analysis

Analyzing proteins as a diagnostic parameter in clinical practice was introduced with the development of the traditional techniques that combined methods based on protein precipitation and colored reactions. Since the introduction of electrophoresis in routine protein profiling in patients with neurological diseases, the main goal is developing novel methods for protein analyses that will offer more information and onset into the intrinsic protein characteristics. In recent years, almost every approach used to describe a method or technique applied to study protein diversity is termed "proteomics"(Nedelkov 2005). Analyses in proteomics, especially when human plasma proteome is considered, are technically challenging because the circulating proteome is a complex mixture of diverse proteins that spans approximately 10 orders of magnitude in concentration (Anderson and Anderson 2002). Routine techniques in protein profiling include mainly electrophoretic methods and can be distinguished as: gel-based proteomics approaches, fractionation or separation with other media and support material, which are based toward the identification of abundant proteins. For these types of assays, experimental designs need to involve enrichment strategies such as immunoisolation of protein complexes of interest to reduce sample complexity and increase sensitivity of detection.

The development of non-gel-based approaches for quantitative proteomics, together with advances made to detect posttranslational modification guide progress toward delineating the mechanisms involved in nerve regeneration and degeneration dysfunctions. Such neuroproteomics approaches lay the foundation for further detailed functional studies (Sun and Cavalli 2010). Both of these approaches relay on a two stage mechanism of protein analysis: *protein separation* followed by *identification and analysis* (Turck, Maccarrone et al. 2005). Classical proteomic approaches employ fractionation on the protein level with the help of 2D-PAGE. This technique produces high resolution protein separations resulting in the display of potentially thousands of protein spots. Identification of these spots is rather difficult and requires additional informatics-based approaches in order to derive relevant conclusions. Some of the limitations of 2D-PAGE have currently been overcome with the implementation of 2D-DIGE (Difference Gel Electrophoresis) where fluorescent dyes are used to distinguish between proteins from control samples and one from individuals with certain disease (Alban, David et al. 2003). It is therefore evident that at this point in proteomic technology development the broadest proteome coverage comes from a combination of multidimensional fractionation, advanced instrumentation and additional computational techniques.

Introducing mass spectrometry in protein analysis contributes towards overcoming several of the disadvantages common for standard techniques. The most efficient and most widely used protein identification method in proteomics are MALDI-TOF-MS, SELDI-TOF-MS, ESI-MS/MS and other methods (Lahm and Langen 2000; Issaq, Veenstra et al. 2002). Using shot-gun mass spectrometry approach proteins are digested by specific enzymes into small peptides and analyzed on-line by MS. This technique allows low abundant proteins to be identified despite the presence of high abundant proteins in the samples. Further advantage was done by Aebersold and co-workers (Gygi, Rist et al. 1999). They have developed a novel isotope-coded affinity tag (ICAT) strategy that permits the stable-isotope labeling of cysteine residues in proteins, thus facilitating a quantitative global analysis of differences in protein expression. A more common approach is combining chromatography separation (usually liquid chromatography, since proteins are high molecular mass compounds) with mass spectrometry detection. Chromatographic methods reduce the complexity of protein mixtures on the basis of different binding principles, and every approach adds a unique resolving power. The proteins are usually separated on the basis of affinity, charge, hydrophobicity, or size (Fountoulakis, Takacs et al. 1999; Takacs, Rakhely et al. 2001). The choice of the chromatographic method best-suited to fulfill the experimental requirements is essential for the success of the experiment (Fountoulakis and Takacs 1998). There are several methodologies that use liquid chromatography (mainly HPLC) as a tool for protein separation. Basic LC-MS/MS techniques generally employ ion-pair reversed-phase chromatography followed by electrospray ionization and mass spectrometry analysis. Depending on the ionization technique, LC –MS/MS coupling can be done either "on-line" (where HPLC is directly coupled to the ESI source of the tandem MS) or "off-line" (where, after being resolved in the HPLC process, samples are deposited directly onto a MALDI target, mixed with corresponding matrix and analyzed via MALDI-TOF MS) (Mallick and Kuster 2010). In the last 15 years combined approaches coupling immunoaffinity separation and mass spectrometry detection have been implemented (Nedelkov 2006). Also, a new approach that is considered promising in the efforts of proteome analysis is the use of aptamers as an alternative class of reagents to use for highly multiplexed protein measurements (Brody, Gold et al. 2010).

All of the above mentioned protein composition studies can be extended to two main approaches - analyzing either individual proteins or obtaining protein profile ("group" protein analysis).

1.2.1 Protein profiling approach

In the "group" protein analysis, termed as protein profiling, our main focus is to detect and identify as many proteins as possible, perform qualitative analyses, and obtain protein pattern for each sample analyzed (Fig.1/a).

Electrophoresis techniques have been the hub of laboratory testing and a component of almost all diagnostic panels (McCudden, Voorhees et al. 2010). A rather intriguing fact is however, that electrophoresis has come only a short way in advancing during the years, when used for protein profiling in patients with neurological diseases. Since it was implemented as a method in routine clinical practice, electrophoresis has come only a short way in actually progressing. In routine clinical practice discontinuous polyacrylamide gel electrophoresis (DISC-PAGE) is usually applied for determining the protein profile (Monteoliva and Albar 2004). More detailed information can be obtained using denaturing sodium dodecylsulphate polyacrylamide gel electrophoresis (SDS-PAGE) (Hu, Huang et al. 2004). In diagnosing some specific neurological diseases, isoelectric focusing (IEF) and immunofixation can be used to confirm the presence of specific oligoclonal, monoclonal or polyclonal immunoglobulin. Determination of these protein components is in many cases necessary to delineate between differential diagnoses. By combining IEF with gel electrophoresis, two dimensional gel electrophoresis is created (2D-GE), a technique, which is probably the most frequently used methodology for protein profiling. When applied into clinical practice, this methodology is used to analyze the complete proteome present in tissue samples, biological fluids and cell lysates. The result is an electrophoregram (for 1D-GE techniques) or pattern plot (for 2D-GE) fingerprinting the specific protein composition in the analyzed sample.

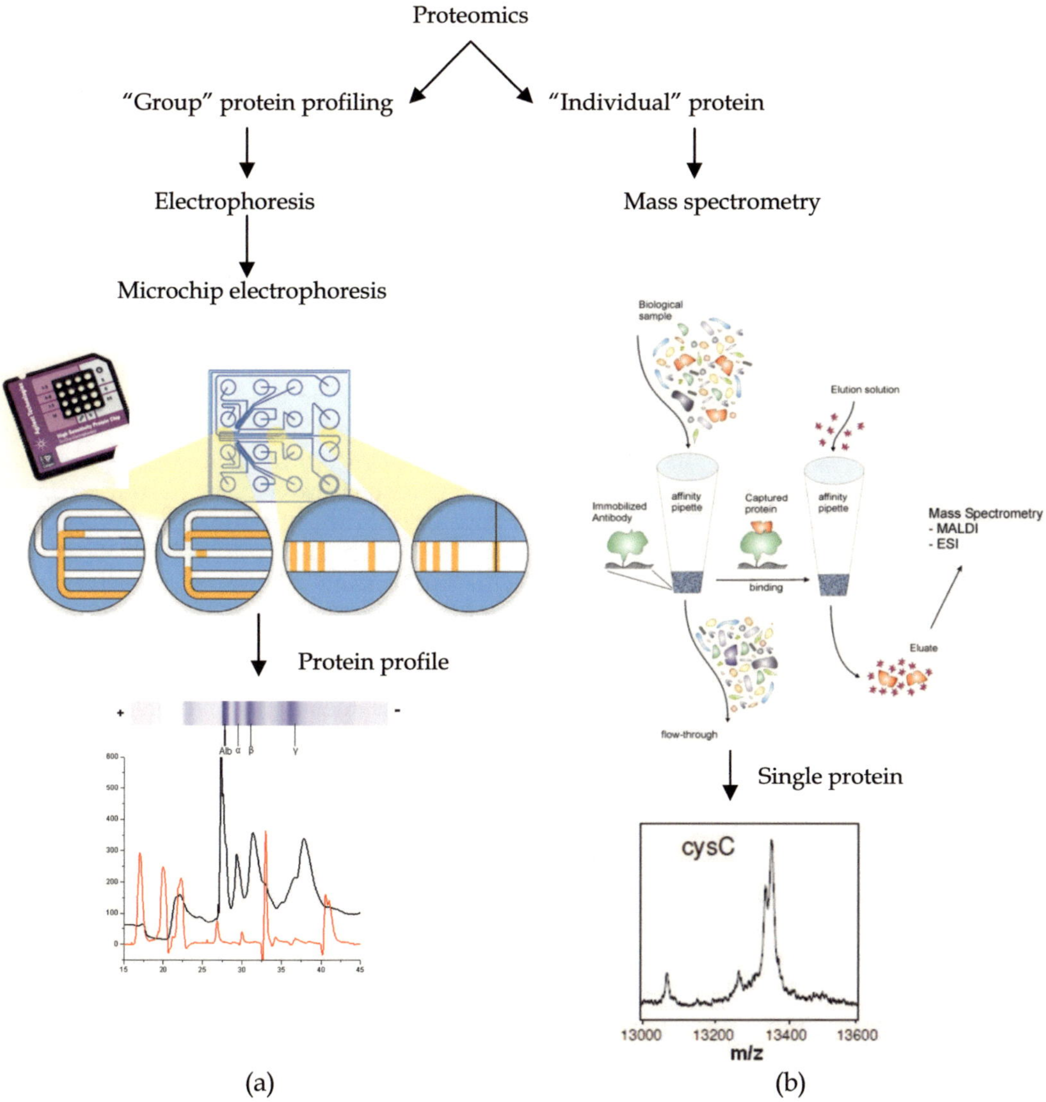

Fig. 1. Methods for protein analyses a) protein profiling using microchip electrophoresis, b) single protein analysis using mass spectrometry immunoassay (MSIA)

The general goal when using these types of qualitative group approaches is obtaining complete protein profiles both, from control samples and samples from patients with different (neurological) diseases. By comparing the obtained protein profile from the control subject (normal reference sample) to a profile originating from a patient we are able to construct a certain pattern based on the principal of similarity analysis (Trenchevska, Aleksovski et al. 2009). In our work, using this approach, we have been able to implement microchip electrophoresis method to distinguish a specific pattern for several neurological diseases (multiple sclerosis, blood-brain barrier dysfunction diseases, inflammatory conditions and autoimmune disorders) which will be discussed further in details.

1.2.2 Single protein assays

Although, the classical proteomics efforts are geared towards the analysis of the protein constitutes in both CSF and serum (Maccarrone, Birg et al. 2004; Maccarrone, Milfay et al. 2004), alternative strategies have been established for the identification of novel disease markers for neurological disorders. When it comes to protein analyses, often the concentration plays a significant role in contributing to diagnosis (example - determination of IgG concentration in multiple sclerosis). However, quantitation of all proteins in a sample is a Herculean task itself, due to the fact that the outcome of a proteome profiling experiment results in a content-rich and convoluted data that require powerful approaches to discover the subtle differences between the healthy and diseased samples (Figure 1a). In this regard, mass spectrometry has found its way as a sensitive technique for quantitative protein analyses. Although mass spectrometry has been a golden standard for proteomics from the very beginning, its complexity, cost, maintenance and other analytical characteristics are the underlying reason why this technique is rarely used in routine clinical practice (Rabilloud 2002). A step forward has been done with introducing immunoaffinity approaches (Engvall and Perlmann 1971; Ritchie 1999; Craig, Ledue et al. 2001; Yan, Lee et al. 2004). The pilot work has been done with introducing ELISA as a technique for quantification single proteins from biological samples. This technique is currently the most common abandoned method used in routine screening of known proteins and is commonly used as a laboratory test for detecting antibodies or rapidly screen and quantify antigens in biological samples. Several advantages have made this technique favorable; it follows simple sample preparation, it does not require specific conditions and data acquisition is relatively simple (Dufva and Christensen 2005). However, it can only be applied in analyzing known proteins, and, what is more, a suitable antibody must exist for retrieving the antigens from the sample. Also, ELISA based methods determine the total protein concentration and are lacking the ability to detect, identify or quantify protein variants, post-translational modifications or point mutations. Therefore, advances in this area are directed in developing assays that use combined techniques in order to obtain more detailed information about each protein intrinsic characteristics. Combined techniques have been conceptualized in the mid-nineties, via the SELDI (Hutchens and Yip, US patent No.5,719,060) (Engwegen, Gast et al. 2006; Poon 2007), and later by MSIA (Nelson et al., US patent No.6,974,704)(Nelson, Krone et al. 1995; Krone, Nelson et al. 1996) approach. The newly developed methodologies are the platform for biomarker discovery assays. These assays target "individual" proteins and use specific antibody towards the protein of interest. These specific proteins from the proteome are considered to be potential diagnostic markers for certain neurological diseases. MSIA methodology, which will be further discussed in details, bridges between the selectivity that can be obtained with immunoassays and the specificity of mass spectrometry detection (Fig. 1/b).

2. Electrophoresis in protein profiling

Identification and determination of different types of proteins play an important role in medical diagnosis. Conventional electrophoresis methods are well known for protein detection and analysis in several biological fluids, primarily blood serum and plasma and cerebrospinal fluid. CSF analysis, coupled with other methods, remains the cornerstone of diagnosis of various neurological diseases, including multiple sclerosis (Reiber, Otto et al. 2001; Sindic, Van Antwerpen et al. 2001). Even though electrophoresis is practically the basic technique in protein profiling, both in routine and scientific clinical practice, it provides only semi-quantitative information about the concentration of a certain protein. Regarding the protein profiling, these techniques still offer significant amount of information, especially about the abundance of specific protein classes, such as immunoglobulins. This is of great importance in demyelization neurological diseases. Additional criteria for this and other types of neurological diseases are presence of oligoclonal immunoglobulins. For detection of oligoclonal IgG in serum and unconcentrated CSF, several techniques can be used, primarily isoelectric focusing (IEF) combined with polyethylene-enhanced gel immunofixation and silver staining, CSF:serum quotient diagram and body index (Tourtellote, Povin et al. 1980; Sandic, Monteyne et al. 1994; Mitrevski, Stojanoski et al. 2001). Combining IEF and PAGE, 2D-GE methods are developed, optimizing techniques for detailed protein mapping, as mentioned previously. Introducing bioinformatics tools is further implemented in order to obtain more information from the protein profile. This approach necessitates usage of protein standards in each run. Using additional computational programs and following the advances in the field of bioinformatics, more information can be obtained from each protein profile spectra.

2.1 Conventional DISC-PAGE and IEF

Discontinuous polyacrylamide gel electrophoresis (DISC-PAGE) is one of the most widely used techniques for analytical separation of proteins and peptides. DISC-PAGE separations are based upon the intrinsic protein charge-to-mass ratio and the molecular mass of the protein (Chiou 1999). Polyacrylamide gels are thermostable, transparent, strong and chemically inert, can be prepared in different pore concentration and are non-ionic, therefore making them convenient for protein analyses (Ornstein 1964). Presented in Fig.2 are electrophoregrams obtained from normal samples (Fig.2/a) and sample from patient with blood-brain barrier disfunction (Fig.2/b) using DISC-PAGE classical method, implemented in routine clinical practice. Each protein zone can be identified and quantified according to the peak area and when compared to standard. The obtained results for the basic parameters in protein profiling using DISC-PAGE are presented in Table 1.

Protein fraction	Optical density	Peak area	Band %	Rf	Protein fraction	Optical density	Peak area	Band %	Rf
Prealbumin	44.97	1.984	2.31	0.071	Prealbumin	52.91	4.026	4.72	0.095
Albumin	240.97	5.332	46.92	0.201	Albumin	207.6	6.138	37.97	0.299
α - globulins	45.73	1.984	3.58	0.368	α - globulins	70.89	2.640	5.93	0.442
β1 -globulins	52.44	1.736	4.03	0.461	β1 -globulins	187.8	4.686	22.01	0.620
β2 -globulins	186.52	3.534	20.27	0.594	β2 -globulins	133.2	1.650	7.45	0.694
γ -globulins	106.48	2.046	7.85	0.683	γ -globulins	158.8	4.092	21.93	0.817
		a)					b)		

Table 1. Characteristic parameters for protein profile obtained using DISC-PAGE from a) control group (normal sample) and b) sample from patient with neurological disorder.

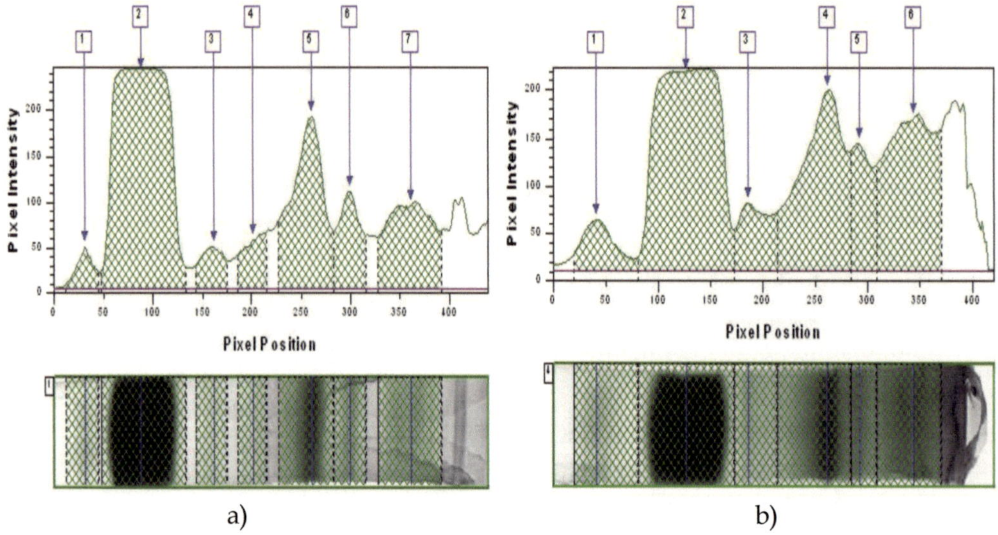

Fig. 2. Electrophoregrams presenting protein profile from CSF samples obtained from a) control group (normal sample) and b) sample from patients with disfunction in blood-brain barrier

2.2 Miniaturization in electrophoresis

The miniaturization processes have been implemented in all spheres of protein research, resulting in newly developed techniques that follow the concept of microchip electrophoresis. The onset of miniaturization electrophoresis dates from 1954 when the first microchip used in the semiconductors structure was created (Manz, Graber et al. 1990). It took more than 20 years to introduce the first microchip in gas chromatography analyses in 1975. However, the great leap in applying miniaturization in biomedical sciences and research was in the beginning of 1990s, when the first commercial microchip was constructed (Woolley and Mathies 1994; Keramas, Perozziello et al. 2004; Balslev, Jorgensen et al. 2006; Geschke 2006; Geschke 2009). This pioneer technique was introduced for the first time in genomic and DNA analysis in the mid-1990s, when the first commercially available microchip for DNA and RNA analyses was produced. Protein microchips were used for the first time in 1999, when 6 fluorescent labeled proteins with molecular mass ranging between 9 and 116 kDa were successfully separated on a microchip in less than 35 s (Yao, Anex et al. 1999). Another step forward was done in 2001 when a method for fluorescent labeled protein-SDS complexes (where proteins were non-covalently bounded to the denaturing agent) separation was optimized (Jin, Giordano et al. 2001). The first commercially available microchip was known as LabChip and produced by Bousse et al. (Bousse, Mouradian et al. 2001) in Caliper Technologies, Mountain View, CA. At the same time, Agilent 2100 Bioanalyzer appears on the market, as the first commercial instrument for microchip electrophoresis separation platforms. The preliminary results using microchip technology indicated great potential, especially for implementation in routine clinical practice, which was the basic goal of developing such methods.

2.3 Use of lab-on-a-chip electrophoresis in protein profiling

Miniaturized lab-on-a-chip electrophoresis is a novel technique in protein profile analyses, introduced with the development of Agilent 2100 Bioanalyzer (Woolley and Mathies 1994). The microchip system includes system of microchannels through where gel is rushed by applying pressure. The gel contains fluorescent dye which serves as a label; therefore protein detection is done by fluorescence analysis. By running the chip, proteins can be separated according to their size, and, as a result, protein profile can be obtained. Looking into the basics of lab-on-a-chip electrophoresis it can be noted that the basis of analysis is denaturing SDS-PAGE; therefore proteins separate only according to their molecular mass and not their charge. The microchip platform consists of a system of micro-channels ranging in width from 20 to 100 μm and height of 10-25 μm. Protein separation is performed in a solid media (polyacrylamide gel) both in native and denaturing conditions. Gel preparation is performed in a buffered solution, therefore presenting the necessary ions for the protein separation. Created potential difference indicated protein movement through the system of channels. During their passing through the system, proteins form an affinity bond to a fluorescent dye, therefore becoming visible for detection. Using a highly sensitive fluorescent detector, signals from the proteins are noted and protein profile can be obtained from a single sample in less than one minute (Trenchevska, Aleksovski et al. 2009). LiF detector is commonly used due to its high selectivity and sensitivity - it can detect fluorescein concentration in 300 fM quantities (Ocvirk, Tang et al. 1998). This detection method is actually the critical point that allows protein analysis in such a short time.

Lab-on-a-chip protein electrophoresis employs several advantages when compared to other types of electrophoresis. It is significantly faster, shortening the time required per analysis, which is of great importance, especially for application in clinical laboratories where a large cohort of samples is analyzed on daily basis. Further, the amount of sample required for the analysis is only 5 μL, which is convenient especially when proteins in CSF are analyzed. Also, unlike traditional electrophoresis techniques, lab-on-a-chip method uses fluorescent detector, which has higher sensitivity. The microchip is designed in a specific manner depending on the analysis required, whether it is DNA, RNA or protein. Regarding the proteins in neurological diseases, using this technique under optimized conditions, we were able to analyze both low molecular mass proteins (MW<50 000 Da) and high molecular mass proteins (50 000 Da < MW < 250 000 Da) (Auroux, Iossifidis et al. 2002).

2.3.1 Method development

In order to obtain better resolution and assay characterization, several modifications can be made. Lab-on-a-chip electrophoresis platform does not usually allow many modifications; however, several optimizations can contribute to obtaining better results. This technique so far is very well implemented in DNA and RNA assays, but its application in protein analyses is rather limited for several reasons. Lab-on-a-chip electrophoresis system uses fluorescent detector, therefore require fluorescent dyes for protein labeling. These types of dyes, however, do not form covalent bond with the labeled protein; therefore require longer incubation times in order to allow high-efficient specific binding (Floriano, Acosta et al. 2007). Having this in mind, Giordano et al. introduced a concept that significantly reduces these effects. It was noted that using SDS as denaturing agent incorporated in the gel, besides uniformly charging the proteins, favorizes their binding with the fluorescent dye, further producing higher signal to the detector (Christodoulides, Floriano et al. 2007; Floriano, Acosta et al. 2007; Sloat, Roper et al. 2008). When biological samples are analyzed, further problems in developing the assay occur, due to the intrinsic complexity of the specimen itself. In order to obtain the protein profile using lab-on-a-chip electrophoresis, several conditions must be optimized.

Sample preparation for lab-on-a-chip electrophoresis - prior to analysis samples were stored at -20°C for two weeks. Serum and cerebrospinal fluid samples from control group (designated as normal according to their cross-reactivity toward the usual infectious agents and donor information), and from patients with different neurological diseases (primarily multiple sclerosis, than blood-brain barrier disfunction and other demyelization diseases) were used for the analyses. Samples were prepared by combing 84 μL sterile water, 4 μL sample and 2 μL denaturing agent (BME). Within each run, protein standard (ladder) was used for calibration and protein fraction identification.

Optimization of denaturing agent concentration – denaturation agents contribute to easier formation of protein-fluorescent dye complex therefore resulting in higher efficiency of the detector. In the sample optimization steps, we have incubated the samples with different concentration of denaturing agent beta-mercaptoethanol (BME). Sample to denaturing agent ratio used for the analysis were – 1:1; 1:1.5; 1:2; 1:2.5; 1:3; 1:3.5 and 1:5. The results have been previously published and have shown optimal protein to BME ratio of 1:3.5 (Trenchevska, Aleksovski et al. 2009).

Optimization of incubation temperature – Temperature is an important parameter in protein analyses due to its effect onto the protein structure (denaturation) and affinity towards the fluorescent dye, which, in turn can cause increase of the signal in the detector. When optimizing incubation temperature, samples were incubated in water bath at five different temperatures – 5°C, 22°C (room temperature), 37°C (normal body temperature), 60°C and 90°C. It was noted that optimal incubation temperature is 90°C (Trenchevska, Aleksovski et al. 2009).

Assay procedure – After sample preparation and following incubation under the optimized conditions, the microchip was placed in the bioanalyzer and run. In the process of electrophoretic separation in the bioanalyzer, the electric current provides ideal conditions for staining and destaining within 45 s per sample analyzed. During the separation process, the sample is initially rushed through the pores in polyacrylamide gel, and then allowed to bind with the fluorescent dye incorporated into the microchannels. When using denaturing conditions, further SDS binding causes proteins to gain net negative charge, therefore separating proteins in a sample only according to the molecular mass.

Results processing – After completion of the separation process, complete numerical analysis is necessary in order to obtain more information from the protein profile for each sample. Analyses regarding statistical parameters are important in clinical practice, because, in a time scale, they provide useful information about the distribution of specific protein fractions and their relation to a specific disease. Collecting such large amount of data is enabled due to the automation and development of microcomputers. Using Web-based databases, data acquisition, manipulation and computation for electrophoresis protein pattern recognition is further performed using standard statistical signal analysis (Spirovski, Stojanoski et al. 2005). In this context, the next promising area of interest is cluster analysis, along with artificial neural networks, bioinformatics techniques that have been successfully applied to various areas in medical practice, as diagnostic systems (Vogt and Nagel 1992; Jerez-Aragones 2003), biomedical analysis (Lisboa 2002) and neuroimaging (Aizenberg, Aizenberg et al. 2001).

In our work, using the optimized lab-on-a-chip electrophoresis method, we were able to obtain the protein profile from patients with multiple sclerosis, neurodegenerative diseases and blood-brain dysfunction and further perform statistical analysis on the obtained data.

2.3.2 Application in clinical practice (profiling in patients with different neurological disorders)

Lab-on-a-chip electrophoresis was used in order to confirm the "group" aspect approach in protein profiling that is of great significance in every day clinical practice. Protein profiles from patients were classified in one of the four major types according to the distribution of the five basic protein zones: prealbumin, albumin, α-globulin, β-globulin and γ-globulin – normal (N), transudative (T), gamaglobuline (γ) and transudative-gamaglobuline (Tγ). When compared to protein standard, in each of the zones, different proteins can be identified. This identification, however, offers only qualitative details, and cannot be used in quantifying separate proteins with high accuracy. We have previously reported using the optimized lab-on-a-chip electrophoresis to analyze serum and cerebrospinal fluid samples from control group and patients with neurological diseases (Trenchevska, Aleksovski et al. 2009). It was noted that using this advanced technique, protein profiles can be used to obtain satisfactory qualitative analyses, therefore contributing to precise clinical diagnosis. In patients with multiple sclerosis, for example, characteristic electrophoretic patterns were noted, characterized by high IgG concentration (which is evident in 46% of all MS cases, where intrathecal IgG synthesis occurs), and normal total protein levels (Fishman 1992; Daskalovska 2000). Examples of the electrophoregrams for both normal samples and samples from patient with multiple sclerosis are presented in Figure 3.

3. Mass spectrometry-based protein identification protocols

Mass spectrometry has been used in clinical practice mainly for detection of small molecules (MW<1 kDa) aiming to detect inborn errors in metabolism, or monitoring toxicity, drug and doping abuse (Ahmed 2008). Introduction to mass spectrometry in proteomics was made possible in recent years thanks to the discovery of the so called soft ionization techniques (ESI and MALDI) that were recognized by the Nobel Prize in chemistry 2002 (Tanaka, Waki et al. 1988; Fenn, Mann et al. 1989). Using either ESI or MALDI, a molecular mass with a precision and accuracy of ±0.05% or better can be achieved. This depends heavily on the purity of the protein sample, the relative size of the protein, the presence or absence of post-translational modifications, the resolution of the mass spectrometer itself and so on. Mass spectrometry has been broadly used in determination of protein amino acid sequence using either tandem mass spectrometry MS/MS sequencing of enzymatically derived peptide fragments of the original protein, or sometimes direct MS/MS on the intact protein. Using these approaches, post translational modifications such as protein phosphorylation, sulfonation, oxidation and terminal amino acid cleavage can be identifyed. Over the past few years, the sensitivity and specificity of mass spectrometry coupled with liquid chromatography, have improved to a degree such that protein quantification can be derived from very complex mixtures (tissues, biofluids, cell lysates etc.). Recent publications contribute to the newly developed methods for protein characterization, identification and quantification, especially regarding low abundant proteins in biological specimen (Gygi, Rist et al. 1999; Kiernan, Nedelkov et al. 2006)

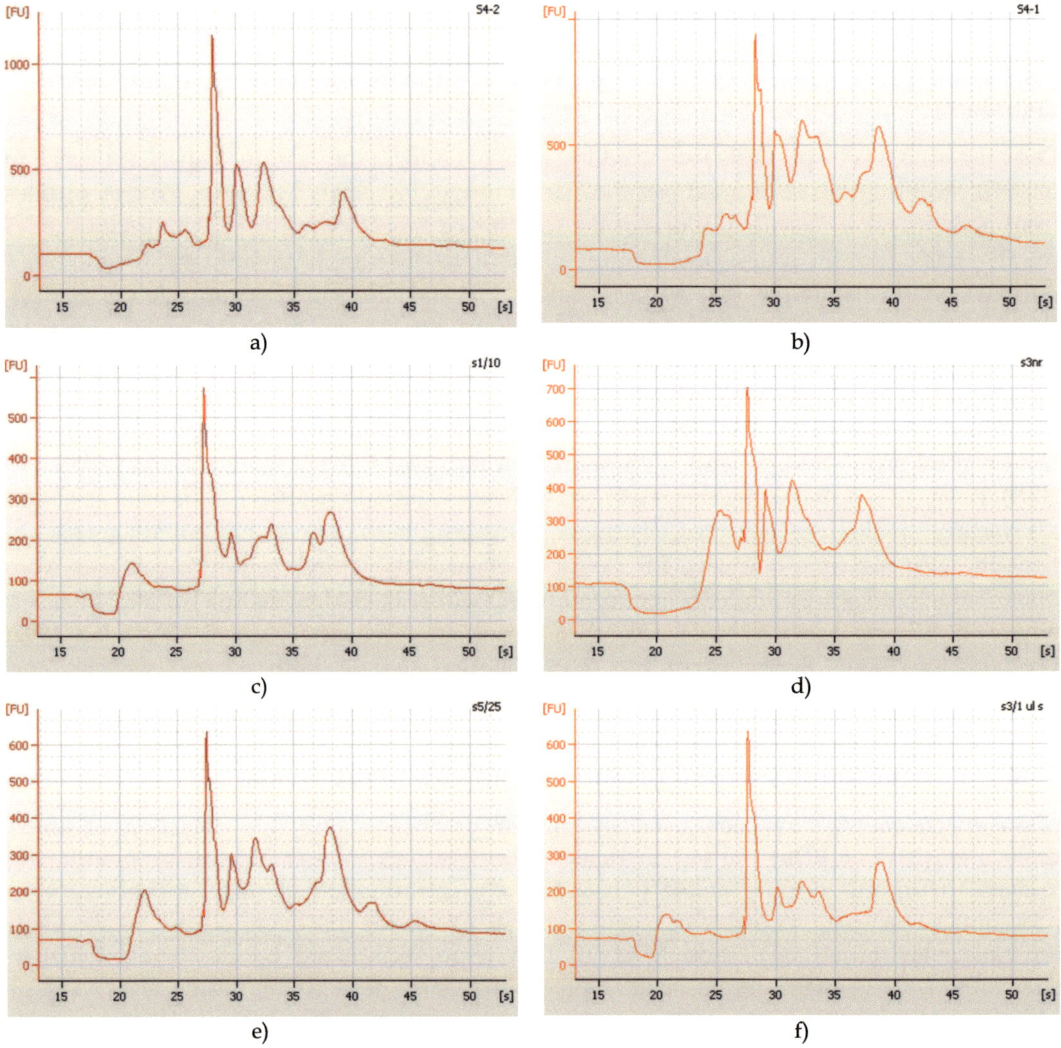

Fig. 3. Characteristic electrophoregrams obtained using lab-on-a-chip protein electrophoresis in samples from a) control group (normal sample); b) sample from patient with multiple sclerosis; c) sample from patient with polyradiculoneuropathy; d) sample from patient after ictus cerebralis; e) sample from patient with blood-brain barrier disfunction and f) control sample. Noted in the electrophoregrams are differences in the protein distribution primarily in the γ-globulin region, which is expected in samples from patients with demyelization processes, where intrathecal IgG synthesis is dominant.

To use mass spectrometry for biomarker discovery in clinical proteomics is conceptually simple. What we do is compare obtained spectral peaks from specific protein or proteins in body fluids or tissue extracts in a diseased group, with those from the control group. These peaks correspond to potential biomarker molecules. MS biomarker discovery efforts have focused on four subsets of the proteome: (i) polypeptides and whole proteins in tissues or body fluids separated by electrophoresis or chromatography, with or without prefragmentation; (ii) enzymatic peptide fragments separated by HPLC and analyzed by ESI or MALDI; (iii) proteins in tissue or body fluids that are adsorbed on surface protein ships in a matrix, analyzed by SELDI and (iv) naturally occurring fragmented peptides in blood that represent low range of the plasma/serum proteome, analyzed by MALDI (van der Merwe, Oikonomopoulou et al. 2007). In our work, we mainly concentrate in analyzing intact proteins as potential biomarkers using one of the basic approaches - top down proteomic analysis.

3.1 Top-down proteomics analysis

As a tool for proteins and peptides separated by electrophoresis or chromatography, and with or without previous fragmentation, mass spectrometry has been applied in several different ways; the two approaches are top-down and bottom-up MS. Top-down MS is the direct analysis of proteins on the intact level. Bottom-up approach identifies proteins following enzymatic or chemical digestion of the sample resulting in the formation of much smaller peptide fragments. These smaller protein segments are much easier to analyze with low resolution MS instruments and therefore bottom-up peptide analysis is currently the most popular MS-based proteomics approach (Han, Jin et al. 2006).

The strength of top-down proteomics approach lies in the direct detection of the native molecular mass of biological protein species. Mass spectrometry detection provides information for the native protein, and also for the natively occurring small peptides, biologically generated protein cleavages, post-translational modifications or point mutations - all of which are postulated to be relevant in many diseases and other biological processes occurring in cells. Other major advantage of top-down approach is the simplified sample preparation that does not necessitate enzymatic or chemical digestion prior to analysis. Scientist using top-down approach in studying proteins are mainly oriented towards addressing clinical questions - using population screening in the complicated process of identification and validation of potential biomarkers (Whitelegge, Halgand et al. 2006).

Several techniques are favored in top-down proteomics research platform. SELDI-TOF MS is a widely used biomarker discovery method that combines the selectivity of chromatography and sensitivity of mass spectrometry detection. The major challenge for this approach is the requirement for off-line enrichment and purification of the selected biomarker candidates, followed by MS/MS identification using different MS platform(Reid and McLuckey 2002).

MALDI-TOF MS has also found its way in implementing in top-down proteomics quest for novel biomarkers. One of the disadvantages of the methods used in routine clinical biomarker discovery techniques is the complicated sample preparation which requires chromatographic or electrophoretic separation of the targeted protein. Immunoaffinity capture of a protein directly from a biological sample is a base method used in all immunoassays (such as ELISA). Therefore, by combining the selectivity of immunoaffinity capture and the specificity of mass spectrometry, a novel methodology has been developed in recent years– Mass Spectrometry Immunoassay (MSIA).

In our work we have developed several assays using MSIA approach. Using this novel platform we were able to analyze several proteins, some of which have been introduced as potential biomarkers for several neurological diseases. An introduction to the overall procedure and application of this technique will be introduced through the development of Cystatin C MSIA assay.

3.2 Mass spectrometry immunoassay (MSIA)

Mass Spectrometry Immunoassay (MSIA) is a novel approach that has been employed for both, qualitative and quantitative characterization of body fluid proteins. From the methodology point of view, it is a combination of today's predominant technology involved in routine clinical practice - immunoassay for targeted protein affinity extraction assessment and uses mass spectrometry detection (MALDI-TOF-MS) for achieving the specificity necessary for this type of analyses. This approach lacks the disadvantage demonstrated by the immunoassays - inability to detect protein variants, post translational modifications or mutations. On the contrary, MSIA gives onset into the detailed intrinsic protein characteristics, both for high or low abandoned proteins. One great advantage of this hybrid methodology is the simplicity of protein extraction from complicated biological samples. The basic concept of the analysis includes a two-step approach; first, proteins are captured by a principle of microscale affinity by aspiration/dispense cycles on an antibody-derivatized affinity pipette, and in the second step eluted proteins are subsequently analyzed using MALDI-TOF-MS (Fig.4)

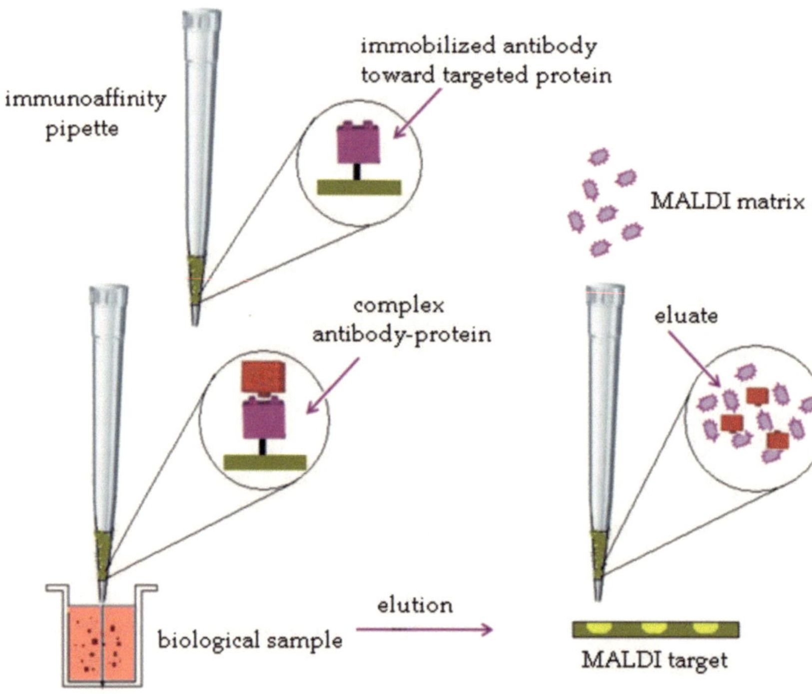

Fig. 4. Mass spectrometry immunoassay scheme

In the initial stage of this method's development, agarose beads derivatized with an affinity ligand (e.g. polyclonal antibodies) were used to create a μL-scale column inside a micropipette tip (Krone, Nelson et al. 1996). These columns are further derivatized with a corresponding antibody toward the targeted protein. Additional activation of the beads is necessary prior to the derivatization process. A summary of the consecutive steps in activation and derivatization of the affinity pipettes is presented in Figure 5.

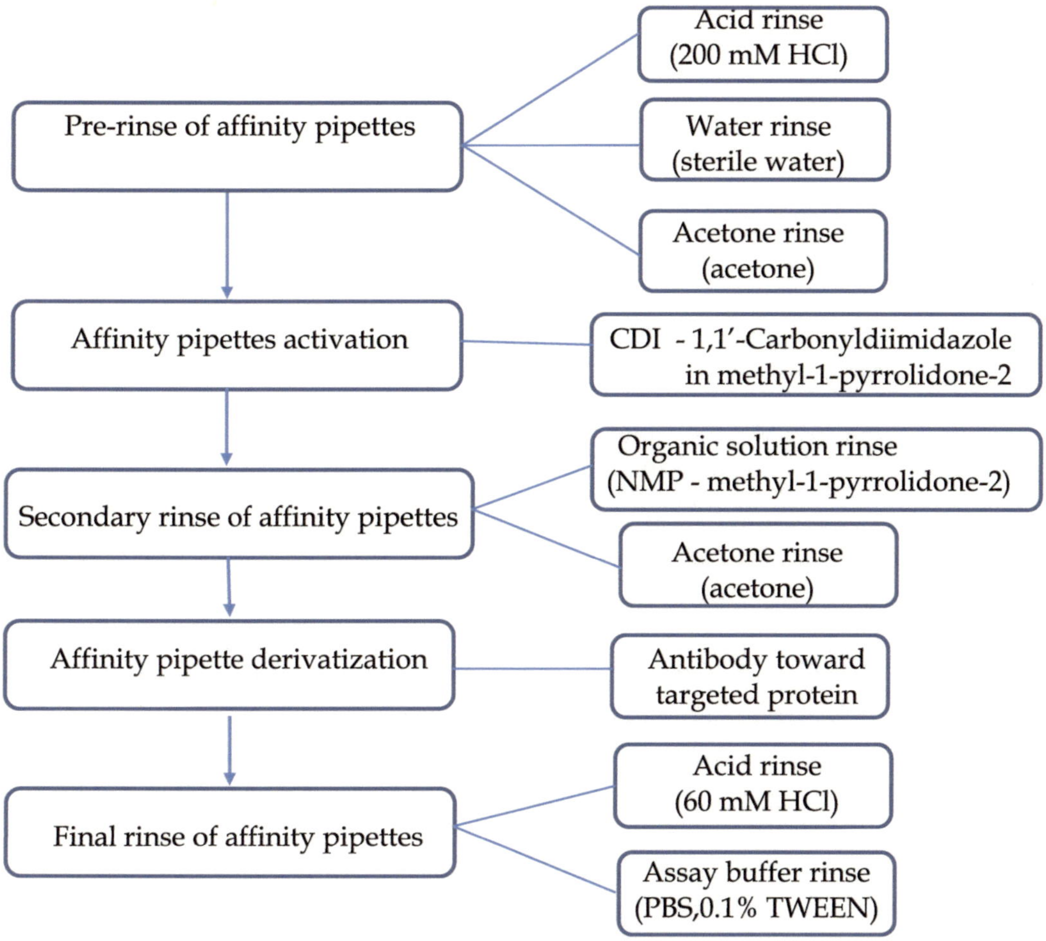

Fig. 5. Affinity pipettes activation and derivatization procedure

When the affinity pipettes are coated with the corresponding antibody, further activation of the surface is needed in order to favor protein binding. Using Multimek 96 automated 96-channel pipettor (Beckman Coulter, Brea, CA, USA), the antibody coated affinity pipettes were rinsed with buffer (PBS, with 0,1%TWEEN) in 10 aspiration/dispense cycles. Next, pipettes were immersed into a microplate containing the sample (serum, plasma, urine or CSF). Following additional buffer rinse (in order to elute the non-specific bounded proteins or other constitutes origin from the sample) and two water rinse cycles, retrieved targeted protein on the affinity pipette is ready for discharge. Figure 6 illustrates the steps in this analysis.

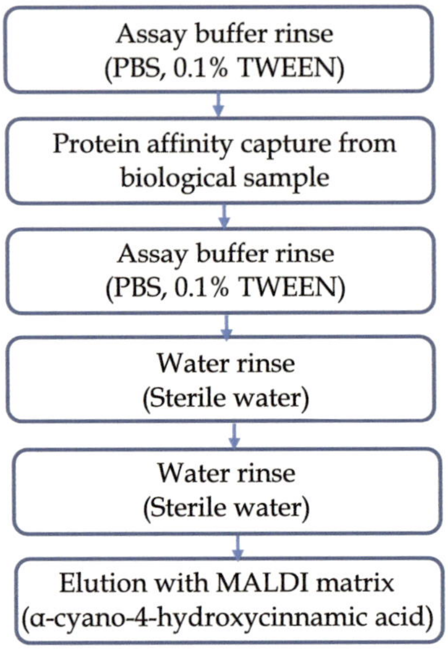

Fig. 6. Steps in MSIA protein analysis

Preparing for the second step of detection - the mass spectrometry detection, captured protein is eluted directly on the MALDI target, by 6 μL aliquots of MALDI matrix (α-cyano-4-hydroxycinnamic acid in aqueous solution containing 33% (v/v) acetonitrile and 0.4% (v/v) trifluoroacetic acid). Using this acidic matrix, captured protein are dissociated from the antibodies and eventually dispensed onto the target. Following drying and visual inspection of the sample spots, linear mass spectra were acquired using delayed extraction mode with 1.7 kV draw out pulse, 200 ns delay and a full accelerating potential of 20 kV.

	MSIA	
	Qualtitative MSIA	Quantitative MSIA
Primary goal	Population proteomic studies	Biomarker discovery and validation
Samples	Large cohort of samples	Control and disease samples spiked with reference protein
Assay development	Affinity pipettes immobilized with antibody toward targeted protein	Affinity pipettes immobilized with two antibodies - toward targeted protein and IRS
Immunoaffinity separation	Retrieval of targeted protein	Retrieval of targeted protein and the IRS
Mass spectrometry detection	MALDI-TOF MS	MALDI-TOF MS
Results	Detection of protein variants, post-translational modification and point mutation	Calculating concentration of native protein and protein variants
Additional analyses	Enzymatic digestion	/

Table 2. Differences between qualitative and quantitative MSIA approaches

Although introduced in the recent years, this technique has already been implemented in developing qualitative and quantitative assays for several protein and protein variants using different biological samples as medium. There is one basic difference regarding these two approaches (Table 2). When using MSIA platform for qualitative analysis, affinity pipettes are derivatized only with antibody towards the targeted protein; additional antibody must be fitted into the affinity micocolumn in order to retrieve another protein in the quantitative assay. In quantitative MSIA, affinity pipettes are derivatized with a secondary antibody, toward a protein termed as internal reference standard (IRS). Choosing the IRS is one of the critical steps in developing of the assay, due to the high criteria required for such a protein. An important prerequisite for an IRS is that it should not be present in human plasma or serum (or other biological fluids, as well), so that its spiked concentration in the analytical samples is always constant. Also, the signal on the mass spectrometer produced by the IRS should be in close proximity to the signal of the targeted protein, in order to be able to use the same MS acquisition parameters for both proteins. The goal in developing qualitative assays is determination and identification of existing or novel protein variants and point mutations. In these type of analyses, a large cohort of samples is required for analyses in order to delineate between the "wild" isoforms (post-translational modifications, or additional derivatization) present in majority of samples, and which subsequently are termed as "normal" and the pathological variants which are only present in a small number of samples or in samples from patients with certain diseases. In quantitative assays we are able to calculate the exact concentration of each variant, which, again, by screening populations, can provide information about the range of "normal" concentration distribution of the variant and the protein in general. These correlations can further be used in discussing the potential biomarker capacity of a certain protein or variant. Presented here are results of the developed MSIA qualitative and quantitative assays for determination of cystatin C and its variants.

3.2.1 Qualitative CysC MSIA assay in CSF and serum

Cystatin C is a serine proteinase inhibitor belonging to the type 2 cystatin gene family (Jarvinen, Rinne et al. 1987; Mussap and Plebani 2004). It inhibits both endogenous proteases, such as liposomal cathepsins, and proteases of parasites and microorganisms. It is a non-glycosilated single chain protein with a molecular weight of 13,343. Due to the important function, cystatin C is expressed at the stable levels in most nuclear cells. Its amino acid sequence consists of 120 amino acid residues encoded by a 7.3 kb gene located in chromosome 20 (Schnittger, Rao et al. 1993). Cystatin C has been indicated in numerous pathological states (Henskens, Veerman et al. 1996; Grubb 2000; Reed 2000), most notably in renal failure (Randers, Kristensen et al. 1998; Randers and Erlandsen 1999). There are a growing number of reports demonstrating that cystatin C is more preferable than creatinine for measurement of GFR (Naruse, Ishii et al. 2009). Also, a variant of human cystatin C (L68Q) is an amyloidogenic protein deposited in the cerebral vasculature of patients with hereditary cerebral hemorrhage with amyloidosis in which patients suffer from repeated cerebral hemorrhages (Ghiso, Jensson et al. 1986; Olafsson and Grubb 2000; Calero, Pawlik et al. 2001). In the clinical practice, cysC is well-desribed serum marker of renal failure that is not dependent of age, sex or lean muscle mass (Seronie-Vivien, Delanaye et al. 2008; Naruse, Ishii et al. 2009). At the same time, cystatin C is becoming acknowledged as a marker for elevated risk of death from myocardial infraction and stroke(Naruse, Ishii et al.

2009). The concentration of cystatin C in healthy individuals range from 0.8 to 1.2 mg/L, depending on the measurement method (Roos, Doust et al. 2007). Increased serum levels are almost always associated with reduction in GFR. The role of cystatin C as potential biomarker for multiple scleroses was introduced in the work of Irani et al. They have reported a correlation between the ratio of one cysC truncated form des-SSPGKPPR and native cysC peak, and the occurrence of multiple sclerosis(Irani, Anderson et al. 2006). Other research groups do not support this concept, claiming that the cleaved peptide occurs as a result of sample storage, not exclusively MS existence (Del Boccio, Pieragostino et al. 2006; Hansson, Hviid Simonsen et al. 2006; Nakashima, Fujinoki et al. 2006).

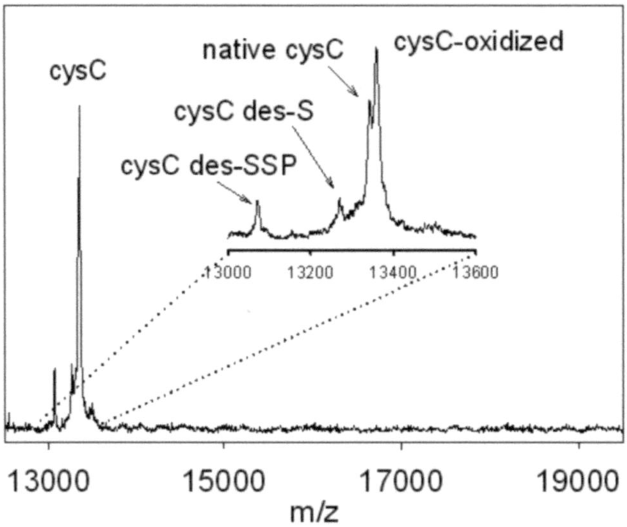

Fig. 7. Cystatin C mass spectra showing signal from native form and additional "wild type" protein variants

In previous work MSIA assays have been developed for qualitative identification of cystatin C from human plasma (Kiernan, Nedelkov et al. 2006) and urine samples (Kiernan, Tubbs et al. 2003). After several assay optimization we were able to develop MSIA assay for determination of cysC in cerebrospinal fluid both from control group and a couple of matched serum/CSF samples obtained from patients with multiple sclerosis(Trenchevska, Aleksovski et al. 2009).

MSIA provides excellent results for this type of single protein analysis, because it preserves the protein in its native form during the sample preparation procedure, and using the MALDI-TOF MS, allows an insight into the detailed protein structure, presence and distribution of isoforms. When completing MSIA data from analyzed cysC in human plasma sample, besides the native peak (CysC native MW=13 343), several protein variants can be noted: oxidation peak (MW=13 359), des-S variant (MW=13 260) and des-SSP variant (MW= 13 076) (Fig.7)

These isoforms were noted in all samples analyzed, and also in a large population proteomics study where 1000 samples were screened using the developed MSIA cystatin C assay (Nedelkov, Tubbs et al. 2004; Nelson, Nedelkov et al. 2004). The goal of the further research was to develop MSIA method for cysC identification in CSF. For utilization of this assay, a critical step was sample preparation in terms of optimizing the dilution. In this analysis, both control CSF samples and samples from patients diagnosed with MS were analyzed. Moreover, paired serum/CSF samples origin from same individuals was screened. As presented in the previous studies, using the optimized MSIA qualitative assay, cysC and its wild type isoforms were detected in the analyzed CSF samples (Nedelkov, Shaik et al. 2008). However, several correlations were observed when matched serum/CSF samples were analyzed. The sample that consisted most extensive truncations in the serum cysC, exploits most variants in the CSF sample as well (Fig.8/c,d). Also, additional peaks not common in serum cysC analysis were noted both in the control CSF samples and the samples from patients with MS. These are mainly truncated cysC isoforms missing 3, 4, 7, 8, 9, 10, 11, 14 and 17 *N*-terminal amino acids; some of which have been reported for the first time by our group (Fig. 8/a,b).

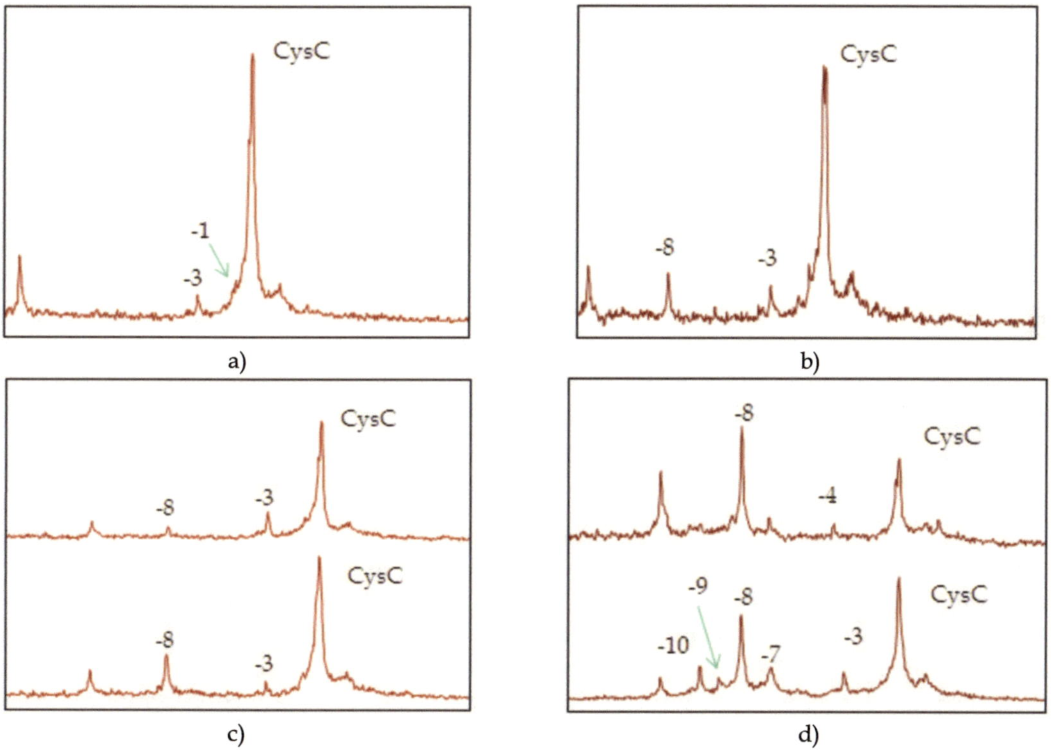

Fig. 8. MALDI-TOF MS spectra obtained after cystatin C MSIA in a) serum sample (control); b) CSF sample (control); c) paired serum/CSF sample (control) and d) paired serum/CSF sample (patients with diagnosed multiple sclerosis) (reprinted with permission from (Nedelkov, Shaik et al. 2008))

3.2.2 Developing quantitative MSIA assay for CysC and its variants

Developing quantitative assays for protein determination can contribute to the diagnosis and prognosis in clinical proteomics studies due to the fact that oftentimes, not only the occurrence, but also the concentration distinguishes between "normal" and "diseased" condition. Using conventional ELISA and other immunologically based quantitative assays, we can obtain information about the total protein concentration. All these techniques, however, lack the ability to quantify specific protein variants and isoforms, which in turn, are more probable biomarker candidates.

Using MSIA, we have been able to develop and validate several fully quantitative assays, both for quantitation of intact proteins, as well as protein isoforms.

There are several possible approaches regarding mass spectrometry quantitation of proteins and protein variants. One requires usage of isotope labels, whereas, second uses different protein, termed as internal reference standard for quantitation. The goal of developing platforms to be implemented in every-day clinical practice requires simplified sample preparation procedure and handling. In our work we present the developed quantitative assay for determination and quantitation of cystatin C and its variants in biological samples. Results from this quantitative assay have recently been published (Trenchevska and Nedelkov 2011). In this chapter we summarize the basic concepts and "hot spots" that need to be considered when developing this type of assay in clinical practice. The procedure includes several steps:

Choice of internal reference standard - There are several approaches in the process of choosing an adequate internal reference standard for a quantitative assay. An important prerequisite that an internal standard must possess is not to be present in human plasma or serum, so that its spiked concentration in the analytical sample remains constant in each analysis. Also, the signals that the IRS produces in the mass spectra should be in close proximity to the signal of the targeted protein, so that the same MS acquisition parameters can be used for analysis of both proteins. For developing quantitative assay for cysC we have used beta-lactoglobulin (BL), the major whey protein in cow's milk, which has molecular weight of 18 281 (it is close to the MW of cysC = 13 343), and is present in many mammalian species, but not in human. In Figure 9, signals from cystatin C and the internal reference standard BL can be noted.

Optimization of standard curve concentration range - In this step first it is necessary to determine the ratios of immobilized cysC and BL antibodies immobilized on the affinity pipettes. In general, concentration of cysC antibody should be higher in order to accurately quantify the various amounts of cysC in the examined analytical samples. Since we can control the concentration of BL in the samples, the antibody concentration can be lower in the affinity pipettes. For the analysis we have used the following antibody ratio - cysC:BL=8.5:1 (m/m). Next, we determine the optimal concentration and volume of spiked BL in the samples, and last, we determine the concentration range for the standard curve. It is important to construct the curve in its linear range concentration and then dilute the samples if necessary, because of the greater accuracy. In this assay we have constructed a six point cysC standard curve, spanning the range from 0.0312 to 1.0 mg/L cystatin C (Fig.10).

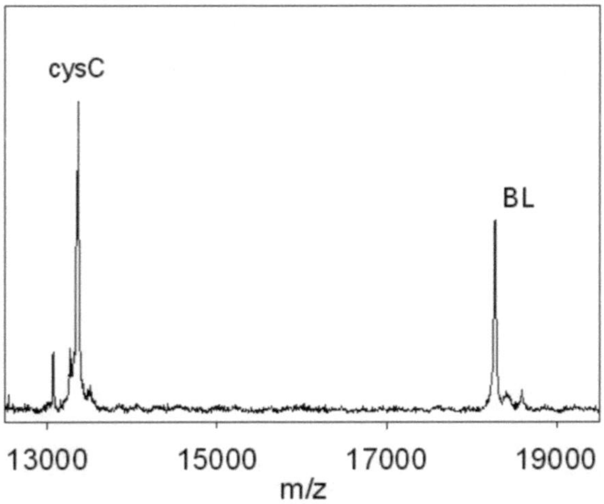

Fig. 9. Mass spectra from cystatin C and Beta lactoglobulin used as internal reference standard for quantitation

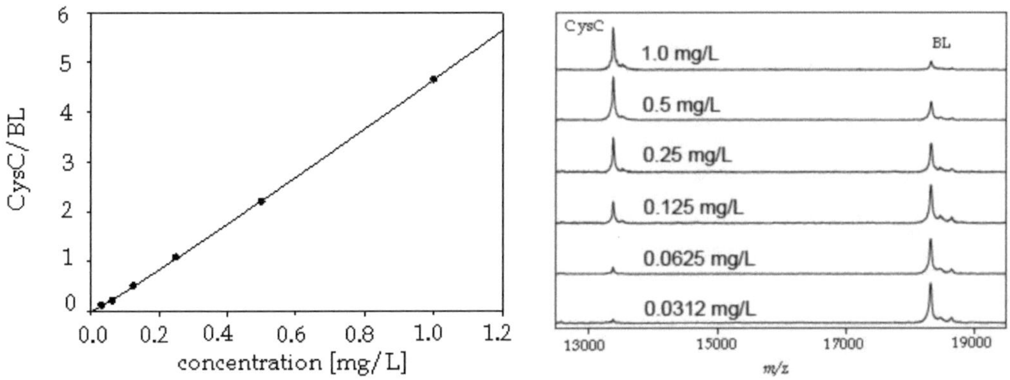

Fig. 10. Presented is a typical standard curve used for cysC quantitation (left); representative cysC mass spectra used for standard curve generation (right) (reprinted with permission from (Trenchevska and Nedelkov 2011).

Sample preparation - Prior to the analysis, the analytical samples were diluted twice in the assay buffer and spiked with 5 μL BL (c (BL) =10 mg/L).

Assay parameters - For this quantitative assay several characteristic parameters were analyzed in order to check the reproducibility and quality of assessment. Intra-assay precision was done by analyzing three plasma samples in replicates, each with a single standard curve. Inter-assay precision was determined by analyzing one plasma sample three times on different days with separate standard curve. Linearity of the assay was determined by analyzing serial dilutions of a sample with known cysC concentration and comparing the observed with the expected concentrations. Also, spiking-recovery experiments were performed by adding cysC standard in known concentration into the analytical sample, again with a known cysC concentration. By comparing the expected with the observed results we were able to recover the spiked cysC concentration.

Assay validation – In order to further validate the newly developed assay, a comparison with a well-established method was performed. Several samples were analyzed both with commercially available ELISA and with the developed MSIA method. The good correlation between both assays validated the results obtained with the new cystatin C assay (ref. statija cysC).

Assay application – The next phase, and practically the last step between the method and its application in the full potential is actually screening many samples and quantifying not only the native protein, but the isoforms present. Using this assay, we were able to quantify cystatin C and its variants in a total of 500 plasma samples. For all the samples, concentrations of cystatin C and its variants was determined, and averaged (average cysC concentration = 0.94 mg/L) which corresponds to the average CysC concentration previously established using ELISA (Erlandsen, Randers et al. 1998). In all the samples the "wild type" variants were noted; CysC 3Pro-OH and two truncated forms lacking one (des-S) and three (des-SSP) N-terminal amino acids respectably (Fig.11).

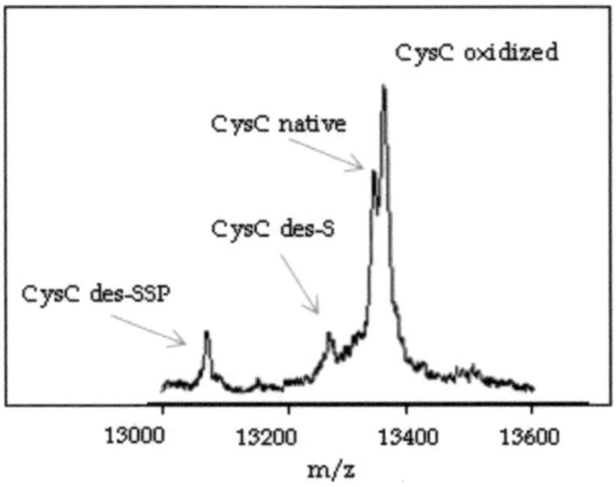

Fig. 11. Typical MALDI-TOF spectra from cystatin C showing the detected variants

Presented in Table 3 are partial results from the quantitative analysis of cystatin C, where we were able to calculate the concentration of each variant present in the analytical sample.

sample	Native cysC [mg/L]	Hydroxyl cysC [mg/L]	cysC des-S [mg/L]	cysC des-SSP [mg/L]	Total cysC [mg/L]
1	0.25	0.33	0.07	0.07	0.71
2	0.32	0.41	0.08	0.03	0.84
3	0.39	0.48	0.09	0.08	1.04
4	0.42	0.54	0.08	0.08	1.11
5	0.35	0.46	0.11	0.11	1.02
6	0.27	0.35	0.07	0.09	0.79
7	0.24	0.34	0.06	0.04	0.68
8	0.69	0.83	0.15	0.18	1.85
9	0.45	0.58	0.12	0.11	1.27
10	0.29	0.38	0.08	0.09	0.85

Table 3. Example of quantitative data obtained for cystatin C protein variants

4. Further strategies in clinical proteomics

From a diagnostic point of view, it is of great advantage to analyze and assess biological markers of disease from several biological fluids from the same individual. Albeit on a small scale, the results shown here indicate that such studies are possible if the right assays are utilized. The developed MSIA method provides a unique way of delineating protein isoforms and their abundance in serum and CSF. This way, additional population proteomics studies can be done, that will provide with further insight into the physiology of biological processes and diseases. Group protein profiling still remains an irreplaceable method in clinical practice, due to the amount of information that can be provided in a single analysis. When combined with the advanced methods for statistical classification and analysis and using the tools of bioinformatics, analyses at a large scale can be performed. Obtained data can further be used in creating software programs and data bases for recognition and identification of specific protein profiles.

Further analyses regarding our group will progress in several directions: (1) develop quantitative assays for other proteins that are considered to be potential diagnostic markers for specific neurological diseases; (2) implement these assays to fully quantify proteins and protein isoforms in serum and cerebrospinal fluid samples; (3) introduce the concept of immunoaffinity separation techniques into clinical practice (4) develop algorithms for protein profile data base creation and pattern recognition and (5) investigate the possibility to implement the novel methods to analyze proteins using other media such as tears and saliva.

5. Conclusions

Analyzing proteins is a complicated task since many approaches can be followed (Andersson, Alvarez-Cermeno et al. 1994; Anderson and Anderson 1998; Bakhtiar and Nelson 2001; Diamandis 2003; Conrads, Hood et al. 2004; Bons, Wodzig et al. 2005; Anderson 2010). There are two majorly differentiated approaches that can be applied in routine clinical practice, analyzing protein profile (protein profiling) and choosing single protein (biomarker discovery) and optimizing methods for identification and determination. Regarding these remarks, there is a quite divergence between the "group" protein screening and "individual" protein determination. However, by combining different novel techniques we are able to bridge the gap in between. In addition, we can discuss the necessary development both in the methodology and techniques in order to have the highest impact on the study of the molecular composition of CSF proteins.

The application of these novel techniques to the study of neurological disorders is providing an insight into the pathogenesis of neurodegeneration, and is fueling major efforts in biomarker discovery.In the protein profiling concept we are able to analyze patterns obtained from the proteome of a patient with a certain disease, and compare it with a sample from a control group. This approach is still widely used in screening patients with neurological diseases, using electrophoresis techniques as a basic technique. By comparing these profiles, a typical prototype pattern is created for separate conditions, and by simply comparing these patterns (nowadays with the use of informatics tools and statistics programs) differential diagnosis is possible.

This approach, however, only presents the big picture. It is the single protein biomarker assays that are more and more abundant in clinical laboratories. The quest for novel biomarkers results in developing techniques and mechanisms of investigating protein intrinsic characteristics at a molecular level.

From the obtained results we can conclude that even though in routine clinical practice enzymatic immunoassays are still dominant, especially for quantitative protein analysis, they have one crucial disadvantage. These assays are oblivious to protein modifications, unless there is an antibody toward that exact modification. The mass spectrometry immunoassay, on the other hand, is designed to detect protein modifications and intact proteins in a single assay. This qualitative determination is already a way to delineate between control subjects and diseased samples. With the added quantitative feature, this and similar assays are poised to change the way we look proteins and protein modifications and their role in health and disease.

An integrated evaluation of the data that are obtained by all the holistic approaches, in combination with clinical and epidemiological data will eventually not only increase our understanding of disease mechanisms, but subsequently also enable us to develop more specific and individualized medicines and therapies.

All our efforts are oriented toward the main goal - to aid in the process of revealing the protein complexity of neurological disorders and contribute to its better understanding.

6. Acknowledgements

This work was supported in part by Grant No. 094505 from the Ministry of Education and Science of the Republic of Macedonia, and Grant Number 1 R43 RR025701 from the National Center for Research Resources (NCRR), a component of the National Institutes of Health (NIH). Its contents are solely the responsibility of the authors and do not necessarily represent the official views of NCRR or NIH. Support from the Clinic of Neurology and the Department of Clinical Biochemistry, PhD Angel Mitrevski, as well as the CEEPUS program and coordinators at the Department of Physical and Macromolecular Chemistry at the Charles University in Prague are gratefully acknowledged.

7. References

Aebersold, R. and D. R. Goodlett (2001). "Mass spectrometry in proteomics." *Chem Rev* 101(2): 269-95.

Ahmed, F. E. (2008). "Mining the oncoproteome and studying molecular interactions for biomarker development by 2DE, ChIP and SPR technologies." *Expert Rev Proteomics* 5(3): 469-96.

Aizenberg, I., N. Aizenberg, et al. (2001). "Cellular neural networks and computational intelligence in medical image processing." *Immage Vision Comp.* 19: 177-183.

Alban, A., S. O. David, et al. (2003). "A novel experimental design for comparative two-dimensional gel analysis: two-dimensional difference gel electrophoresis incorporating a pooled internal standard." *Proteomics* 3(1): 36-44.

Anderson, N. L. (2010). "The clinical plasma proteome: a survey of clinical assays for proteins in plasma and serum." *Clin Chem* 56(2): 177-85.

Anderson, N. L. and N. G. Anderson (1998). "Proteome and proteomics: new technologies, new concepts, and new words." *Electrophoresis* 19(11): 1853-61.

Anderson, N. L. and N. G. Anderson (2002). "The human plasma proteome: history, character, and diagnostic prospects." *Mol. Cell. Proteomics* 1(11): 845-67.

Andersson, M., J. Alvarez-Cermeno, et al. (1994). "Cerebrospinal fluid in the diagnosis of multiple sclerosis: a consensus report." *J Neurol Neurosurg Psychiatry* 57(8): 897-902.

Auroux, P. A., D. Iossifidis, et al. (2002). "Micro total analysis systems. 2. Analytical standard operations and applications." *Anal Chem* 74(12): 2637-52.

Bakhtiar, R. and R. W. Nelson (2001). "Mass spectrometry of the proteome." *Mol Pharmacol* 60(3): 405-15.

Balslev, S., A. M. Jorgensen, et al. (2006). "Lab-on-a-chip with integrated optical transducers." *Lab Chip* 6(2): 213-7.

Bons, J. A., W. K. Wodzig, et al. (2005). "Protein profiling as a diagnostic tool in clinical chemistry: a review." *Clin Chem Lab Med* 43(12): 1281-90.

Bousse, L., S. Mouradian, et al. (2001). "Protein sizing on a microchip." *Anal Chem* 73(6): 1207-12.

Brody, E. N., L. Gold, et al. (2010). "High-content affinity-based proteomics: unlocking protein biomarker discovery." *Expert Rev Mol Diagn* 10(8): 1013-22.

Calero, M., M. Pawlik, et al. (2001). "Distinct properties of wild-type and the amyloidogenic human cystatin C variant of hereditary cerebral hemorrhage with amyloidosis, Icelandic type." *J Neurochem* 77(2): 628-37.

Chevalier-Larsen, E. and E. L. Holzbaur (2006). "Axonal transport and neurodegenerative disease." *Biochim Biophys Acta* 1762(11-12): 1094-108.

Chiou, S.-H., Wu, S-H. (1999). "Evaluation of commonly used electrophoretic methodds for the analysis of proteins and peptides and their applicaion to biotechnology." *Analytica Chimica Acta* 383: 47-60.

Christodoulides, N., P. N. Floriano, et al. (2007). "Lab-on-a-chip methods for point-of-care measurements of salivary biomarkers of periodontitis." *Ann N Y Acad Sci* 1098: 411-28.

Conrads, T. P., B. L. Hood, et al. (2004). "Proteomic patterns as a diagnostic tool for early-stage cancer: a review of its progress to a clinically relevant tool." *Mol Diagn* 8(2): 77-85.

Craig, W. Y., T. B. Ledue, et al. (2001). *Plasma proteins: Clinical utility and interpretation.* Scarborough, ME, Foundation for Blood Research.

Daskalovska, V. (2000). *Multipla skleroza.* Skopje.

De Vos, K. J., A. J. Grierson, et al. (2008). "Role of axonal transport in neurodegenerative diseases." *Annu Rev Neurosci* 31: 151-73.

Del Boccio, P., D. Pieragostino, et al. (2006). "Cleavage of cystatin C is not associated with multiple sclerosis." *Ann Neurol.*

Diamandis, E. P. (2003). "Point: Proteomic patterns in biological fluids: do they represent the future of cancer diagnostics?" *Clin. Chem.* 49(8): 1272-5.

Dufva, M. and C. B. Christensen (2005). "Diagnostic and analytical applications of protein microarrays." *Expert Rev Proteomics* 2(1): 41-8.

Engvall, E. and P. Perlmann (1971). "Enzyme-linked immunosorbent assay (ELISA). Quantitative assay of immunoglobulin G." *Immunochemistry* 8(9): 871-4.

Engwegen, J. Y., M. C. Gast, et al. (2006). "Clinical proteomics: searching for better tumour markers with SELDI-TOF mass spectrometry." *Trends Pharmacol Sci* 27(5): 251-9.

Erlandsen, E. J., E. Randers, et al. (1998). "Reference intervals for serum cystatin C and serum creatinine in adults." *Clin Chem Lab Med* 36(6): 393-7.

Fenn, J. B., M. Mann, et al. (1989). "Electrospray ionization for mass spectrometry of large biomolecules." *Science* 246(4926): 64-71.

Fishman, R. A. (1992). *Cerebrospinal fluid in diseases of the nervous system*. Philadelphia, W.B.Saunders Corp.

Floriano, P. N., S. Acosta, et al. (2007). "Microchip-based enumeration of human white blood cells." *Methods Mol Biol* 385: 53-64.

Fountoulakis, M. and B. Takacs (1998). "Design of protein purification pathways: application to the proteome of Haemophilus influenzae using heparin chromatography." *Protein Expr Purif* 14(1): 113-9.

Fountoulakis, M., M. F. Takacs, et al. (1999). "Enrichment of low abundance proteins of Escherichia coli by hydroxyapatite chromatography." *Electrophoresis* 20(11): 2181-95.

Geschke, O. (2006). "Miniaturization--not just a matter of size." *Anal Bioanal Chem* 385(8): 1350.

Geschke, O. (2009). "Microfluidics for bioapplications." *Anal Bioanal Chem* 395(3): 619.

Ghiso, J., O. Jensson, et al. (1986). "Amyloid fibrils in hereditary cerebral hemorrhage with amyloidosis of Icelandic type is a variant of gamma-trace basic protein (cystatin C)." *Proc Natl Acad Sci U S A* 83(9): 2974-8.

Grubb, A. O. (2000). "Cystatin C--properties and use as diagnostic marker." *Adv Clin Chem* 35: 63-99.

Gygi, S. P., B. Rist, et al. (1999). "Quantitative analysis of complex protein mixtures using isotope-coded affinity tags." *Nat Biotechnol* 17(10): 994-999.

Han, X., M. Jin, et al. (2006). "Extending top-down mass spectrometry to proteins with masses greater than 200 kilodaltons." *Science* 314(5796): 109-12.

Hansson, S. F., A. Hviid Simonsen, et al. (2006). "Cystatin C in cerebrospinal fluid and multiple sclerosis." *Ann Neurol*.

Hein Nee Maier, K., A. Kohler, et al. (2008). "Biological markers for axonal degeneration in CSF and blood of patients with the first event indicative for multiple sclerosis." *Neurosci Lett* 436(1): 72-6.

Henskens, Y. M., E. C. Veerman, et al. (1996). "Cystatins in health and disease." *Biol. Chem. Hoppe Seyler* 377(2): 71-86.

Hu, Y., X. Huang, et al. (2004). "Recent advances in gel-based proteome profiling techniques." *Mol Biotechnol* 28(1): 63-76.

Irani, D. N., C. Anderson, et al. (2006). "Cleavage of cystatin C in the cerebrospinal fluid of patients with multiple sclerosis." *Ann Neurol* 59(2): 237-47.

Issaq, H. J., T. D. Veenstra, et al. (2002). "The SELDI-TOF MS approach to proteomics: protein profiling and biomarker identification." *Biochem Biophys Res Commun* 292(3): 587-92.

Jarvinen, M., A. Rinne, et al. (1987). "Human cystatins in normal and diseased tissues--a review." *Acta Histochem* 82(1): 5-18.

Jerez-Aragones, J. M. (2003). "A combined neural network and decision trees model for prognosis of breast cancer relapse." *Artf.Intell.Med.* 27: 45-63.

Jin, L. J., B. C. Giordano, et al. (2001). "Dynamic labeling during capillary or microchip electrophoresis for laser-induced fluorescence detection of protein-SDS complexes without pre- or postcolumn labeling." *Anal Chem* 73(20): 4994-9.

Keramas, G., G. Perozziello, et al. (2004). "Development of a multiplex microarray microsystem." *Lab Chip* 4(2): 152-8.

Kiernan, U. A., D. Nedelkov, et al. (2006). "Multiplexed mass spectrometric immunoassay in biomarker research: a novel approach to the determination of a myocardial infarct." *J Proteome Res* 5(11): 2928-34.

Kiernan, U. A., D. Nedelkov, et al. (2006). "High-throughput affinity mass spectrometry." *Methods Mol Biol* 328: 141-50.

Kiernan, U. A., K. A. Tubbs, et al. (2003). "Comparative urine protein phenotyping using mass spectrometric immunoassay." *J. Proteome Res.* 2(2): 191-7.

Krone, J. R., R. W. Nelson, et al. (1996). "Mass spectrometric immunoassay." *SPIE* 2680: 415-421.

Lahm, H. W. and H. Langen (2000). "Mass spectrometry: a tool for the identification of proteins separated by gels." *Electrophoresis* 21(11): 2105-14.

Link, H. and R. Muller (1971). "Immunoglobulins in multiple sclerosis and infections of the nervous system." *Arch Neurol* 25(4): 326-44.

Lisboa, P. J. G. (2002). "A review of evidence of health benefit from artificial neural networks in medical intervention." *Neural.Net.* 15: 11-39.

Maccarrone, G., I. Birg, et al. (2004). "In-depth analysis of the human CSF proteome using protien prefractionaltion." *Clin.Proteomics* 1: 333-364.

Maccarrone, G., D. Milfay, et al. (2004). "Mining the human cerebrospinal fluid proteome by immunodepletion and shotgun mass spectrometry." *Electrophoresis* 25(14): 2402-12.

Mallick, P. and B. Kuster (2010). "Proteomics: a pragmatic perspective." *Nat Biotechnol* 28(7): 695-709.

Manz, A., N. Graber, et al. (1990). "Miniaturized total Chemical Analysis systems: A Novel Concept for Chemical Sensing, Sensors and Actuators." 244-248.

McCudden, C. R., P. M. Voorhees, et al. (2010). "Interference of monoclonal antibody therapies with serum protein electrophoresis tests." *Clin Chem* 56(12): 1897-9.

Mitrevski, A., K. Stojanoski, et al. (2001). "Detection of oligoclonal IgG bands in cerebrospinal fluid on polyacrylamide support media: comparisson of isoelectric focusing and disc electrophoresis." *Acta Pharm.* 51(3): 163-171.

Monteoliva, L. and J. P. Albar (2004). "Differential proteomics: an overview of gel and non-gel based approaches." *Brief Funct Genomic Proteomic* 3(3): 220-39.

Mussap, M. and M. Plebani (2004). "Biochemistry and clinical role of human cystatin C." *Crit Rev Clin Lab Sci* 41(5-6): 467-550.

Nakashima, I., M. Fujinoki, et al. (2006). "Alteration of cystatin C in the cerebrospinal fluid of multiple sclerosis." *Ann Neurol.*

Naruse, H., J. Ishii, et al. (2009). "Cystatin C in acute heart failure without advanced renal impairment." *Am J Med* 122(6): 566-73.

Nedelkov, D. (2005). "Population proteomics: addressing protein diversity in humans." *Expert Rev Proteomics* 2(3): 315-24.

Nedelkov, D. (2006). "Mass spectrometry-based immunoassays for the next phase of clinical applications." *Expert Rev Proteomics* 3(6): 631-40.

Nedelkov, D., S. Shaik, et al. (2008). "Targeted Mass Spectrometric Immunoassay for DEtection of Cystatin C Isoforms in Cerebrospinal Fluid." *The Open Proteomics Journal* 1: 54-58.

Nedelkov, D., K. A. Tubbs, et al. (2004). "High-Throughput Comprehensive Analysis of Human Plasma Proteins: A Step toward Population Proteomics." *Anal. Chem.* 76(6): 1733-7.

Nelson, R. W., J. R. Krone, et al. (1995). "Mass-Spectrometric Immunoassay." *Anal. Chem.* 67(7): 1153-1158.

Nelson, R. W., D. Nedelkov, et al. (2004). "Quantitative mass spectrometric immunoasay of insulin like growth factor 1." *J. Proteome Res.* 3(4): 851-855.

Ocvirk, G., T. Tang, et al. (1998). *Analyst* 123: 1429-1434.

Olafsson, I. and A. Grubb (2000). "Hereditary cystatin C amyloid angiopathy." *Amyloid* 7(1): 70-9.

Ornstein, L. (1964). "Disc Electrophoresis. I. Background and Theory." *Ann N Y Acad Sci* 121: 321-49.

Poon, T. C. W. (2007). "Opportunities and limitations of SELDI-TOF-MS in biomedical research: practical advices." *Expert rev. Proteomics* 4(1): 51-65.

Rabilloud, T. (2002). "Two-dimensional gel electrophoresis in proteomics: old, old fashioned, but it still climbs up the mountains." *Proteomics* 2(1): 3-10.

Randers, E. and E. J. Erlandsen (1999). "Serum cystatin C as an endogenous marker of the renal function--a review." *Clin. Chem. Lab. Med.* 37(4): 389-95.

Randers, E., J. H. Kristensen, et al. (1998). "Serum cystatin C as a marker of the renal function." *Scand J Clin Lab Invest* 58(7): 585-92.

Reed, C. H. (2000). "Diagnostic applications of cystatin C." *Br J Biomed Sci* 57(4): 323-9.

Reiber, H., M. Otto, et al. (2001). "Reporting cerebrospinal fluid data: knowledge base and interpretation software." *Clin Chem Lab Med* 39(4): 324-32.

Reid, G. E. and S. A. McLuckey (2002). "'Top down' protein characterization via tandem mass spectrometry." *J Mass Spectrom* 37(7): 663-75.

Ritchie, R. F., Ed. (1999). *Serum Proteins in Clinical Medicine*. Scarborough, ME, Foundation for Blood Research.

Roos, J. F., J. Doust, et al. (2007). "Diagnostic accuracy of cystatin C compared to serum creatinine for the estimation of renal dysfunction in adults and children--a meta-analysis." *Clin Biochem* 40(5-6): 383-91.

Sandic, C. J. M., P. Monteyne, et al. (1994). "Polyclonal and oligoclonal IgA synthesis in the cerebrospinal fluid of neurological patients.An immunoaffinity-mediated capillary blot study." *J.Neuroimmunol.* 94: 103-111.

Schnittger, S., V. V. Rao, et al. (1993). "Cystatin C (CST3), the candidate gene for hereditary cystatin C amyloid angiopathy (HCCAA), and other members of the cystatin gene family are clustered on chromosome 20p11.2." *Genomics* 16(1): 50-5.

Seronie-Vivien, S., P. Delanaye, et al. (2008). "Cystatin C: current position and future prospects." *Clin Chem Lab Med* 46(12): 1664-86.

Sindic, C. J., M. P. Van Antwerpen, et al. (2001). "The intrathecal humoral immune response: laboratory analysis and clinical relevance." *Clin Chem Lab Med* 39(4): 333-40.

Sloat, A. L., M. G. Roper, et al. (2008). "Protein determination by microchip capillary electrophoresis using an asymmetric squarylium dye: noncovalent labeling and nonequilibrium measurement of association constants." *Electrophoresis* 29(16): 3446-55.

Spirovski, F., K. Stojanoski, et al. (2005). "Comparison of statistical cluster methods in electrophoretic protein pattern analysis." *Acta Pharm* 55(2): 215-22.

Sun, F. and V. Cavalli (2010). "Neuroproteomics approaches to decipher neuronal regeneration and degeneration." *Mol Cell Proteomics* 9(5): 963-75.

Takacs, M., G. Rakhely, et al. (2001). "Molecular characterization and heterologous expression of hypCD, the first two [NiFe] hydrogenase accessory genes of Thermococcus litoralis." *Arch Microbiol* 176(3): 231-5.

Tanaka, K., H. Waki, et al. (1988). "Protein and polymer analyses of up to m/z 100,000 by laser ionization time-of-flight mass spectrometry." *Rapid Commun. Mass Spectrom.* 2: 151-153.

Tourtellote, W. W., A. R. Povin, et al. (1980). "Multiple sclerosis: measurement and validation of central nervous system IgG synthesis rate." *Neurology* 30: 240-244.

Trenchevska, O., Aleksovski, V., Stojanoski, K., (2009) "Advanced techniques in clinical practice: Use of lab-on-a-chip electrophoresis and other methods in protein profiling." *Journal of Medical Biochemistry* 29: 1-5.

Trenchevska, O., Aleksovski, V., Stojanoski, K., (2009) (2009). "Temperature and denaturing substances influence on lab-on-a-chip electrophoresis." *Journal of Medical Biochemistry* 28: 1-5.

Trenchevska, O. and D. Nedelkov (2011). "Targeted quantitative mass spectrometric immunoassay for human protein variants." *Proteome Sci* 9(1): 19.

Turck, C. W., G. Maccarrone, et al. (2005). "The quest for brain disorder biomarkers." *J Med Invest* 52 Suppl: 231-5.

van der Merwe, D. E., K. Oikonomopoulou, et al. (2007). "Mass spectrometry: uncovering the cancer proteome for diagnostics." *Adv Cancer Res* 96: 23-50.

Vesterberg, O. (1989). "History of electrophoretic methods." *J Chromatogr* 480: 3-19.

Vogt, W. and D. Nagel (1992). "Cluster analysis in diagnosis." *Clin Chem* 38(2): 182-98.

W. Bruno, M. D. V., M.S. Abraham Saifer, M. Abraham, M.D. Rabiner, (1956). *A.M.A. Arch. Neurol. Psychiatry,* 75(5): 472-487.

Whitelegge, J., F. Halgand, et al. (2006). "Top-down mass spectrometry of integral membrane proteins." *Expert Rev Proteomics* 3(6): 585-96.

Woolley, A. T. and R. A. Mathies (1994). "Ultra-high-speed DNA fragment separations using microfabricated capillary array electrophoresis chips." *Proc Natl Acad Sci U S A* 91(24): 11348-52.

Yan, W., H. Lee, et al. (2004). "A dataset of human liver proteins identified by protein profiling via isotope-coded affinity tag (ICAT) and tandem mass spectrometry." *Mol. Cell. Proteomics* 3(10): 1039-41.

Yao, S., D. S. Anex, et al. (1999). "SDS capillary gel electrophoresis of proteins in microfabricated channels." *Proc Natl Acad Sci U S A* 96(10): 5372-7.

7

Angelman Syndrome: Proteomics Analysis of an *UBE3A* Knockout Mouse and Its Implications

Low Hai Loon[1], Chi-Fung Jennifer Chen[2], Chi-Chen Kevin Chen, Tew Wai Loon[1], Hew Choy Sin[3] and Ken-Shiung Chen[1,3,*]

[1] *School of Biological Sciences, Nanyang Technological University,*
[2]*University of Texas, Southwestern Medical School, Dallas, TX,*
[3]*Institute of Advanced Studies, Nanyang Technological University*
[1,3]*Singapore*
[2]*USA*

1. Introduction

Angelman syndrome (AS) is a genetic disorder with an incidence of 1 in 15,000, and it was first described in 1965 by Harry Angelman (1,2). It is characterized by a severe developmental delay together with mental disorders, movement disorders and behavioral abnormalities. Early severe epilepsy, sleep alteration, ataxia, important gait, absence of language and craniofacial dysmorphism are phenotypic characteristics used as diagnostic criteria of AS (3).

Several genetic mechanisms are known to associate with the development of Angelman syndrome including the deletion of 4 Mb region in chromosome 15q11-13, uniparental disomy (UPD), imprinting centre defects, and mutation in *UBE3A* (4). The loss of expression of imprinted genes causes multiple human genetic disorders, including AS and Prader-Willi syndrome (PWS). Although these two diseases are associated with the lack of gene expression from the same chromosome 15q11-q13 region, the clinical features of the two disorders are distinct. Deletion or loss of paternally inherited gene expression results in PWS, while loss of maternally inherited gene expression causes AS (4).

Multiple mouse models have been developed for the study of AS (Table 1). The first reported AS mouse model generated was a mouse with paternal UPD for chromosome 7 (5), followed by another mouse model generated by radiation-induced deletion of *p* locus and *Ube3a* (6). However, these two models carried a large deletion of mouse chromosome 7C that could affect multiple loci (1). In the current study, we used a mouse model which carried an exon 2 deletion of the *Ube3a* gene resulting in a shift in the reading frame, thereby inactivating all putative isoforms of Ube3a (7). If the offspring mice inherited the mutated *Ube3a* allele of maternal origin, the mice will have no Ube3a expression in the cerebellum, Purkinje cells and hippocampus, as *Ube3a* on the paternal chromosome is silenced by genomic imprinting. This mouse model exhibits symptoms similar to that of Angelman syndrome patients, including motor dysfunction, seizures, context-dependant learning deficiency and severely impaired long-term potentiation (LTP) (7).

*Corresponding author

Several proteins that are involved in REDOX (oxidation-reduction reactions) were identified in the 2-D DIGE, including LDH, MDH, GSTs-Mu1, SOD2, and ATP5a1. The result suggested that loss of Ube3a may lead to mitochondrial dysfunction. In addition, the accumulation of Chaperone protein Hsp70 was observed and mRNA levels remained unchanged, suggesting that Hsp70 might be a substrate of Ube3a. Furthermore, NSF, which is known to be involved in neuronal signal transmission, was reduced at protein levels but unaffected at mRNA levels. Finally, CaBP is responsible for binding free calcium ions and may play an inductive role in seizures observed in AS mouse models and patients. TPI1, Triosephosphate isomerase 1, is one of the key enzymes in the glycolysis pathway, while CFL1, Cofilin 1, is known to be a potent regulator of actin filament dynamics. It remains to be determined how differential expression of these proteins may contribute to the development of AS.

	Mutation	Phenotype	Reference
1	*Ube3a* exon 2 deletion	AS	(7)
2	LacZ insertion inactivation of *Ube3a*	AS	(8)
3	insertion/duplication located 13 kb upstream of Snrpn exon 1	AS imprinting mutation	(9)
4	80-kb deletion located upstream of Snrpn exon 1	AS imprinting mutation	(9)
5	*Ube3a-Gabrb3 –Atp10a* deletion	AS	(10)
6	Replacement of mouse PWS-IC with human PWS-IC	PWS and AS imprinting mutation	(11)
7	UPD	AS	(5)
8	GABRB3 inactivation	Some clinical features of AS; 90% of $\beta 3^{-/-}$ mice die within 24 h of birth, survived mice exhibit hyperactive, epileptic seizures, neurological impairments	(12)
9	Transgenic insertion induced deletion; *Zfp127-Herc2* deletion	PWS/AS	(13)

Table 1. Angelman syndrome mouse models

2. Materials and methods

2.1 Protein extraction

Tissue was homogenized in extraction buffer containing 7 M Urea (Cat. No. U5128, Sigma), 2 M Thiourea (Cat. No. RPN 6301, Amersham), 30 mM Tris (Cat. No. 75825, USB), 4% CHAPS (Cat. No. 13361, USB), adjusted to pH 8.5 with HCl. Complete protease inhibitor cocktail (Cat. No. 1697498, Roche) and nuclease mix (Cat. No. 80-6501-42, Amersham) were added into extraction buffer before use. Tissue was homogenized with 3-s pulses followed by 5-s of cooling on ice between the pulses, until no visible tissue could be observed. The homogenized sample was then transferred to the centrifuge tube and centrifuged at 20,000 x g for 20 min. The supernatant was transferred into a new centrifuge tube and centrifuged for another 20 min at 20,000 x g. The supernatant was then aliquoted and stored at -80ºC. The protein concentration was determined by using Bio-Rad protein assay (Cat. No. 500-0002, Bio-Rad) based on Bradford's method according to the manufacturer's protocol.

2.2 CyDye labelling

Cy2 minimal dye, Cy3 minimal dye, Cy5 minimal dye (Cat. No. 25-8008-60, Cat. No. 25-8008-61, Cat. No. 25-8008-62, Amersham) are the three cyanine dyes used in the experiment. CyDye was reconstituted by using N-N-Dimethylformamide (Cat. No. 22,705-6, Aldrich). 400 pmol of CyDye was used to label 50 µg of protein as recommended by the manufacturer. The labelling reaction was performed on ice for 30 min, quenched with 1 µl of 10 mM lysine (Cat. No. L5501, Sigma) and incubated on ice for 10 min. Cy2 was always used to label the internal control as recommended by the manufacturer. Alternative use of Cy3 and Cy5 for the labelling of wild type and diseased samples prevented labelling bias. In the labelling reaction, the ratio of "dye: protein" was kept low to ensure optimal labelling efficiency.

2.3 1-D isoelectric focusing

Immobiline™ Dry strip, pH 3-11NL, 24 cm strip (Cat. No. 17-6003-77, Amersham) was used for the isoelectric focusing. The strip was rehydrated using rehydration buffer containing 8 M Urea, 4% CHAPS, 1% Pharmalyte 3-11 (Cat. No. 17-6004-40, Amersham), 13 mM DTT (Cat. No. 17-1318-02, Amersham), Destreak solution (Cat. No. 71-5025-39 Amersham). Rehydration was done for 16-18 hr. The rehydrated strip was then transferred to a strip holder and placed on the IPGphor (Cat. No. 80-6414-02, Amersham) that was used for isoelectic focusing. The protein lysate was then applied to the strip by cup loading method, and an equal volume of sample buffer (8 M Urea, 130 mM DTT, 4% CHAPS, 2% Pharmalyte 3-11) was added into the labelled protein sample. The protein was focused on 200 Vhr for each 10 µl of sample applied, followed by 500 Vhr, 1000 Vhr, 1000-8000 V gradient increment for 1hr, and 8000 V for 32,000 Vhr. The strip was equilibrated before it was applied to the 2D electrophoresis unit, first with DTT (Cat. No. 17-1318-02, Amersham) in 10 ml equilibration buffer (6 M Urea, 50 mM Tris-Cl, 30% glycerol, 2% SDS, Bromophenol blue; Glycerol Cat. No. 16374, USB) for 20 min and followed with IAA (Cat. No. RPN 6302, Amersham) for another 20 min.

2.4 2-D gel electrophoresis

The equilibrated strip was transferred to SDS-PAGE and sealed with 1% agarose sealing solution with bromophenol blue (Cat. No. 12370, USB) as trace dye. Gel electrophoresis was performed on 12% acrylamide SDS-PAGE (40% stock, Cat. No. 17-1310-01, Amersham) casted one night before usage, in 2X SDS running buffer (50 mM Tris, 384 mM Glycine, 0.4% SDS; Glycine Cat. No. 161-0718 Bio-Rad, SDS Cat. No. 75819, USB) at 15ºC. 5 W per gel was applied for protein entry, and 10 W per gel for protein separation. The electrophoresis run was stopped when the dye front reached the bottom of the gel. The electrophoresis run was performed on Ettan DALT *six* system (Cat. No. 80-6485-27, Amersham). The 2-D spot pattern comparison was then made by using Decyder software (Amersham) to figure out protein candidates with significant different steady state levels and those differences in expression were consistent in all 2-D DIGE sample analyzed.

2.5 Silver staining proteins visualization

The acrylamide gel was fixed in 50% Methanol (Cat. No. A-454-4, Fisher), 12% Acetic acid (Cat. No. 1.00063.2511, Merck) overnight with mild shaking. The silver staining was performed using Silver Stain Plus kit (Cat. No. 161-0449, Bio-Rad) according to manufacturer's protocol. The stained gel was then stored in 1% acetic acid solution.

2.6 MALDI-TOF protein identification

Stained gel spots were excised by scalpels and cut into 1 mm^3 cubes. Silver stained gel spots were then destained by using 100 mM Sodium Thiosulfate (Cat. No. A3525, Applichem) and 30 mM Potassium Ferricyanide (III) (Cat. No. 24.402-3, Aldrich) with gentle vortexing. The gel spots were then washed with double distilled water and equilibrated with 100 mM Ammonium Bicarbonate (Cat. No. A6141, Sigma). Gel spots were then dehydrated in Acetonitrile (Cat. No. 34967, Riedel-de Haën). DTT and IAA were added respectively into dehydrated gel spots. The gel spots were then dehydrated again with acetonitrile before 10 ng/µl Trypsin (Cat. No. V5280, Promega) was added for digestion overnight at 37°C. Peptides were extracted using 50% ACN/5% Trifluoroacetic Acid (TFA). The peptides were then dried using vacuum dry method and cleaned with ZipTip® C_{18} (Cat. No. ZTC 18S 096, Millipore) according to manufacturer's instruction.

2.7 Mouse genomic DNA extraction

Mouse tail was cut and digested in 495 µl NTES buffer (50 mM Tris-Cl, 50 mM EDTA, 100 mM NaCl, 5 mM DTT, 0.5 mM spermidine and 2% SDS) and 5 µl of proteinase K (Cat. No. 13215100, Roche) overnight at 55°C in a rotary oven. The next day, equilibrated phenol (Cat. No. C2432, Sigma), phenol:chloroform:isomyl alcohol (Cat. No. 75831, USB) and chloroform (Cat. No. 75829, USB) were sequentially used for purification of protein from DNA extract. The genomic DNA was then precipitated by isopropyl alcohol (Cat. No. A415-4, Fisher) and dissolved in TE buffer.

2.8 Mouse genotyping

Three primers named oIMR1965, oIMR1966 and oIMR1967 were used to determine the genotype of the mouse. Primer oIMR1965 was the common primer; when it paired with primer oIMR1966, a 700 bp fragment from the wild type allele would be amplified. On the other hand, when primer oIMR1965 paired with primer oIMR1967, a 320 bp fragment from mutant allele would be amplified. The PCR cycling condition was heat activation at 95°C for 3 min, followed by 40 cycles of 95°C for 30 s, 67°C for 1 min and 72°C for 1 min; the final extension step was done at 72°C for 2 min. The PCR product was analyzed by electrophoresis on 1.5% agarose gel.

2.9 Real time RT-PCR

The reaction was performed using iTaq™ SYBR® Green Supermix with ROX (Cat. No. 172-5850, Bio-Rad) containing 2X reaction buffer, 0.4 mM dATP, 0.4 mM dCTP, 0.4 mM dGTP, 0.8 mM dUTP, iTaq DNA polymerase, 6 mM Mg^{+2}, SYBR Green I dye, 1 µM ROX internal reference dye and stabilizers. Reaction volume used was 25 µl, including 12.5 µl of 2X SYBR® Green Supermix, 1 µl of synthesized cDNA, 1 µl of 10 µM forward primer, 1 µl of 10 µM reverse primer [Table 2], topping up with nuclease free water.

Cycling was performed on 7500 Real Time RT-PCR system (Applied Biosystem). Cycling conditions were machine warm up at 50°C for 2 min, hot initiation at 95°C for 10 min, cycling condition (45 cycles) of 95°C for 30 s, 60°C for 30 s and 72°C for 2 min, followed by a dissociation stage to generate a melting curve. ΔΔCT method was employed to calculate the differential expression of mRNA in samples examined, by comparing cycling results between target gene and basal control Glyceraldehyde-3-phosphate dehydrogenase (GADPH).

Name	Sequence
HSP70	Sense: 5'-AAG AAC GCG CTC GAG TCC TAT GC-3' Anti-sense: 5'-CAC CCT GGT ACA GCC CAC TGA TGA T-3'
CaBP	Sense: 5'-GAT GGC AAC GGA TAC ATA GAT GAA-3' Anti-sense: 5'-TCC ATC CGA CAA GGC CAT TAT GTT C-3'
GADPH	Sense: 5'-AGT CTA CTG GTG TCT TCA CCA CCA TGG-3' Anti-sense: 5'-TTC TCG TGG TTA ACA CCC ATC AC-3'
VDR	Sense: 5'-AGG TGC AGC GTA AGC GAG AGA T-3' Anti-sense: 5'-CCT CAA TGG CAC TTG ACT TAA GC-3'
NeuroD	Sense: 5'-CTC AGT TCT CAG GAC GAG GA-3' Anti-sense: 5'-TAG TTC TTG GCC AAG CGC AG-3'
Pax6	Sense: 5'-AGT CAC AGC GGA GTG AAT CAG-3' Anti-sense: 5'-AGC CAG GTT GCG AAG AAC-3'
Mash1	Sense: 5'-AGC AGC TGC GGA CGA GCA-3' Anti-sense: 5'-CCT GCT TCC AAA GTC CAT TC-3'
LDH	Sense: 5′-AGC AAA GAC TAC TGT GTA ACT GCG A-3′ Anti-sense: 5′-ACC TCG TAG GCA CTG TCC AC-3′
MDH	Sense: 5′-AGG CTA CCT TGG ACC GGA GCA GTT-3′ Anti-sense: 5′-GTG GCA GAA CCT GCT CCA GCC TT-3′
Glutathione S-Transferase Mu1	Sense: 5′-TGA CGC TCC CGA CTT TGA CAG AA-3′ Anti-sense: 5′-TAA GCA AGG AAA TCC ACA TAG GTG-3′
ATP synthase 5a1	Sense: 5′-AGA AGA CTG GCA CAG CTG AGA TGT-3′ Anti-sense: 5′-CCA GTC TGT CTG TCA CCA AT-3′
SOD2	Sense: 5′-ATG AAA GCC ATC TGC ATC ATT AGC-3′ Anti-sense: 5′-GCA ATT ATT CCG CAT CCC AAA CG-3′
NSF	Sense: 5'- TGG GGC AGC AGC TTG TCT TTA -3' Anti-sense: 5'- TTA GCA CCA AGC CTC CTT TGC -3'

Table 2. Primer sequences used in Real Time RT-PCR analysis:

2.10 Western blot analysis

Protein homogenates were heated in Laemmli sample buffer (Cat. No. 161-0737, Bio-Rad), at 95°C for 10 min. The heated samples were resolved on 12% SDS-PAGE gel and transferred to Immun-Blot PVDF membrane (Cat. No. 162-0177, Bio-Rad) at 100 V for at least 1 hr. The membrane was then blocked with 5% non-fat milk in 0.1% T-TBS (10 mM Tris-Cl, pH 7.5, 150 mM NaCl and 0.1% Tween-20; NaCl Cat. No. 1.06404, Merck, Tween-20 Cat. No. 161-0781, Bio-Rad) for 1 hr at RT. The membrane was then washed three times in 0.1% T-TBS, followed by incubation with primary antibody [Table 3] for 1 hr. The membrane was then washed again three times in 0.1% T-TBS and incubated for 1 hr with HRP conjugated secondary antibody. The membrane was then washed again three times in 0.1% T-TBS before being developed by ECL method (Cat. No. RPN 2108, ECL Western blotting analysis system, Amersham). The blot was stripped with 0.1% T-TBS overnight on an orbital shaker for second antibody detection. The intensity of protein bands detected by Western blot analysis was determined by calibrated densitometer GS-800 and Quantity One 1-D analysis software (Cat. No. 170-7983, Bio-Rad).

Antibody name	Dilution factors used in experiment
Anti-E6AP (Cat. No. A300-352A, Bethyl)	1:2500-5000
Anti Calbindin D-28k (Cat. No. AB1778, Chemicon)	1:2500-5000
Anti-Actin (Cat. No. MAB1501, Chemicon)	1:1000-2500
Secondary HRP conjugated anti-mouse/anti-rabbit (GE Healthcare)	1:2500-5000
Anti-Hsp70 (Cat. No. sc32239 , Santa Cruz)	1:2500-5000
Anti-SOD2 (Cat. No. sc-30080, Santa Cruz)	1:2500-5000
Anti-NSF (Cat. No. ab16681, abcam)	1:10000
Anti-Mash1 (Cat. No. AB155582, Chemicon)	1:2500-5000
Anti-NeuroD (Cat. No. AB155580, Chemicon)	1:2500-5000

Table 3. Antibodies used in experiments

3. Results

In this project, the effects of the loss of UBE3A proteins were investigated using *Ube3a* knockout mice. Two-D DIGE method [Figure 1] was used to identify candidate substrates of Ube3a in the cerebellum and hippocampus; a total of 94 proteins and 74 proteins were initially found differentially expressed in the cerebellum or hippocampus of the *Ube3a* knockout mice, respectively. Next, the protein candidates were tested with the following filtering criteria: 1) proteins appeared in all 2-D DIGE runs examined and 2) the one-way Analysis of Variance (ANOVA) compared protein expression level between the wild type and AS mice indicating the difference is statistically significant. The differentially expressed proteins were then identified by MALDI-TOF with a threshold score of 63. A total of 10 proteins that were successfully identified and fulfilled the filtering criteria are listed in Table 4. An additional 4

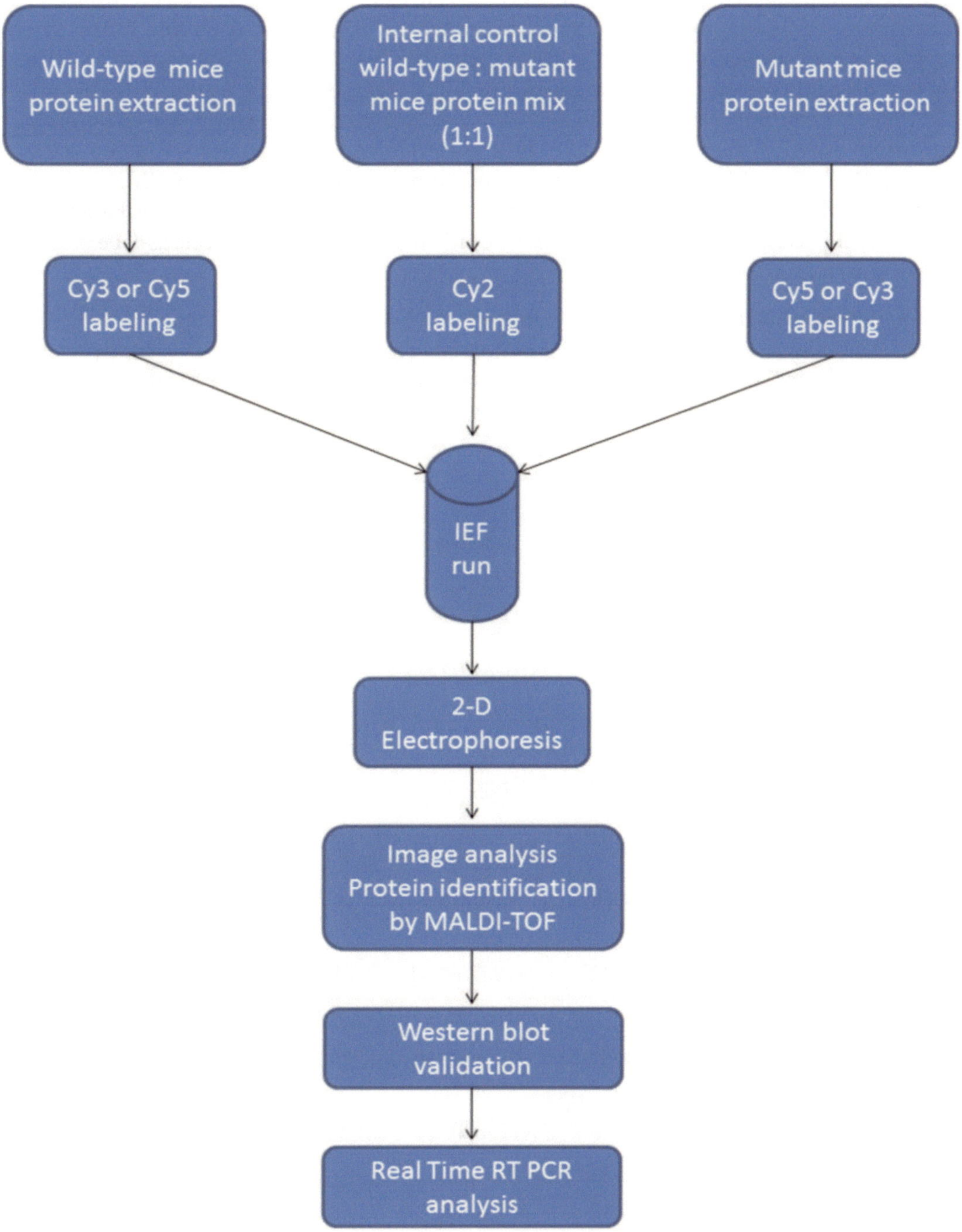

Fig. 1. Work flow of project

proteins, including Mash1, NeuroD, Pax6 and VDR, were not detected in 2-D DIGE runs but were investigated in this project due to the fact that these proteins were shown to be highly associated with one of the proteins identified in this project, CaBP (14). Differentially expressed proteins identified by the 2-D DIGE could be due to the direct, indirect or both direct and indirect effects from the loss of Ube3a expression. Ube3a is known to be involved in proteasome-dependent as well as proteasome-independent functions. Therefore, Western blot analysis was performed to verify the differentially expressed proteins identified by 2-D DIGE analysis and further studied at the mRNA level by Real-Time RT-PCR. It helps to understand that these protein candidates may be affected at the protein level due to impaired protein degradation mechanism (4). Alternatively, these proteins may be affected at the transcriptional level, as Ube3a is also involved in transcriptional regulation (15).

By comparing protein samples from wild type mice and AS mice in the 2-D DIGE study, protein candidates that showed differential expression were found and identified by the MALDI-TOF method. Western blot was then employed to confirm the differential expression observed in 2-D DIGE. Real time RT-PCR was used to detect any differences at the transcriptional level in the protein candidates identified.

Protein identified by MALDI-TOF	pI	Molecular Weight	Accession number	Sequence coverage %	Score	Function
CABP	4.82	25943	P12658	50%	375	Calcium ion buffer
HSP70	5.52	70079	NP_034609.2	24%	358	Protein folding and degradation
SOD2	8.80	24602	P09671	30%	219	REDOX
LDH	7.61	36498	P06151	7%	134	REDOX
MDH	6.16	36477	gi|92087001	30%	365	REDOX
GSTs-Mu1	7.72	25969	P10649	35%	319	REDOX
NSF	6.52	82613	gi|29789104	29%	162	Docking and fusion of synaptic vesicles
ATP5a1	9.22	59752	gi|6680748	49%	436	ATP synthesis
Cofilin 1, non muscle	8.22	18776	gi|6680924	22%	116	Disassembles actin filaments
TPI1 (Triosephosphate isomerase 1)	6.90	27038	gi|6678413	56%	489	Glycolysis, energy production

Table 4. Differentially expressed proteins detected by 2-D DIGE

3.1 2-D DIGE and silver staining

After the Decyder software analysis was performed by using analytical gel (CyDye labelled), another set of protein electrophoresis (preparative gel) were performed using 600 µg of unlabelled protein sample. The protein samples used in the preparative gel were the same as those used for 2-D DIGE analysis. After electrophoresis, silver staining was conducted to visualize protein spots on the gel. Typically, 800-1000 protein spots were visualized on each gel [Figure 2].

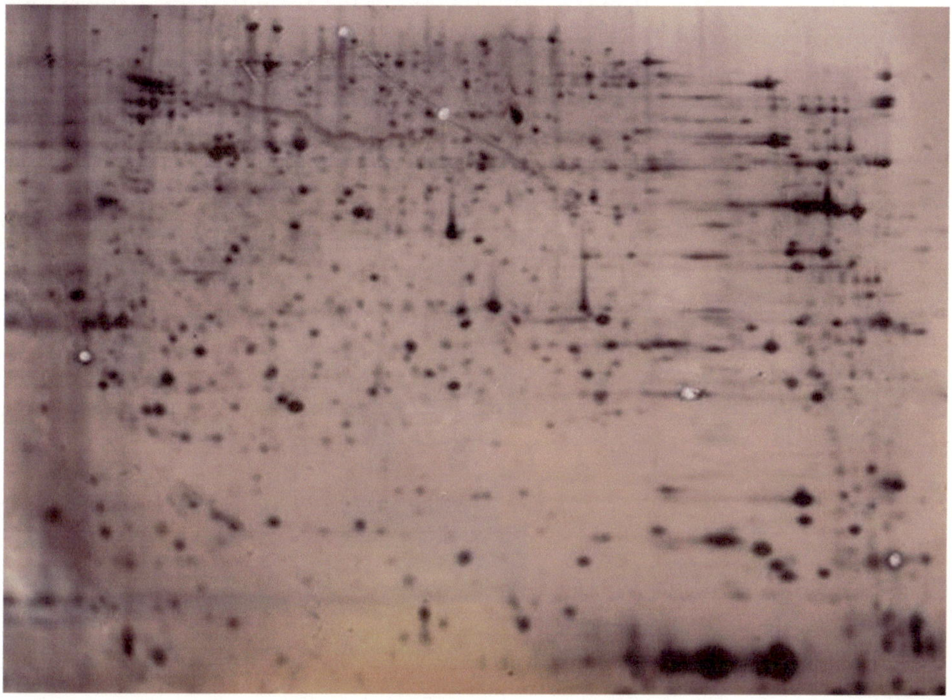

Fig. 2. Silver staining of acrylamide gel after SDS-electrophoresis
Protein extract (600 µg) from cerebellum was loaded in a first dimension IPG strip (pH3-11, NL, 24 cm; Running time: 15.5 hr, approx 47 kVh) and resolved in 12.5% acrylamide gel (Running time: 5.15 hr, 10 W per gel). Proteins were visualized by silver staining. These gels are called preparative gels, and they contain more protein content to allow for subsequent analyses including silver staining and MALDI-TOF. CyDye labelled proteins were run on analytical gels which are scanned by lasers and thus do not require a high quantity of proteins.

3.2 Detection and identification of differentially expressed protein in AS versus wild type brain tissue

A total of ten differentially expressed proteins were detected by using 2-D DIGE from protein samples extracted from the cerebellum or hippocampus of wild type mice and AS mice (*Ube3a* knockout). The protein spots were recovered from silver-stained acrylamide gels run in parallel, and identification was made based on the protein profile generated by MALDI-TOF [Figure 3] with a threshold score of 63. All candidates were confirmed at least twice in separate 2-D DIGE runs and MALDI-TOF identification. Another four bHLH proteins, including Mash1, NeuroD, Pax6 and VDR, were also studied in this project, as the proteins are highly related to CaBP (14).

A total of eight proteins studied are involved in REDOX reactions, including HSP70, SOD2, MDH, LDH, VDR, GSTs-Mu1, ATP5a1 and CaBP. Four of the bHLH proteins, VDR, Pax6, Mash1 and NeuroD are involved in neuronal cell differentiation, while NSF is crucial in synaptic vesicle transmission and learning processes that are controlled by the hippocampus [Figure 4]. TPI1 is involved in energy production, while Cofilin 1 is involved in actin disassembly and may also be involved in neuronal signal transduction.

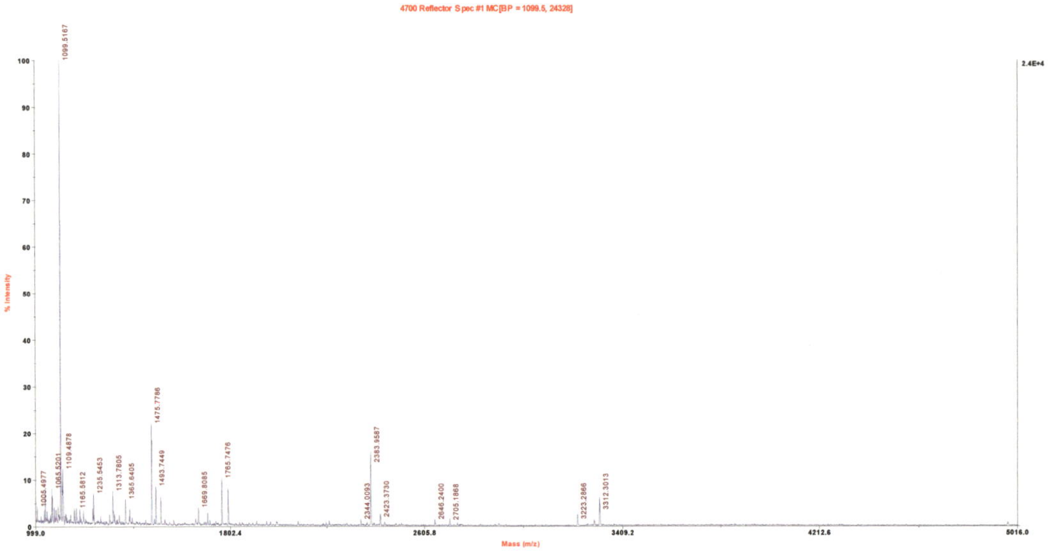

Fig. 3. Protein identification by MALDI-TOF
MS spectrum for one of the proteins identified- CaBP. After peptide detection, the peptide profile was used to match the NCBI database for protein identification.

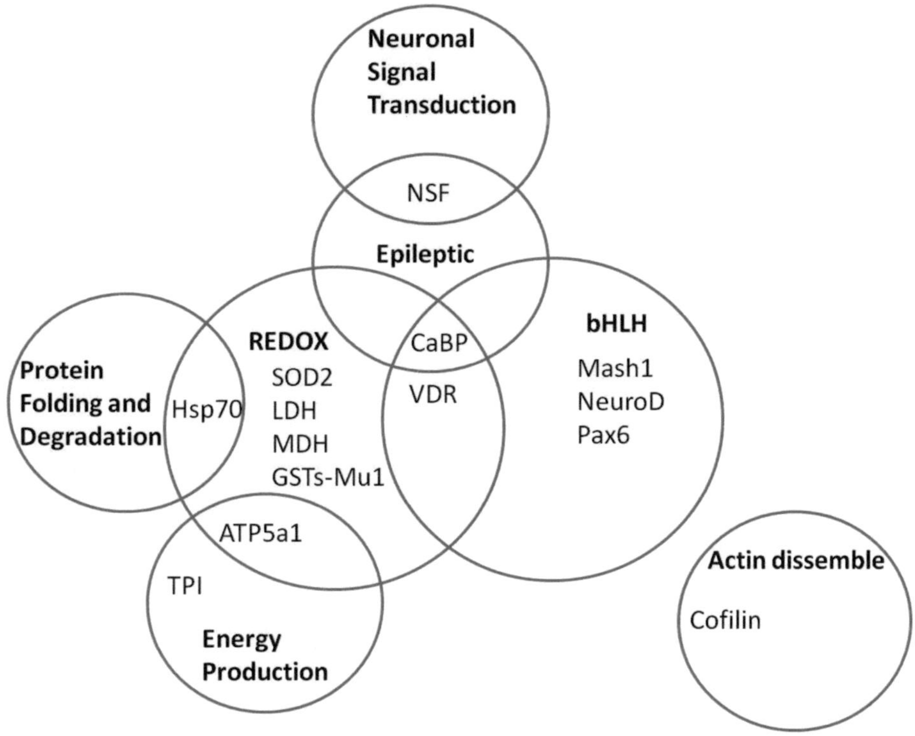

Fig. 4. 2-D DIGE results and inter-connected functions of the identified proteins. This figure shows differentially expressed proteins categorized by their functions. Some proteins are known to be involved in multiple pathways and functions.

3.3 Validation of 2-D DIGE/MS results by Western blot analysis

Western blot was conducted to validate the differentially expressed proteins that were identified in 2-D DIGE/MS. In the cerebellum, three proteins, including SOD2, CaBP and Mash1, were down-regulated in Ube3a knockout mice [Figure 5], while Hsp70, NSF and NeuroD were accumulated in knockout mice [Figure 6]. However, SOD2, Mash1, CaBP, NeuroD and NSF were down-regulated [Figure 7] and HSP70 was accumulated [Figure 8] in the hippocampus of *Ube3a* knockout mice. The Western blots were repeated at least three times by using different sets of cerebellum and hippocampus tissues [Figures 5-8].

In the cerebellum, Hsp70 was found to be up-regulated by approximately 120% based on the densitometer scan results. NSF and NeuroD were up-regulated by 85% and 50%, respectively. SOD2 was down-regulated by 45% in the cerebellum of *Ube3a* knockout mice. Based on densitometer scan results, CaBP and Mash1 were both found to be reduced by approximately 75% in defective mice.

In the hippocampus, Hsp70 was increased by 50% when samples from wild type mice were compared to defective mice. SOD2 and Mash1 were both reduced by approximately 80% in *Ube3a* knockout mice; CaBP and NeuroD were found down-regulated by 40% and 45%, respectively, when compared to the wild type sample. Lastly, NSF was reduced by nearly 50% in *Ube3a* knockout mice.

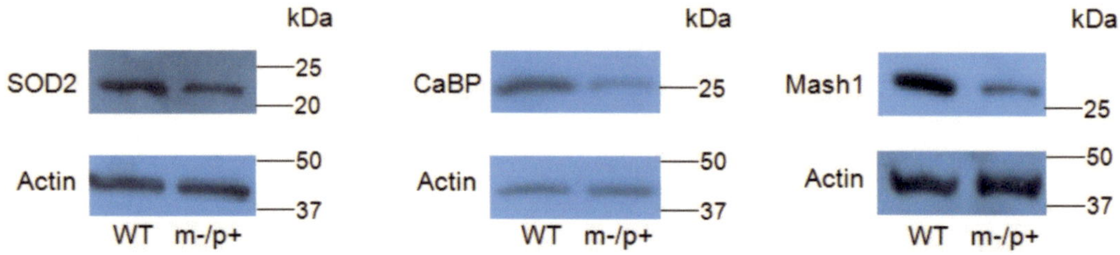

Fig. 5. Validation of down-regulation of SOD2, CaBP and Mash1 in the cerebellum of *Ube3a* knockout mice. SOD2, CaBP and Mash1 are down-regulated in AS mouse model. Antibody dilution factor used for Western blotting were- SOD2, 1:5000; CaBP, 1:5000; Mash1, 1:5000.

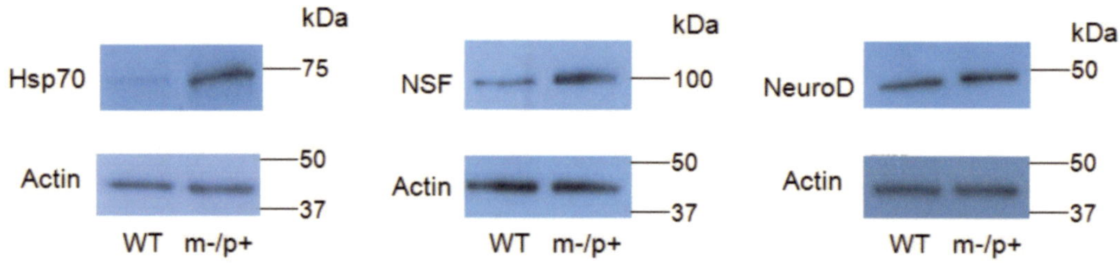

Fig. 6. Validation of proteins accumulated in the cerebellum of *Ube3a* knockout mice. Three proteins, including HSP70, NSF and NeuroD, are accumulated in AS mice. Antibody dilution factors used for Western blotting were- HSP70, 1:5000; NSF, 1:5000; and NeuroD, 1:5000.

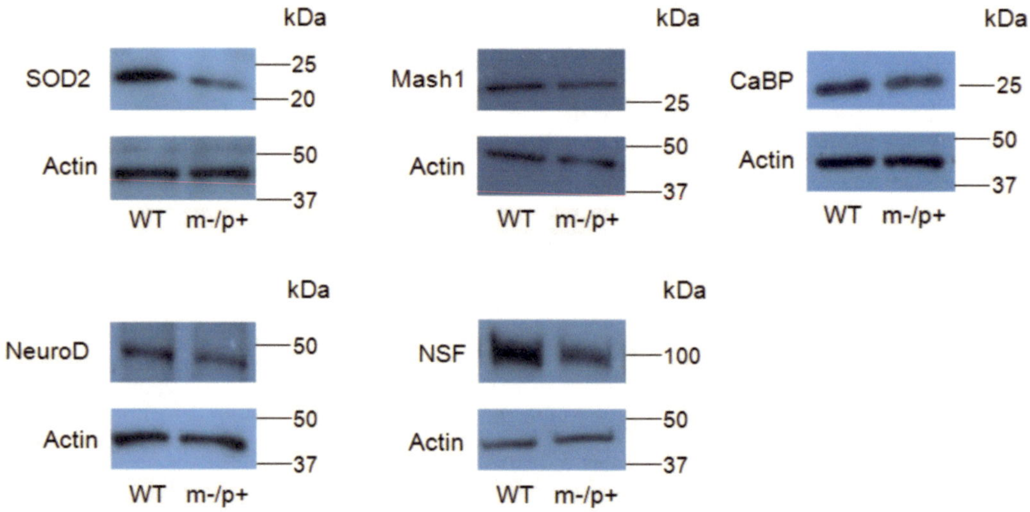

Fig. 7. Validation of down-regulated proteins in the hippocampus of *Ube3a* knockout mice. Five proteins, including SOD2, Mash1, CaBP, NeuroD and NSF, are down-regulated in AS mice. Antibody dilution factors used for Western blotting were-SOD2, 1:5000; Mash1, 1: NSF, 1:5000; NeuroD, 1:2500.

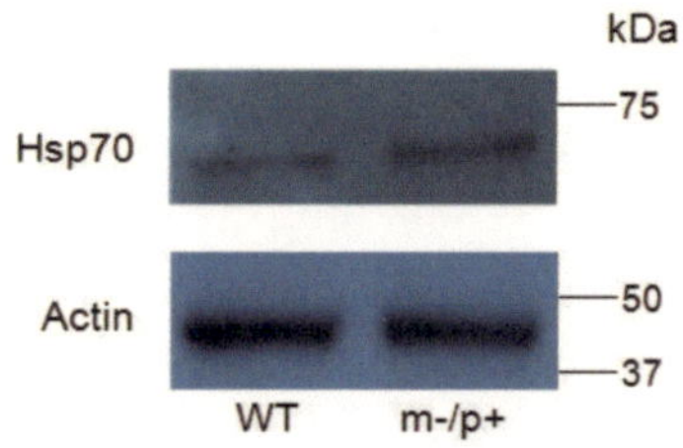

Fig. 8. Validation of Hsp70 accumulation in the hippocampus of *Ube3a* knockout mice. Hsp70 showed accumulation in AS mice among protein candidates detected by 2-D DIGE/MS. Antibody dilution factor used for Western blotting was- HSP70, 1:5000.

The major differences in the Western blot validation are the differential expressions of NeuroD and NSF in these two tissues. These two proteins were found to be up-regulated in the cerebellum but down-regulated in the hippocampus [Figure 9]. This suggests that the expression of these two proteins might be tissue specific. Western blot analysis for protein candidates VDR, LDH, MDH, GSTs-Mu1 and ATP5a1 has not been conducted due to the unavailability of antibodies when this study was conducted.

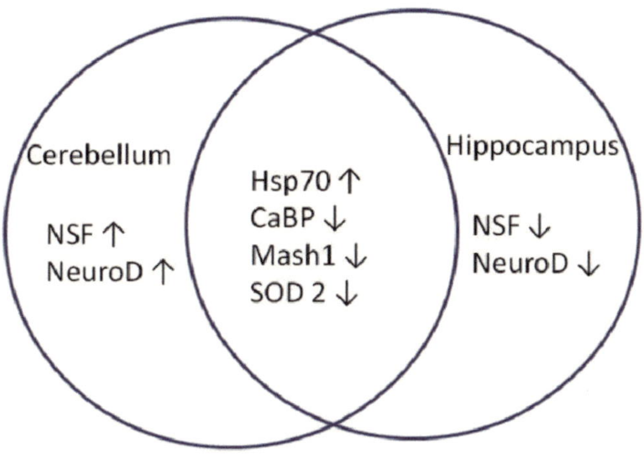

Fig. 9. A summary of the validation of 2-D DIGE/MS results by Western blot analysis. A total of 6 proteins from the cerebellum and hippocampus were tested by Western blot. Three of them, including CaBP, Nash1 and SOD2, were down-regulated and one (Hsp70) was up-regulated in both tissues, while both NSF and NeuroD showed tissue-specific expression patterns.

3.4 Transcriptional analysis of the differentially expressed proteins verified by Western blot analysis

Since variation of steady state protein level between wild type and mutant mice can be caused by enhancing transcriptional activity instead of enhancing protein half life, Real Time RT-PCR was conducted to quantify mRNA levels of proteins detected by 2-D DIGE. mRNA extracted from the cerebellum and hippocampus of wild type mice as well as *Ube3a* knockout mice were used in this study. Real Time RT-PCR was conducted at least three times for individual sets of mice. The Student's T-test was applied for this study.

Based on results of Real Time RT-PCR obtained from the cerebellum sample [Table 5], mRNA levels of *CaBP, NeuroD* and *VDR* were down-regulated by 57%, 33% and 55%, respectively. The mRNA levels of other proteins, including *Hsp70, SOD2, Mash1, Pax6, NSF, ATP5a1, LDH, MDH* and *Glutathione S-transferase Mu1,*were not affected in the AS mouse. Real Time RT-PCR revealed that mRNA levels of *CaBP, NeuroD, Pax6, VDR* and *LDH* were down-regulated in the hippocampus of *Ube3a* knockout mice by 80%, 85%, 82%, 72% and 45%, respectively, while the mRNA level of *Glutathione S-transferase Mu1* was up-regulated by 107% [Table 5]. In contrast, mRNA levels of *MDH, ATP5a1, NSF, Mash1, SOD2* and *Hsp70* were not affected in the hippocampus of *Ube3a* knockout mice.

Cerebellum		
Percentage changes (protein level)	Candidates	Percentage changes (mRNA level)
75% ↓	CaBP	57% ↓
75% ↓	Mash1	6% -
45% ↓	SOD2	13% -
120% ↑	HSP70	17% -
50% ↑	NeuroD	33% ↓
85% ↑	NSF	2% -
n/a	LDH	17% -
n/a	MDH	15% -
n/a	GSTs-Mu1	1% -
n/a	VDR	55% ↓
n/a	ATP5a1	12% -
n/a	Pax6	21% -
Hippocampus		
Percentage changes (protein level)	Candidates	Percentage changes (mRNA level)
40% ↓	CaBP	80% ↓
80% ↓	Mash1	12% -
80% ↓	SOD2	22% -
50% ↑	HSP70	25% -
45% ↓	NeuroD	85% ↓
50% ↓	NSF	6% -
n/a	LDH	45% ↓
n/a	MDH	14% -
n/a	GSTs-Mu1	107% ↑
n/a	VDR	72% ↓
n/a	ATP5a1	15% -
n/a	Pax6	82% ↓

Table 5. A summary of Western blot validation and Real Time RT-PCR analysis of candidates tested in the cerebellum and hippocampus of *Ube3a* knockout mice.

4. Discussion

When Ube3a was first identified as an E3 ligase, little was known about its targeting substrates besides p53 (1). However, as techniques improved over the years, additional substrates of Ube3a were identified [Table 6].

	Gene / Protein	Function	Reference
1	Src Family of Tyrosine Kinase Blk	Regulators of cytoskeletal organization, cell-cell contact, cell-matrix adhesion, DNA synthesis, cellular proliferation	(16)
2	Cystic fibrosis transmembrane regulator-associated ligand (CAL)	Facilitate of lysosomal degradation of other proteins, intracellular trafficking, autophagy of neuronal cells, vesicular trafficking pathways	(17)
3	Trihydrophobin 1 (TH1)	Assembly of functional human negative transcription elongation factor (NELF) complex	(18)
4	Epithelial call transforming sequence 2 oncogene (ECT2)	Cytokinesis, cytoskeletal remodelling in response to neurite guidance cues	(19)
5	Polyglutamine aggregation	Protein aggregation associated to cell death and neurodegenerative diseases	(20-22)

Table 6. Recently identified substrates of Ube3a

Among these proteins, Blk, from the tightly regulated Src family of non-receptor tyrosine kinase, is important in cytoskeletal organization, cell-cell contact, and cell-matrix adhesion; a few other proteins from the Src family are also interacting partners of Ube3a (16). Cystic fibrosis transmembrane regulator-associated ligands (CAL), which serve as membrane-associated scaffolds, are involved in the targeting of other plasma membrane proteins and autophagy in neuronal cells (17). Trihydrophobin 1 (TH1) is another interacting partner and target of Ube3a that was recently identified; it is an integral subunit of the human negative transcription elongation factor (NELF) complex, which is important in transcriptional pausing *in vitro* (18). ECT2 is involved in cytokinesis and cytoskeletal remodelling in response to all known neurite guidance cues (19). Its dysregulation may explain the general learning and behaviour defects in AS patients (4). Polyglutamine inclusion, which is translated from the expansion of a CAG trinucleotide repeat, causes several human neurodegenerative diseases, including spino-bulbar muscular atrophy (SBMA), Huntington's disease (HD) and the spinocerebellar ataxias (20-22).

In this study, we intended to examine the differential expression of proteins caused by the knockout of *Ube3a* in the AS model. By 2-D DIGE/MS, we identified proteins that are differentially expressed in the mutant mice, which may serve as the target substrates of Ube3a. The accumulation or reduction of these proteins may correlate with the phenotypes observed among AS patients.

From our 2-D DIGE/MS experiment and Western blot analysis using cerebellum [Figure 6] and hippocampus [Figure 8] tissue samples, up-regulation of Hsp70 was observed in *Ube3a* knockout mice. However, Real-Time RT-PCR analysis [Table 5] using RNA samples extracted from mice showed that Hsp70 mRNA levels were not significantly affected in the cerebellum and hippocampus when comparing *Ube3a* knockout and wild type mice. In conclusion, the differential expression of Hsp70 was observed only at the translational or protein level. It is conceivable that Hsp70 is the target of Ube3a, as Hsp70 is a multi-functional protein; its most prominent task is to serve as a chaperone in the ubiquitin proteasome system. Parkin and CHIP are two other E3-ligases that are known to interact with Hsp70 for protein quality control tasks (21). To perform its quality control task, Hsp70 serves as a chaperone that binds to misfolded proteins during translation or after stress-mediated protein damage. Studies have shown that Hsp70 interacts with co-chaperone CHIP, which functions as a RING domain E3-ligase, and together they serve as the protein quality control system that clears stress-damaged proteins from cells. Such proteins include tau in Alzheimer's disease and expanded polyglutamate protein in Huntington's disease (23,24). A recent study also demonstrated that E6AP reduces polyglutamate protein aggregation, which induces cell death. Results also showed that E6AP is over-expressed correlated with HSP70. The author suggested that HSP70 may play a modulatory role on the function of E6AP (20). Another study has also shown that Hsp70 is degraded through CHIP-dependent targeting to the ubiquitin-proteasome system (21). If E6AP does interact with Hsp70 to perform protein quality control, one of the possible scenarios might be that HSP70 is targeted by E6AP after the substrates have depleted. In the AS mouse model used in this study, *Ube3a* was knocked out; this might result in the accumulation of HSP70 after the target substrates have depleted. Ube3a may be acting in the positive feedback system, by promoting the degradation of HSP70 when HSP70 exceeds its threshold level in the body. The loss of Ube3a in knockout mice may prolong the half-life of Hsp70. As other studies have suggested, Hsp70 normally assists in multi-ubiquitin chain ubiquitination at lysine48 (K48), and such ubiquitination normally leads to the degradation of the protein (25). Even though there are other E3-ligases, all E3-ligases have their own specific targets. In addition, different post-translational modifications by Ube3a may have different effects on the protein and influence the range of functions that it performs (26). Lack of Ube3a may not only affect the half-life of Hsp70 but also affect the functions of Hsp70.

It is possible that Hsp70 might play a role in cell protection. In *Ube3a* knockout mice, there may be accumulation of other proteins that are specific substrates of Ube3a for degradation. Elevated levels of HSP70 may be triggered by accumulation of the substrate proteins or misfolded proteins. Studies have shown that elevated levels of HSP70 may assist in unfolding the misfolded proteins to prevent them from becoming toxins in the brain (27-31). This may also be the reason that protein aggregates commonly seen in other neurodegenerative diseases are absent in AS mouse models and AS patients. It is generally known that overexpression of HSP70 prior to neuronal insult improves cell survival in both stroke and epilepsy models. However according to recent studies, the neuroprotection effect from the expression of HSP70 in other neurodegenerative diseases was not observed in epileptogenic states, and over-expression of HSP70 in such cases only served as an indicator of neuronal stress in the acute phase of epilepsy (27). However, other studies have suggested that the death of neuronal cells is not caused by protein aggregation in the brain, but rather by the soluble intermediates. Accumulation of HSP70 may prevent the formation of protein aggregation but allow soluble intermediates to cause toxic effects in AS patients. Both soluble intermediates and protein aggregates attribute to the clinical features of neurodegenerative diseases (32).

Expression of VDR is found to be reduced in *Ube3a* knockout mice at the protein level in this 2-D DIGE/MS study. We have also examined the mRNA level of VDR in the cerebellum and hippocampus of *Ube3a* knockout mice, and it is found to be down-regulated by 55% and 72%, respectively. Its ligand, vitamin-D_3, controls calcium homeostasis, bone formation, cell differentiation and apoptosis (33,34). The down-regulation of VDR may affect calcium homeostasis in mutant mice, as epilepsy is highly correlated with the disruption of calcium levels in cells and is one of the most well-known characteristics observed in Angelman syndrome patients. VDR is a transcriptional regulator that interacts with specific DNA sequences composed of hexanucleotide direct repeats and binds as either a homodimer or heterodimer with retinoid X receptors (RXRs); cell cycle inhibitors p21 and p27 are two known genes that VDR regulates (35,36). If VDR is down-regulated in *Ube3a* knockout mice, its upstream regulator BAG1L may also be affected. BAG1L, along with BAG1, BAG1M (Rap46), and BAG1S, are four protein isomers that the human BAG1 gene encodes. Recently, Hsp70 has been identified as a partner of BAGL1 in enhancing the trans-activation function of VDR in a concentration-dependent manner; this interaction has been speculated to improve tumor cell responses (37,38). Since BAG1L couples with Hsp70 to perform its functions, the accumulation of Hsp70 detected in the AS mouse model may be related to the down-regulation of VDR. VDR is a multifunctional protein that is known to regulate calcium homeostasis (33,34) and immunity (39). Therefore, the correlation between BAG1L, accumulation of Hsp70 and down-regulation VDR may be an interesting area to study in the *Ube3a* knockout model.

The homeostasis of Ca^{2+} in neurons can be achieved by the transportation of Ca^{2+} across the membrane, sequestration by cellular organelles, or with cytosolic buffering proteins such as pavalbumin and CaBP. Calcium ions, in turn, are actively involved in signal transduction, the development of regulatory proteins that modulate calcium ion transients, neurogenesis and many other functions. Lack of cytoplasmic CaBP severely impairs Ca^{2+} homeostasis and causes nerve cells to be selectively vulnerable to Ca^{2+} related injury (40,41). In the 2-D DIGE/MS study and Western blot analysis, CaBP was one of the proteins that was down-regulated in both cerebellum and hippocampus tissue of *Ube3a* knockout mice. It is known that the decline of CaBP in hippocampal dentate granule cells correlates with the kindling model for epilepsy; this may help to explain the frequent seizures observed among Angelman syndrome patients, as excess levels of intracellular Ca^{2+} may disrupt neuronal signal transduction (42).

Another study has shown that CaBP facilitates neuronal differentiation via up-regulation of genes such as *NeuroD, Pax6, VDR* and *Mash1* in a pathway involving CaMK (14). Mash1 or ASC1 is one of the basic helix-loop-helix (bHLH) transcription factors that heterodimerizes with the ubiquitous Class I bHLH E proteins to form complexes that are crucial in neurogenesis and neural differentiation during development (43). Adult neural progenitor cells continue to generate new neurons, astrocytes and oligodendrocytes in the brain throughout life, under normal turnover circumstances, or after ischemia in status epilepticus. Mash1 and Olig2 stimulate neurogenenesis and differentiation of progenitor cells in the telencephalon, generating the vast array of neurons and glia cells found in the adult cerebral cortex and giving rise to the ganglionic eminence and olfactory epithelium (44,45). A study using Mash1 null mutant mice showed that Mash1 is required for the generation of an early population of oligodendrocyte precursors (OPCs), which is involved in the regulation of synaptic transmission and adult neurogenensis (46). Mice with a targeted deletion in Mash1 also fail to develop pulmonary neuroendocrine cells (PNECs), and they die in the neonatal period due to respiratory failure (47). NeuroD or Beta2 is another basic helix loop helix (bHLH) transcription factor expressed in neurons of the cortical plate, as well as neuroendocrine cells in the stomach, gut, pancreas and adult lung (48,49). It is involved in the differentiation of neurons and the development of the pancreas, inner ear and retina (48,50). Like other bHLH factors, it heterodimerizes with E proteins and controls the transcription of a variety of genes to induce neuron differentiation. When NeuroD is deleted in mice, the early differentiating pancreatic endocrine cells die, and total pancreatic insulin level is only about 5% of normal level. The mutant mice will eventually die within five days after birth due to hyperglycemia. In the hippocampus of NeuroD null mice, when the granule cells reach the dentate gyrus, both cell proliferation and differentiation are severely disturbed, leading to severe cellular depletion in the brain (49). The hippocampal mRNA and protein levels of CaBP have been demonstrated to express concurrently with the expression of these bHLH transcription factors (14). In the Real-Time RT-PCR study, fresh tissue from the AS mouse model was used instead of the progenitor cell cultures that were used in the previous study (14). This was to ensure that the *Ube3a* knockout environment was retained and was able to reflect the complex activity *in vivo*. In this case, *CaBP* mRNA levels were down-regulated by 57% in the cerebellum and 80% in the hippocampus; *NeuroD* mRNA levels were down-regulated concurrently by 33% and 85% in the cerebellum and hippocampus, respectively. However, *Mash1* mRNA levels remained unchanged in the two tissues. *NeuroD* encoding a bHLH protein is involved in neuronal cells development as well as differentiation; the down-regulation of *NeuroD* at mRNA levels may implicate the lack of differentiation in dendritic spines observed in the AS mouse model (51). Even though *Mash1* mRNA levels were unaffected, its protein levels were reduced in both the cerebellum and hippocampus of *Ube3a* knockout mice. On the other hand, *NeuroD* mRNA was down-regulated in the cerebellum and hippocampus, while NeuroD protein was accumulated in the cerebellum and down-regulated in the hippocampus. The deficiency of these two proteins in the hippocampus may not only affect the development and differentiation of cells but also affect neurogenesis after ischemic or neuronal damage.

Vitamin D_3 has been shown to induce the expression of CaBP (52,53), and vitamin D_3 receptor (VDR) and CaBP have been found to co-localize in many tissues, especially in the brain. Reduced *CaBP* and *VDR* mRNA levels in the hippocampus of neurodegenerative Alzheimer's disease have been reported (54). This coincides with our findings in the Real Time RT-PCR experiment that *CaBP* and *VDR* are down-regulated by 57% and 55%, respectively, in the cerebellum, and down-regulated by 80% and 72%, respectively, in the hippocampus of *Ube3a* knockout mice. Since both mRNA levels were affected and VDR protein levels were down-regulated in the 2D-DIGE analysis, this might correlate with the CaBP deficiency observed in the cerebellum and hippocampus. These findings demonstrate a specific association between VDR and CaBP.

Reactive oxygen species (ROS) are electronically activated species that have been shown to behave as signal transduction molecules that modulate protein function, such as facilitating oxidative posttranslational modification on protein chaperones (55,56). The intrinsic mitochondrial apoptotic pathway is the most common form of cell death in neurodegeneration; it controls the activation of caspase-9 by regulating the release of cytochrome c from the mitochondrial intermembrane space (IMS) (57). ROS are normal by-products of mitochondrial respiratory chain activity (58). ROS concentration is mediated by mitochondrial antioxidants such as manganese superoxide dismutase (SOD2) and glutathione peroxidase (59). Over production of ROS (oxidative stress) is a central feature of all neurodegenerative disorders (60). In addition to the generation of ROS, mitochondria are also involved in life-sustaining functions, including calcium homeostasis, mitochondrial fission and fusion, lipid concentration of the mitochondrial membranes and mitochondrial permeability transition (56,57,61). It is known that mice lacking SOD2 die several days after birth, amid massive oxidative stress (62). In our study, we observed that protein levels of SOD2 but not transcriptional levels were down-regulated in AS mice. Since SOD2 is vital for handling oxidative stress in mitochondria, down-regulation of SOD2 may cause a surge of oxidative damage in cells and eventually lead to cell death.

Lactate dehydrogenase (LDH), malate dehydrogenase (MDH) and Glutathione S-transferase Mu1 are found differentially expressed in the AS mice. These are proteins that are known to be involved in REDOX reactions. LDH catalyzes the interconversion of pyruvate and lactate with concomitant interconversion of NADH and NAD. Malate dehydrogenase (MDH) is an enzyme in the citric acid cycle that catalyzes the conversion of malate into oxaloacetate by using NAD^+. Pyruvate in the mitochondria is acted upon by pyruvate carboxylase to form oxaloacetate, a citric acid cycle intermediate (63,64). Glutathione S-transferase (GSTs) families consist of a total of eight sub-classes of isoenzymes, including alpha, kappa, mu, omega, pi, sigma, theta and zeta. These isoenzymes can be cytosolic, mitochondrial, or microsomal proteins depending on the site that they are acting on (65). Glutathione S-transferase Mu1 (GSTM1) is a human glutathione S-transferase. The mu class of enzymes functions mainly in the detoxification of electrophilic compounds, including carcinogens, therapeutic drugs, environmental toxins and products of oxidative stress, by conjugation with glutathione (GST) (66). Genetic variations of GSTM1 can change an individual's susceptibility to carcinogens and toxins, as well as affect the toxicity and efficacy of certain drugs. GSTM1 is essential for cell protection as reports show that GSTM1 null mice are predisposed to increased cancer risk due to increased susceptibility to environmental toxins and carcinogens (65,67,68). When SOD2, LDH, MDH and GSTs class mu1 are reduced in *Ube3a* knockout mice, mitochondrial defects are likely to occur, which may lead to neurodegeneration. Mitochondrial dysfunction and oxidative stress are implicated in the pathogenesis of neurodegenerative disease, which includes Alzheimer's disease, Parkinson's disease, Huntington's disease and Amyotrophic lateral sclerosis (ALS) (60,69). In the case of ALS, there are several proteins reported to have changes in expression that coincide with the *Ube3a* knockout mice used in this study; those proteins include ATP synthase, mitochondrial F1 complex α subunit; glutathione S-transferase class Mu1 and heat shock 70-kda protein (55). Intriguingly, in *parkin* knockout mice, a similar set of proteins is found to be differentially expressed in the cortex and striatum, including ATP synthase α chain mitochondrial, lactate dehydrogenase, malate dehydrogenase, stress-70 protein, glutathione S-transferase P2 and N-ethylmaleimide-sensitive fusion protein (70). In the current study, protein levels of ATP synthase α chain mitochondrial, lactate dehydrogenase, malate dehydrogenase, stress-70 protein, glutathione S-transferase class Mu1, and N-ethylmaleimide-sensitive fusion protein are found to be differentially expressed in the AS mice. The mRNA levels of these proteins remained steady in mutant mice, except for LDH, which had a 55% down-regulation of mRNA levels, and glutathione S-transferase class Mu1, which had a 100% up-regulation of mRNA levels in the hippocampus. This showed that most of the proteins involved in REDOX are affected at the translational or protein level in the absence of functional Ube3a, thus suggesting that down-regulation of LDH, MDH and glutathione S-transferase class Mu1 at the protein level may play a crucial role in the pathogenesis of AS.

NSF is not affected at the transcriptional level in the cerebellum and hippocampus of *Ube3a* knockout mice, but it is specifically affected at the protein level. NSF is up-regulated in the cerebellum but down-regulated in the hippocampus of AS mice. NSF protein is thought to be involved in the docking and fusion of synaptic vesicles at the plasma membrane. It is known that transportation of neurotransmitters at the synapse, which involves synaptic vesicles fusing with the pre-synaptic membrane, relies on such processes to perform neuronal function. Studies have also shown that mutation of *NSF* in *Drosophila* can result in coma, presumably because neuronal functions have been blocked in the absence of NSF (71). AS patients exhibit symptoms such as tremor, ataxia and motor incoordination; a study has also shown motor dysfunction in *Ube3a* knockout mice (7). Since NSF is expressed abundantly in the hippocampus under normal circumstances (72), it is of interest to study the relationship between NSF deficiency in the hippocampus and movement incoordination in mutant mice. *NSF* has also been discovered as an epilepsy gene (73,74). Along with the discovery of CaBP deficiency in *Ube3a* knockout mice, these two proteins are crucial to the study of clinical features such as inducible seizures that are commonly found in AS patients.

In this study, we used the proteomic approach to study the effects of Ube3a deficiencies. Our results unveil that multiple proteins involved in redox reactions are affected and suggest that oxidative stress is associated with AS. Our results also indicated that proteins involved in neuronal cell differentiation, learning process, energy production, actin disassembly and likely neuronal signal transduction are affected in AS. Our findings provides clues for identification of therapeutic targets and for understanding of the detailed molecular mechanism of AS and other related neurological disorders.

5. Acknowledgements

The authors acknowledge financial support from the Academic Research Fund (M52080023) awarded to Ken-Shiung Chen and the grant from IAS Research Project (M58A40001).

6. References

[1] Jiang, Y., Lev-Lehman, E., Bressler, J., Tsai, T.F. and Beaudet, A.L. (1999) Genetics of Angelman syndrome. *Am J Hum Genet*, 65, 1-6.

[2] Witte, W., Nobel, C. and Hilpert, J. (2011) [Anesthesia and Angelman syndrome.]. *Anaesthesist.*

[3] Lalande, M. and Calciano, M.A. (2007) Molecular epigenetics of Angelman syndrome. *Cell Mol Life Sci*, 64, 947-960.

[4] Nicholls, R.D., Saitoh, S. and Horsthemke, B. (1998) Imprinting in Prader-Willi and Angelman syndromes. *Trends Genet*, 14, 194-200.

[5] Cattanach, B.M., Barr, J.A., Beechey, C.V., Martin, J., Noebels, J. and Jones, J. (1997) A candidate model for Angelman syndrome in the mouse. *Mamm Genome*, 8, 472-478.

[6] Culiat, C.T., Stubbs, L.J., Montgomery, C.S., Russell, L.B. and Rinchik, E.M. (1994) Phenotypic consequences of deletion of the gamma 3, alpha 5, or beta 3 subunit of the type A gamma-aminobutyric acid receptor in mice. *Proc Natl Acad Sci U S A*, 91, 2815-2818.

[7] Jiang, Y.H., Armstrong, D., Albrecht, U., Atkins, C.M., Noebels, J.L., Eichele, G., Sweatt, J.D. and Beaudet, A.L. (1998) Mutation of the Angelman ubiquitin ligase in mice causes increased cytoplasmic p53 and deficits of contextual learning and long-term potentiation. *Neuron*, 21, 799-811.

[8] Miura, K., Kishino, T., Li, E., Webber, H., Dikkes, P., Holmes, G.L. and Wagstaff, J. (2002) Neurobehavioral and electroencephalographic abnormalities in Ube3a maternal-deficient mice. *Neurobiol Dis*, 9, 149-159.

[9] Wu, M.Y., Chen, K.S., Bressler, J., Hou, A., Tsai, T.F. and Beaudet, A.L. (2006) Mouse imprinting defect mutations that model Angelman syndrome. *Genesis*, 44, 12-22.

[10] Jiang, Y.H., Pan, Y., Zhu, L., Landa, L., Yoo, J., Spencer, C., Lorenzo, I., Brilliant, M., Noebels, J. and Beaudet, A.L. (2010) Altered ultrasonic vocalization and impaired learning and memory in Angelman syndrome mouse model with a large maternal deletion from Ube3a to Gabrb3. *PLoS One*, 5, e12278.

[11] Johnstone, K.A., DuBose, A.J., Futtner, C.R., Elmore, M.D., Brannan, C.I. and Resnick, J.L. (2006) A human imprinting centre demonstrates conserved acquisition but diverged maintenance of imprinting in a mouse model for Angelman syndrome imprinting defects. *Hum Mol Genet*, 15, 393-404.

[12] Homanics, G.E., DeLorey, T.M., Firestone, L.L., Quinlan, J.J., Handforth, A., Harrison, N.L., Krasowski, M.D., Rick, C.E., Korpi, E.R., Makela, R. *et al.* (1997) Mice devoid of gamma-aminobutyrate type A receptor beta3 subunit have epilepsy, cleft palate, and hypersensitive behavior. *Proc Natl Acad Sci U S A*, 94, 4143-4148.

[13] Gabriel, J.M., Merchant, M., Ohta, T., Ji, Y., Caldwell, R.G., Ramsey, M.J., Tucker, J.D., Longnecker, R. and Nicholls, R.D. (1999) A transgene insertion creating a heritable chromosome deletion mouse model of Prader-Willi and angelman syndromes. *Proc Natl Acad Sci U S A*, 96, 9258-9263.

[14] Kim, J.H., Lee, J.A., Song, Y.M., Park, C.H., Hwang, S.J., Kim, Y.S., Kaang, B.K. and Son, H. (2006) Overexpression of calbindin-D28K in hippocampal progenitor cells increases neuronal differentiation and neurite outgrowth. *FASEB J*, 20, 109-111.

[15] Nawaz, Z., Lonard, D.M., Smith, C.L., Lev-Lehman, E., Tsai, S.Y., Tsai, M.J. and O'Malley, B.W. (1999) The Angelman syndrome-associated protein, E6-AP, is a coactivator for the nuclear hormone receptor superfamily. *Mol Cell Biol*, 19, 1182-1189.

[16] Oda, H., Kumar, S. and Howley, P.M. (1999) Regulation of the Src family tyrosine kinase Blk through E6AP-mediated ubiquitination. *Proc Natl Acad Sci U S A*, 96, 9557-9562.

[17] Jeong, K.W., Kim, H.Z., Kim, S., Kim, Y.S. and Choe, J. (2007) Human papillomavirus type 16 E6 protein interacts with cystic fibrosis transmembrane regulator-associated ligand and promotes E6-associated protein-mediated ubiquitination and proteasomal degradation. *Oncogene*, 26, 487-499.

[18] Yang, Y., Liu, W., Zou, W., Wang, H., Zong, H., Jiang, J., Wang, Y. and Gu, J. (2007) Ubiquitin-dependent proteolysis of trihydrophobin 1 (TH1) by the human papilloma virus E6-associated protein (E6-AP). *J Cell Biochem*, 101, 167-180.

[19] Reiter, L.T., Seagroves, T.N., Bowers, M. and Bier, E. (2006) Expression of the Rho-GEF Pbl/ECT2 is regulated by the UBE3A E3 ubiquitin ligase. *Hum Mol Genet*, 15, 2825-2835.

[20] Mishra, A., Dikshit, P., Purkayastha, S., Sharma, J., Nukina, N. and Jana, N.R. (2008) E6-AP promotes misfolded polyglutamine proteins for proteasomal degradation and suppresses polyglutamine protein aggregation and toxicity. *J Biol Chem*, 283, 7648-7656.

[21] Mishra, A., Godavarthi, S.K., Maheshwari, M., Goswami, A. and Jana, N.R. (2009) The ubiquitin ligase E6-AP is induced and recruited to aggresomes in response to proteasome inhibition and may be involved in the ubiquitination of Hsp70-bound misfolded proteins. *J Biol Chem*, 284, 10537-10545.

[22] Cummings, C.J., Reinstein, E., Sun, Y., Antalffy, B., Jiang, Y., Ciechanover, A., Orr, H.T., Beaudet, A.L. and Zoghbi, H.Y. (1999) Mutation of the E6-AP ubiquitin ligase reduces nuclear inclusion frequency while accelerating polyglutamine-induced pathology in SCA1 mice. *Neuron*, 24, 879-892.

[23] Rujano, M.A., Kampinga, H.H. and Salomons, F.A. (2007) Modulation of polyglutamine inclusion formation by the Hsp70 chaperone machine. *Exp Cell Res*, 313, 3568-3578.

[24] Rosser, M.F., Washburn, E., Muchowski, P.J., Patterson, C. and Cyr, D.M. (2007) Chaperone functions of the E3 ubiquitin ligase CHIP. *J Biol Chem*, 282, 22267-22277.

[25] Lim, K.L. and Lim, G.G. (2011) K63-linked ubiquitination and neurodegeneration. *Neurobiol Dis*, 43, 9-16.

[26] Yi, J.J. and Ehlers, M.D. (2007) Emerging roles for ubiquitin and protein degradation in neuronal function. *Pharmacol Rev*, 59, 14-39.

[27] Turturici, G., Sconzo, G. and Geraci, F. (2011) Hsp70 and its molecular role in nervous system diseases. *Biochem Res Int*, 2011, 618127.

[28] Magrane, J., Smith, R.C., Walsh, K. and Querfurth, H.W. (2004) Heat shock protein 70 participates in the neuroprotective response to intracellularly expressed beta-amyloid in neurons. *J Neurosci*, 24, 1700-1706.

[29] Cummings, C.J., Sun, Y., Opal, P., Antalffy, B., Mestril, R., Orr, H.T., Dillmann, W.H. and Zoghbi, H.Y. (2001) Over-expression of inducible HSP70 chaperone suppresses neuropathology and improves motor function in SCA1 mice. *Hum Mol Genet*, 10, 1511-1518.

[30] Jana, N.R., Tanaka, M., Wang, G. and Nukina, N. (2000) Polyglutamine length-dependent interaction of Hsp40 and Hsp70 family chaperones with truncated N-terminal huntingtin: their role in suppression of aggregation and cellular toxicity. *Hum Mol Genet*, 9, 2009-2018.

[31] Nagel, F., Falkenburger, B.H., Tonges, L., Kowsky, S., Poppelmeyer, C., Schulz, J.B., Bahr, M. and Dietz, G.P. (2008) Tat-Hsp70 protects dopaminergic neurons in midbrain cultures and in the substantia nigra in models of Parkinson's disease. *J Neurochem*, 105, 853-864.

[32] Yamamoto, A. and Simonsen, A. (2011) The elimination of accumulated and aggregated proteins: a role for aggrephagy in neurodegeneration. *Neurobiol Dis*, 43, 17-28.

[33] MacDonald, P.N., Haussler, C.A., Terpening, C.M., Galligan, M.A., Reeder, M.C., Whitfield, G.K. and Haussler, M.R. (1991) Baculovirus-mediated expression of the human vitamin D receptor. Functional characterization, vitamin D response element interactions, and evidence for a receptor auxiliary factor. *J Biol Chem*, 266, 18808-18813.

[34] Zinser, G., Packman, K. and Welsh, J. (2002) Vitamin D(3) receptor ablation alters mammary gland morphogenesis. *Development*, 129, 3067-3076.

[35] Glass, C.K. (1994) Differential recognition of target genes by nuclear receptor monomers, dimers, and heterodimers. *Endocr Rev*, 15, 391-407.

[36] Liu, M., Lee, M.H., Cohen, M., Bommakanti, M. and Freedman, L.P. (1996) Transcriptional activation of the Cdk inhibitor p21 by vitamin D3 leads to the induced differentiation of the myelomonocytic cell line U937. *Genes Dev*, 10, 142-153.

[37] Kudoh, M., Knee, D.A., Takayama, S. and Reed, J.C. (2002) Bag1 proteins regulate growth and survival of ZR-75-1 human breast cancer cells. *Cancer Res*, 62, 1904-1909.

[38] Guzey, M., Takayama, S. and Reed, J.C. (2000) BAG1L enhances trans-activation function of the vitamin D receptor. *J Biol Chem*, 275, 40749-40756.

[39] Welsh, J., Zinser, L.N., Mianecki-Morton, L., Martin, J., Waltz, S.E., James, H. and Zinser, G.M. (2011) Age-related changes in the epithelial and stromal compartments of the mammary gland in normocalcemic mice lacking the vitamin D3 receptor. *PLoS One*, 6, e16479.

[40] Dong, Z., Saikumar, P., Weinberg, J.M. and Venkatachalam, M.A. (2006) Calcium in cell injury and death. *Annu Rev Pathol*, 1, 405-434.

[41] Squier, T.C. and Bigelow, D.J. (2000) Protein oxidation and age-dependent alterations in calcium homeostasis. *Front Biosci*, 5, D504-526.

[42] Kohr, G., Lambert, C.E. and Mody, I. (1991) Calbindin-D28K (CaBP) levels and calcium currents in acutely dissociated epileptic neurons. *Exp Brain Res*, 85, 543-551.

[43] Henke, R.M., Meredith, D.M., Borromeo, M.D., Savage, T.K. and Johnson, J.E. (2009) Ascl1 and Neurog2 form novel complexes and regulate Delta-like3 (Dll3) expression in the neural tube. *Dev Biol*, 328, 529-540.

[44] Uchida, Y., Nakano, S., Gomi, F. and Takahashi, H. (2007) Differential regulation of basic helix-loop-helix factors Mash1 and Olig2 by beta-amyloid accelerates both differentiation and death of cultured neural stem/progenitor cells. *J Biol Chem*, 282, 19700-19709.

[45] Parras, C.M., Galli, R., Britz, O., Soares, S., Galichet, C., Battiste, J., Johnson, J.E., Nakafuku, M., Vescovi, A. and Guillemot, F. (2004) Mash1 specifies neurons and oligodendrocytes in the postnatal brain. *EMBO J*, 23, 4495-4505.

[46] Parras, C.M., Hunt, C., Sugimori, M., Nakafuku, M., Rowitch, D. and Guillemot, F. (2007) The proneural gene Mash1 specifies an early population of telencephalic oligodendrocytes. *J Neurosci*, 27, 4233-4242.

[47] Neptune, E.R., Podowski, M., Calvi, C., Cho, J.H., Garcia, J.G., Tuder, R., Linnoila, R.I., Tsai, M.J. and Dietz, H.C. (2008) Targeted disruption of NeuroD, a proneural basic helix-loop-helix factor, impairs distal lung formation and neuroendocrine morphology in the neonatal lung. *J Biol Chem*, 283, 21160-21169.

[48] Ross, S.E., Greenberg, M.E. and Stiles, C.D. (2003) Basic helix-loop-helix factors in cortical development. *Neuron*, 39, 13-25.

[49] Chae, J.H., Stein, G.H. and Lee, J.E. (2004) NeuroD: the predicted and the surprising. *Mol Cells*, 18, 271-288.

[50] Ochocinska, M.J. and Hitchcock, P.F. (2009) NeuroD regulates proliferation of photoreceptor progenitors in the retina of the zebrafish. *Mech Dev*, 126, 128-141.

[51] Ramocki, M.B. and Zoghbi, H.Y. (2008) Failure of neuronal homeostasis results in common neuropsychiatric phenotypes. *Nature*, 455, 912-918.

[52] Wasserman, R.H. and Taylor, A.N. (1966) Vitamin d3-induced calcium-binding protein in chick intestinal mucosa. *Science*, 152, 791-793.

[53] Thomasset, M., Parkes, C.O. and Cuisinier-Gleizes, P. (1982) Rat calcium-binding proteins: distribution, development, and vitamin D dependence. *Am J Physiol*, 243, E483-488.

[54] Sutherland, M.K., Somerville, M.J., Yoong, L.K., Bergeron, C., Haussler, M.R. and McLachlan, D.R. (1992) Reduction of vitamin D hormone receptor mRNA levels in Alzheimer as compared to Huntington hippocampus: correlation with calbindin-28k mRNA levels. *Brain Res Mol Brain Res*, 13, 239-250.

[55] Jain, M.R., Ge, W.W., Elkabes, S. and Li, H. (2008) Amyotrophic lateral sclerosis: Protein chaperone dysfunction revealed by proteomic studies of animal models. *Proteomics Clin Appl*, 2, 670-684.

[56] Squier, T.C. (2001) Oxidative stress and protein aggregation during biological aging. *Exp Gerontol*, 36, 1539-1550.

[57] Rego, A.C. and Oliveira, C.R. (2003) Mitochondrial dysfunction and reactive oxygen species in excitotoxicity and apoptosis: implications for the pathogenesis of neurodegenerative diseases. *Neurochem Res*, 28, 1563-1574.

[58] Sugawara, T., Noshita, N., Lewen, A., Gasche, Y., Ferrand-Drake, M., Fujimura, M., Morita-Fujimura, Y. and Chan, P.H. (2002) Overexpression of copper/zinc

superoxide dismutase in transgenic rats protects vulnerable neurons against ischemic damage by blocking the mitochondrial pathway of caspase activation. *J Neurosci*, 22, 209-217.

[59] Li, Q., Zhang, M., Chen, Y.J., Wang, Y.J., Huang, F. and Liu, J. (2011) Oxidative damage and HSP70 expression in masseter muscle induced by psychological stress in rats. *Physiol Behav.*

[60] Andersen, J.K. (2004) Oxidative stress in neurodegeneration: cause or consequence? *Nat Med*, 10 Suppl, S18-25.

[61] Scandalios, J.G. (1993) Oxygen Stress and Superoxide Dismutases. *Plant Physiol*, 101, 7-12.

[62] Zelko, I.N., Mariani, T.J. and Folz, R.J. (2002) Superoxide dismutase multigene family: a comparison of the CuZn-SOD (SOD1), Mn-SOD (SOD2), and EC-SOD (SOD3) gene structures, evolution, and expression. *Free Radic Biol Med*, 33, 337-349.

[63] Park, S.J., Cotter, P.A. and Gunsalus, R.P. (1995) Regulation of malate dehydrogenase (mdh) gene expression in Escherichia coli in response to oxygen, carbon, and heme availability. *J Bacteriol*, 177, 6652-6656.

[64] Courtright, J.B. and Henning, U. (1970) Malate dehydrogenase mutants in Escherichia coli K-12. *J Bacteriol*, 102, 722-728.

[65] Morari, E.C., Leite, J.L., Granja, F., da Assumpcao, L.V. and Ward, L.S. (2002) The null genotype of glutathione s-transferase M1 and T1 locus increases the risk for thyroid cancer. *Cancer Epidemiol Biomarkers Prev*, 11, 1485-1488.

[66] Berhane, K., Widersten, M., Engstrom, A., Kozarich, J.W. and Mannervik, B. (1994) Detoxication of base propenals and other alpha, beta-unsaturated aldehyde products of radical reactions and lipid peroxidation by human glutathione transferases. *Proc Natl Acad Sci U S A*, 91, 1480-1484.

[67] Tew, K.D. (1994) Glutathione-associated enzymes in anticancer drug resistance. *Cancer Res*, 54, 4313-4320.

[68] Parl, F.F. (2005) Glutathione S-transferase genotypes and cancer risk. *Cancer Lett*, 221, 123-129.

[69] Sorolla, M.A., Reverter-Branchat, G., Tamarit, J., Ferrer, I., Ros, J. and Cabiscol, E. (2008) Proteomic and oxidative stress analysis in human brain samples of Huntington disease. *Free Radic Biol Med*, 45, 667-678.

[70] Periquet, M., Corti, O., Jacquier, S. and Brice, A. (2005) Proteomic analysis of parkin knockout mice: alterations in energy metabolism, protein handling and synaptic function. *J Neurochem*, 95, 1259-1276.

[71] Pallanck, L., Ordway, R.W. and Ganetzky, B. (1995) A Drosophila NSF mutant. *Nature*, 376, 25.

[72] Puschel, A.W., O'Connor, V. and Betz, H. (1994) The N-ethylmaleimide-sensitive fusion protein (NSF) is preferentially expressed in the nervous system. *FEBS Lett*, 347, 55-58.

[73] Guan, Z., Lu, L., Zheng, Z., Liu, J., Yu, F., Lu, S., Xin, Y., Liu, X., Hong, J. and Zhang, W. (2001) A spontaneous recurrent seizure-related Rattus NSF gene identified by linker capture subtraction. *Brain Res Mol Brain Res*, 87, 117-123.

[74] Yu, F., Guan, Z., Zhuo, M., Sun, L., Zou, W., Zheng, Z. and Liu, X. (2002) Further identification of NSF* as an epilepsy related gene. *Brain research. Molecular brain research*, 99, 141-144.

Part 3

Migraine and the Use of Herbal Medicine as an Alternative Treatment

Migraine: Molecular Basis and Herbal Medicine

Mohammad Ansari[1,2*], Kheirollah Rafiee[1],
Solaleh Emamgholipour[1] and Mohammad-Sadegh Fallah[3]
[1]*Department of Medical Biochemistry, Tehran University of Medical Sciences, Tehran,*
[2]*Araamesh Multi-Professional Pain Clinic, Tehran,*
[3]*Kawsar Human Genetics Research Center (KHGRC), Tehran,*
Iran

1. Introduction

Migraine is a common and disabling brain disorder with no single characteristic which could be used for a definite diagnosis. Usually a combination of different presentations is used as diagnostic criteria which may lead to a challenging feature of under- or misdiagnosis and also under-treatment. Diagnostic criteria for migraine usually emphasize on specificity compared to sensitivity which enhances their research values but reduces their clinical worth. The criteria are subjective and the lack of objective tests to confirm migraine diagnosis raises the need of rule out of other diagnoses. For this reason a potential diagnostic biomarker for migraine would certainly find wide application and may improve current severe deficiencies in migraine diagnosis.

1.1 Definition and classification

The term migraine is originated from Greek word *"hemicrania"* (Silberstein, 2004), meaning "one side of the head". Migraine headache as an episodic neurovascular phenomenon is characterized by recurrent attacks of unilateral headache (Silberstein, 2004) while headache is recognized as the most well-known symptom of migraine, its origin generally remains unclear (Messlinger, 2009). A combination of genetic and environmental factors contributes to the onset, progression, and severity of headache (Pietrobon & Striessnig, 2003). Migraine is classified into two major types – *migraine without aura* and *migraine with aura* (ICHD, 2004).

1.1.1 Migraine without aura

Migraine without aura (previously known as hemicrania simplex, common migraine) is a specific neurological disorder characterized by unilateral, pulsating quality, aggravation on movement, and moderate to severe headache, nausea and photophobia. Most migraineurs suffer from this subtype of migraine, and there are higher frequency and more severe attacks in comparison with migraine with aura. Owing to strong relationship between migraine without aura with menstrual cycle, the menstrual migraine (i.e. pure menstrual migraine and menstrually-related migraine) is categorized in this subtype. In pure menstrual migraine in

* Corresponding author

contrast to other types, migraine headaches are strictly restricted to the perimenstrual phase and do not happen at other times of the menstrual cycle (ICHD, 2004).

1.1.2 Migraine with aura

Migraine with aura (formerly known as classical migraine, ophthalmic, hemiplegic migraine) is defined as a recurrent disorder involving headache attacks appearing gradually over 5-20 minutes and lasting for less than 60 minutes. The aura encompasses focal neurological symptoms that precede or accompany at the onset of migraine attacks. Aura can involve reversible visual and sensory symptoms and speech weakness. Inherited forms of familial hemiplegic migraine and sporadic hemiplegic migraine, in which patients suffer from motor weakness, are classified in this subtype (ICHD, 2004).

1.2 Epidemiology and burden of health

The worldwide prevalence of headache for all age-group is considered to be more than 47%, and of migraine is 10.3% (Jensen & Stovner, 2008). In the United States around 6% of men and 18% of women experience at least one migraine attack in a given year. Before puberty, there is generally no sex difference (Jensen & Stovner, 2008), but incidence rate generally increases with age, especially in girls, until mid-puberty and then declines (Jensen & Stovner, 2008; Silberstein, 2004). In different ethnicity Europeans have the higher incidence rate followed by African-Americans and Asian-Americans (Silberstein, 2004).

It is obvious that migraine has a severe negative influence on quality of life (Silberstein, 2004). Because of its impact on health status, migraine is ranked as one of the top 20 causes of healthy life lost and disability by World Health Organization (WHO) (ICHD, 2004). Migraine annual cost for employers is about 13$ billion in the USA. Direct annual medical cost is over 1$ billion (Silberstein, 2004).

1.3 Comorbidity

In medicine, comorbidity describes the presence of one or more separate conditions that exists simultaneously in the same individuals (Jensen & Stovner, 2008; Scher et al., 2005). In general, the current global prevalence of tension-type headache in patients with migraine is 94%, of which 56% suffer frequent episodic tension-type headache (Jensen & Stovner, 2008). There is a growing evidence for a link between migraine and other diseases, including stroke, hypertension, diabetes, asthma, and obesity (Jensen & Stovner, 2008), as well as epilepsy (Scher et al., 2005). It is noted that migraine has been related to various indefinite disorders such as fibromyalgia, non-headache pain (lower back pain or local muscle pain) (Jensen & Stovner, 2008), some congenital heart defects like patent foramen ovalea, anxiety, and depression (Scher et al., 2005).

2. Molecular basis

2.1 Pathogenesis

Migraine was once considered to be a vascular phenomenon resulting from intracranial vasoconstriction and rebound vasodilation. However, recently it has been suggested that neurogenic process leads to a vascular change and consecutive alteration in cerebral perfusion (neurovascular theory) (Pietrobon & Striessnig, 2003). Historically Ebn-e-sina *(Avicenna,* 980–1037*)* was actually the first medical scientist who addressed neurovascular theory of migraine in the *Canon of Medicine,* which was published centuries ago. It seems that this fact has been ignored in recent articles considering history of theories of pathogenesis of migraine (Abokrysha, 2009).

Although the underlying cause of migraines has remained unknown, many biological events have been associated with migraine attacks. A potential cause of migraine is any change in the stability of pathways either directly or via trigeminocervical pain system. This could be inherited as a low activation threshold.

Cortical spreading depression is another theory that could result in aura by a spreading wave of depolarization (Lauritzen M, 1994). Aura is accompanied with a localized decrease followed by an increase in blood flow in parieto-occipital cortex (Charles, 2009) which leads to activation followed by depression of neurological activity over a cortical area. It could result in the release of some inflammatory mediators that irritates cranial nerves root, mostly the trigeminal nerve that transmits the sense of face and most of the head. There are some experiments supporting involvement of cortical event in the initiation of headache as well (Bartleson & Cutrer, 2010).

Migraine has a strong (up to 50%) genetic component, which is higher in migraine with aura than migraine without aura, with a probable multifactorial polygenic inheritance. Genetic load can be considered as a determinant that is modulated by external and internal factors (migraine triggers) (Pietrobon & Striessnig, 2003). Also, it has been reported that not only genes are involved in migraine, but also their protein encoded by them and their metabolites (known as biomarkers) may be important in its etiology (Loder, 2006).

2.2 Biomarkers in migraine

2.2.1 Definition and classification

Biological markers (biomarkers) have been defined as biological characteristics that can be objectively measured and evaluated as the indicator of normal biological processes, pathogenic processes, or pharmacological responses to a therapeutic intervention (Mayeux, 2004).

It has been shown that changes in the level of some molecules, arising from deficiency, increase or impairments of regulatory processes in their production pathway might be associated with etiology of migraine. Although, it is unknown that these changes can result from or/result in migraine.

In migraine, different biomarkers including genetic, and/or biochemical have been used for diagnosis and/or study of the pathophysiology of the disorder. The term of biomarkers in migraine can be classified in two different categories. Biomarkers of exposure or "antecedent biomarkers" (such as genetic biomarkers) defined as factors that exist before the development of migraine. The levels of these biomarkers are linked to increase or decrease in migraine susceptibility. On the contrary, biomarkers of disease can be defined as factors, used as the indicators of the presence or development of migraine. They can be used to screen the individuals with migraine and prediction of treatment response. In addition, the biomarkers in migraine can be classified into groups, based on the types of measured markers, such as genes, proteins and metabolites patterns in various body fluids (Loder, 2006). According to these categories, all genetic, and proteomic and metabolomic biomarkers are discussed later.

2.2.2 Genetic biomarkers

They are defined as genetic variations (mutations or polymorphisms) that can predict disease susceptibility, and help in early diagnosis of migraine, course of disease, disease severity and/or response to therapy. Some mutations that were found to be related with hemiplegic migraine (de Vries et al., 2006, 2009), and common migraine (Lafrenière et al., 2010), are good examples of mutation biomarkers. Some polymorphisms were also found to be more valuable for screening patients with higher susceptibility into migraine attack in the future (De Vries et al., 2006).

2.2.2.1 The mutation biomarkers in migraine

2.2.2.1.1 Hemiplegic migraine

Apart from familiarity—i.e., no affected relatives vs. affected first degree or second-degree relative(s), familial hemiplegic migraine is comparable in diagnostic criteria to sporadic hemiplegic migraine (Russell & Ducros, 2011).

2.2.2.1.1.1 Familial hemiplegic migraine

The familial hemiplegic migraine phenotype is associated with autosomal dominant mutations in the *CACNA1A*, *ATP1A2* and *SCN1A* genes. These familial forms of migraine caused by mutations in these genes are referred to FHM1, FHM2, and FHM3, respectively (de Vries et al., 2009; Russell & Ducros, 2011). *CACNA1A* gene is located on 19p13 and encodes the main subunit of $Ca_v2.1$ neuronal channels. Most of these mutations are missense which account for 50-75% of mutations in FHM families (De Vries et al., 2006). The *CACNA1A* T666M mutation is the most frequent cause of familial hemiplegic migraine. Interestingly, *CACNA1A* mutations are also found in other disease, such as episodic ataxia type 2 (EA-2) and spinocerebellar ataxia type 6 (SCA-6) (De Vries et al., 2006).

The *ATP1A2* gene is located on 1q23. This gene encodes the α2 subunit of sodium-potassium pumps. Several diseases such as basilar-type migraine and common migraine are associated with mutations in the *ATP1A2* gene (de Vries et al., 2006; 2009).

The *SCN1A* gene is located on 2q24 and encodes the α1 subunit of the neuronal voltage-gated sodium channel $Na_v1.1$. It is suggested that Mutations in this gene account for generalized epilepsy with febrile seizures plus (GEFS+) and severe myoclonic epilepsy of infancy (SMEI) (de Vries et al., 2006; 2009).

Recently it has been shown that mutation in the *SLC1A3*, encoding the glial glutamate transporter EAAT1 is responsible for pure hemiplegic migraine. Also, a homozygous deletion in *SLC4A4*, encoding the electrogenic sodium bicarbonate (Na^+–HCO^{3-}) cotransporter NBCe1 was associated with familial hemiplegic migraine. *SLC1A3* and *SLC4A4* seem to be the fourth and fifth genes (FHM4 and FHM5) which are involved in familial hemiplegic migraine (Russell & Ducros, 2011).

Functional studies have shown that FHM mutations cause (i) an enhancement of Ca^{2+} influx via $Ca_v2.1$ channels leading to an enhanced release of glutamate, at least in the cortex (in the case of *CACNA1A* mutations), (ii) a dysfunction in glial uptake of K^+ and glutamate from the synaptic cleft (in the case of *ATP1A2* mutations), and (iii) an enhanced recovery from fast inactivation and in that way an increased firing rate of neurons (in the case of *SCN1A* mutations). Therefore, as mentioned above, an increase of extracellular glutamate and K^+ levels in the synaptic cleft is associated with FHM mutations. Neurons may depolarize in a more straightforward manner to facilitate cortical spreading depression (de Vries et al., 2006; 2009). It could well explain the aura in these monogenic subtypes (de Vries et al., 2009). The findings in FHM support that dysfunction in ion transport is a crucial factor in migraine pathophysiology and might facilitate the identification of molecular pathways involved in migraine (de Vries et al., 2006; 2009).

2.2.2.1.1.2 Sporadic hemiplegic migraine

Sporadic cases of hemiplegic migraine can result from a de-novo mutation in genes related to the FHMs or by inheritance of a gene mutation from an asymptomatic parent (due to incomplete penetrance) (Russell & Ducros, 2011).

Up to now, only a few *CACNA1A* and *ATP1A2* mutations have been reported in patients with the sporadic hemiplegic migraine. For that reason, it is suggested that these genes have negligible role in pure sporadic hemiplegic migraine. A comparable nomenclature with familial hemiplegic migraine is also used for sporadic hemiplegic migraine, too. Accordingly, mutations in the *CACNA1A* and *ATP1A2* genes are referred to as sporadic hemiplegic migraine (SHM1 and SHM2, respectively) (Russell & Ducros, 2011).

2.2.2.1.2 Common migraine

Contrary to hemiplegic migraine, common forms of migraine are a genetically complex disorder with higher prevalence, genetic and phenotypic heterogeneity. Like other complex genetic traits, finding responsible genes are much more difficult (de Vries et al., 2006). Despite these problems and absence of any evidence of association between genes encoding the ion channels and common migraine in previous studies (Nyholt et al., 2008), it has been reported recently that there is a strong genetic link to common forms of migraine (Lafrenière et al., 2010). Using a candidate gene approach and functional analysis, researchers have identified a mutation, F139wfsX24, in the gene encoding the two-pore domain potassium channel TRESK (TWIK-related spinal cord potassium channel) *KCNK18* in the patients with migraine with aura. The TRESK is involved in pain pathways and regulates neuronal excitability. The mutation can lead to a complete loss of channel function (Lafrenière et al., 2010) and for the first time, a common form of migraine is linked to a genetic mutation (Wood, 2010). The agonist-promoted up-regulation of TRESK activity can act as a beneficial treatment option, either as an acute therapy or as a long-term preventive approach for individuals with migraine (Lafrenière et al., 2010).

Recently, in a genome-wide association study, evidence for association of common forms of migraine and rs1835740 on chromosome 8q22.1 has been reported. It has been claimed that this is the first relationship between genetic and common forms of migraine, particularly migraine with aura. This allele, is located between astrocyte elevated gene 1 (*MTDH/AEG-1)* and plasma glutamate carboxypeptidase (*PGCP*). Due to the role of these two genes in glutamate homeostasis, it seems that complementary pathways such as the glutamate system could fasten mendelian channelopathies with pathogenesis of common forms of migraine (Anttila et al., 2010).

2.2.2.2 Polymorphisms in migraine

Many positive associations have been reported in different linkage studies between common forms of migraine and polymorphisms. However, these results mainly have not been replicated, and are therefore of less clinical value (de Vries et al., 2006; 2009). Methylenetetrahydrofolate reductase gene *MTHFR* 677C>T polymorphism and angiotensin I-converting enzyme *ACE* D/I polymorphism are two good examples for genetic association with migraine. Methylenetetrahydrofolate reductase is a key enzyme in folate and homocysteine metabolism and angiotensin-converting enzyme is an exopeptidase that catalyses the conversion of angiotensin I to angiotensin II, a potent vasoconstrictor (Colson et al., 2006).

A meta-analysis study has shown that the *MTHFR* 677TT genotype was associated with increased risk of migraine with aura and *ACE* II genotype is protective against both migraines with and without aura. Due to high heterogeneity among studies, both variants appeared to be correlated with common forms of migraine only among non-Caucasian populations (Schürks et al., 2010). However, further studies may be required among other ethnicities. Previously it has been shown that *ACE* and *MTHFR* genes act synergistically as a genetic risk of migraine and having at least one copy of the *ACE* D allele beside the *MTHFR* TT genotype increases the risk of migraine with aura by ~3 fold (Roda, 2005).

Another meta-analysis study about serotonin transporter gene (5-HTT) variants (including 5-HTTLPR, VNTR and SNP) indicates that only the VNTR polymorphism is associated with an increased risk of migraine (Liu et al., 2011). Existing evidences indicate that the genetic polymorphisms in serotonergic system, dopaminergic system, gamma amino butyric acid receptor system, inflammation related genes (de Vries et al., 2009), inducible nitric oxide synthase promoter (Jia et al., 2011), hypocretin-1 (also termed orexin-A) receptor (Rainero et al., 2011), and Notch 3 gene (G684A variant) (Menon et al., 2010) are associated with an increased risk of migraine. Other studies suggest that some haplotypes related to endothelial nitric oxide synthase (Gonçalves et al., 2011) and vascular endothelial growth factor (Gonçalves et al., 2010) could affect the susceptibility to migraine. So genotyping of only one polymorphism might not be sufficient and haplotype analysis may be needed to elucidate the association between migraine and these polymorphisms. Future studies with larger sample sizes will be necessary to confirm the present results.

2.2.3 Proteomic and metabolomic biomarkers

Principally, the global analysis of metabolites (metabolomics) and proteins (proteomics) in body fluids and tissues can provide certain advantages in understanding the underlying mechanisms of migraine. The proteomic and metabolomic signature, mostly belong to biochemical markers (such as proteins, peptides, amino acids, and amines), can identify a putative disease fingerprint for migraine in blood, urine and cerebrospinal fluid (Loder, 2006). The list of these biomarkers has been discussed in several reviews (Edvinsson, 2006; Harrington, 2006; Loder et al, 2006).

2.2.3.1 Calcitonin gene-related peptide

Calcitonin gene related peptide is a 37-amino acid neuropeptide that is a member of the *calcitonin* family of peptide. Calcitonin gene related peptide plays an important role in the modulation of physiological functions such as regulation of vascular tone and modulation of pain perception (Durham, 2006; Fischer, 2010).

Calcitonin gene related peptide was originally thought to contribute to migraine and elevated level of this peptide has been reported in this disease (Arulmani et al. 2004; Durham, 2006; Fischer, 2010). Calcitonin gene related peptide can lead to enhancement of cerebral circulation, transmission of pain-related impulses and neurogenic inflammation (Durham, 2006). In fact, in the endothelium dependent and independent (binding to its receptors on the smooth muscle cells) pathways, calcitonin gene related peptide activates adenylate cyclase and enhanced cyclic adenosine mono phosphate production is believed to be involved in increase of blood circulation. Moreover, the cyclic adenosine mono phosphate production can cause enhancement of nitric oxide synthase activity and nitric oxide production followed by increase in cyclic guanosine mono phosphate production as a secondary messenger for nitric oxide. The enhancement of cyclic guanosine mono phosphate production was connected to vasodilation and increase in cerebral circulation (Arulmani et al., 2004). It is believed that the effects of calcitonin gene related peptide on enhancement of substance P release and excitatory amino acids such as glutamate play an important role in transmission of calcitonin gene related peptide- mediated pain impulses. Also, it seems that calcitonin gene related peptide - mediated neurogenic inflammation is followed by degranulation of mast cells and the release of inflammatory agents (Durham, 2006).

2.2.3.2 Serotonin

Serotonin or 5-hydroxytryptamine is synthesized from tryptophan, in various tissues including brain (Hamel, 2007). Additionally, this molecule could be found in some plants (Badria, 2002). The fluctuations of platelet and plasma level of 5-hydroxytryptamine (Panconesi, 2008), change in lymphoblastic serotonin level (Nagata et al., 2007) and number of 5-hydroxytryptamine platelet transporters (as indirect index of 5-hydroxytryptamine recovery) (Panconesi, 2008) have been reported in patients with migraine. There are some controversies regarding the role of serotonin in migraine. It has been shown that there are the gender and seasonal variations of serotonin neurotransmission in human such as 5-hydroxytryptamine receptor hypersensitivity and its decreased cerebrospinal fluid level in women and 5-hydroxytryptamine receptor hyposensitivity in summer. On the other hand, the higher frequency of migraine in women and higher frequency of its attacks in summer compared with winter and autumn has been reported in most studies. Also, nowadays, the triptan, a selective serotonin 5-hydroxytryptamine ($1_B/1_C$) agonist is being used in the treatment of acute migraine attacks. In spite of controversial results about mentioned issues, the importance of the failure of a serotonergic system in migraine pathogenesis is significant. Accordingly, the serotonin system is considered to be involved in migraine (Panconesi, 2008). Moreover, additional studies are necessary to establish its importance in migraine etiology.

2.2.3.3 Melatonin

The synthesis of melatonin or N-acetyl-5-methyoxytryptamine from serotonin occurs in the pineal gland and other tissues in humans (Pandi-Perumal et al., 2006). In addition to the vertebrates, this indnole amine has been identified in numerous taxa including bacteria, unicellular eukaryotes (Hardeland et al., 2011; Pandi-Perumal et al., 2006) and plants (Ansari et al., 2010; Chen et al., 2003). In vertebrates, the production of melatonin reaches to its peak in the darkness and the light inhibits its secretion. Also, age-related decreases in melatonin synthesis and secretion have been reported (Pandi-Perumal et al., 2006). Most studies indicate that melatonin may play a significant role in sleep and circadian rhythm regulation, improvement of immune system (Hardeland et al., 2011) and antioxidant activity (Tan et al., 2007).

It has been found that plasma and urinary levels of melatonin (Peres et al., 2006) and nocturnal urinary 6-sulfatoxymelatonin concentration (Masruha et al., 2008) decrease in patients with migraine. Melatonin receptors are present in trigeminal ganglion and trigeminal nucleus of mammals that could explain its action. Also trigeminovascular nociception that is induced by cortical spreading depression in rats is attenuated by melatonin (Ambriz-Tututi et al., 2009). Therefore, melatonin has been suggested as a possible biomarker for migraine (Loder et al., 2006) and there is a great potential for using melatonin in acute or prophylactic treatment of migraine headache (Miano et al., 2008; Peres et al., 2004). Melatonin seems to be related with migraine pathogenesis in many ways, including its anti-inflammatory and antioxidant effects such as reduction in pro-inflammatory factors and scavenging toxic free radicals, potentiation of gamma amino butyric acid and opioid analgesia, suppression of nitric oxide synthase activity, inhibition of dopamine release, protection against glutamate neurotoxicity, and regulation of neurovascular regulation (Peres, 2005; Peres et al., 2007).

2.2.3.4 Nitric oxide

Nitric oxide as a diatomic molecule is synthesized by nitric oxide synthases from L-arginine. Changes in plasma and platelet (Gallai et al., 1996) levels of nitric oxide in migraine sufferers have been shown. Abnormalities in nitric oxide signaling pathway and increase in activity of nitric oxide synthase has been shown to be associated with enhanced susceptibility to migraine (Olesen, 2008). The oral administration of nitroglycerin as a nitric oxide donor induces headaches, which resembles to spontaneous migraine attacks. Also, in migraineurs, nitroglycerine inhibitors attenuated these nitroglycerin-induced attacks (Olesen, 2008) and as a result nitric oxide is suggested as fundamental biomarker for migraine (Loder et al., 2006). According to this point of view, nitric oxide is thought to be central in the pathophysiology of migraines. It seems likely that nitric oxide functions as the modulator of cellular toxicity, inflammatory responses, release of calcitonin gene related peptides as a potent peptide vasodilator, platelet function, endothelium-dependent vasodilatation, and transmission of pain impulses (Olesen, 2008).

2.2.3.5 Cations

Although, elements have been excluded from metabolome and proteome subclass, their strong connection with biomarkers cannot be ignored. The cations play a key role in cerebrospinal fluid functions and change in their serum levels is associated with pathogenesis of several diseases such as migraine headache (Donma & Donma, 2002). Considering the role of mutation in sodium, calcium and sodium-potassium channels in familial hemiplegic migraine, cations are important in migraine pathogenesis (Harrington et al., 2006). Moreover, nowadays, calcium channel blocker drugs are being used in migraine treatment, more extensively (Goadsby & Sprenger, 2010).

It seems that magnesium has a greater role as a possible biomarker of migraine, than other elements (Loder et al., 2006). It has been reported that serum magnesium concentration decreases in patients with migraine (Roudbari et al., 2005; Sun-Edelstein & Mauskop, 2009). Clearly, decreased magnesium concentration can trigger migraine attack (Mauskop, 1998), probably by promoting cortical spreading depression; alteration in neurotransmitter release and platelet hyperaggregation (Sun-Edelstein & Mauskop, 2009). The blockage of serotonin receptor and/or inducible receptor of glutamate, NMDA, and inhibition of synthesis and release of nitric oxide are believed to be of great physiological importance of magnesium (Sun-Edelstein & Mauskop, 2011).

According to the results of a study, increase in cerebrospinal fluid sodium concentration, independently from other clinical or pharmacological fluctuations of other cations, can participate in pathogenesis of migraine with aura. It is probable that concomitant elevated sodium concentration and normal cerebrospinal fluid potassium concentration, partially can decrease resting membrane potential and lead to decrease of action potential threshold in patients with migraine (Harrington et al., 2006). It has been suggested that salt out acts as potential migraine trigger (Brainard, 1976).

2.2.3.6 Others

Despite the importance of mentioned biomarkers in migraine pathology, several studies have reported changes in level of other biochemical biomarkers such as S100β, a glia-derived cytokine (Papandreou, 2005), dopamine and dopaminergic system (Charbit et al., 2010), endothelin-1 (Kallela et al., 1998), excitatory neurotransmitters such as glutamate and substance P, and pain-related molecules such as met-enkephalin and β-endorphin (Harrington, 2006) in/or between migraine attacks.

2.2.4 Practical considerations

There are some notable issues about mentioned biomarkers: (i) several of these biomarkers have potential interactions with others and have influences on concentration of other biomarkers. For example, melatonin as an imperative antioxidant is considered to be scavenger of nitric oxide and its toxic metabolite peroxynitrite ($ONOO^-$) from body. Additionally, melatonin can indirectly lead to decrease in nitric oxide synthase activity and expression in body (Acuña-Castroviejo et al., 2005); (ii) Results of measurement of a biomarker from two separate samples can be different. For example the concentration of melatonin in urine of patients with migraine is more valuable than its plasma concentration. As a result, assessment of concentration of urine and plasma melatonin were considered as confirmed and probable biomarker, respectively (Loder et al., 2006), and (iii) the levels of some these biomarkers in each person or in each attack are not varied similarly, therefore it seems that contemporary investigation of proteome or metabolome profile in migrainous patients, as has been employed for other conditions such as cancer (Casado-Vela et al., 2011), is necessary.

Despite of wide-ranging list of migraine biomarkers which has been described; it is believed that a complete assessment of clinical features and signs, and careful history taking may be decisive in the migraine diagnosis and these biomarkers, mainly genetic ones, "will be a test, not the mere identification of a marker, which will change clinical practice."(Goadsby, 2006). Nevertheless, migraine symptoms appeared to vary not only in each person but also in each attack. It is noted that after taking a medical history from a patient, one should be sure about absence of any other common headache in this context. To support this diagnosis, a series complementary tests including genetic and biochemical markers appears to be useful. Also, nowadays, instead of treatment of migraine based on pathological mechanisms, it is focused on clinical symptoms. It is evident that current treatments relieve migraine attacks slowly. Treatment strategies based on biomarkers can help us in this field. For example, if a biomarker reaches to normal level or diminishes, it is possible that the choice of the strategy for treatment is successful and/or the patients don't require further treatments. In addition, the investigation about cause of changes in biomarker levels can help us to explore mechanism and underlying environmental factors that trigger migraine. Also, it can be helpful in differentiation of migraine diagnosis (Loder, 2006).

2.3 Trigger factors in migraine

Any factor, that on exposure or withdrawal, alone or in combination, leads to the development of an acute migraine headache, is known as migraine trigger (V.T. Martin & Behbehani, 2001). They also are called precipitating or provoking factors that usually happen before the attack by less than 48 hours (P.R. Martin, 2010). These triggers can be categorized into two identifiable groups: internal and external (V.T. Martin & Behbehani, 2001). Based on twin studies, observed concordance rate for migraine headache in mono- and dizygotic twins are 37-52% and 15-21%, respectively. The fact that concordance rate for migraine in monozygotic twins is not 100%, suggests that environmental factors contribute to the development of migraine headache (V.T. Martin & Behbehani, 2001).

2.3.1 External triggers

External triggers that we hear most often about them, can be classified broadly as environmental, behavioral, dietary, chemical, allergens and some drugs (V.T. Martin & Behbehani, 2001) of which some are listed in Table 1. Stress is the most commonly mentioned migraine trigger, and it seems that can initiate or augment frequency and severity of migraine attack (Hauge et al., 2009; Millichap & Yee, 2003). Most information about prevalence of triggers has been reported in population- or clinical- based studies in a self-report manner by patients own experience which could lead to a significant bias. These studies didn't have the technical or methodological strength and the results are variable and contradictory (P.R. Martin, 2010; V.T. Martin & Behbehani, 2001) and more discussion about the epidemiological studies on external triggers are not necessary, as well.

2.3.1.1 Possible mechanisms

An understanding of the aura and headache components of migraine provides a basis for the potential mechanism of action of dietary triggers. Theoretically, migraine triggers could influence on the cerebral cortex, organizations innervated by the terminal nerve (i.e. dural arteries), the trigeminal pain pathway (trigeminal nerve, thalamic nuclei), and regulatory pathway within the brain stem or the limbic system contribute to migraine. Therefore, migraine triggers aggravate migraine headache in a number of diverse ways, including: (i) direct effect on excitatory or inhibitory neuroreceptors; (ii) release of internal neuropeptides or neurotransmitters and nitric oxide; and (iii) direct excitation of neurons (V.T. Martin & Behbehani, 2001; Millichap & Yee, 2003).

Dietary[a]	Environmental[b]
• Caffeinated beverages	• Bright light/visual stimuli
• Alcoholic beverages	• Odors/smells
• Aged cheeses	• Weather changes
• Chocolate	• Cigarette smoke
• Coffee, tea, cola	Behavioral[b]
• Chocolate	• Stress/tension
• Food allergens (Dairy products, yogurt)	• Hunger/not eating
	• Emotions
• Ice cream	• Lack of sleep and Sleeping late/excess
Chemical[a]	• Fatigue/tiredness
• Monosodium glutamate	• Exercise
• Tyramine	• Hair wash or head bath[c]
• Nitrates	
• Artificial sweetener (Aspartame)	Minor head trauma[d]

[a](V.T. Martin & Behbehani, 2001; Millichap & Yee, 2003); [b](P.R. Martin, 2010; V.T. Martin & Behbehani, 2001); [c] Reported in Indian patients (Ravishankar, 2006), [d] Frequently reported as a trigger for hemiplegic migraine (Russell & Ducros, 2011)

Table 1. External Trigger Factors in Migraine.

2.3.2 Internal triggers

Internal triggers are those that occur in our body. The most common internal triggers are sex hormones (neurosteroids and ovarian steroids). The key stages of reproduction including first menstruation, pregnancy and menopause are associated with frequency or severity of migraine. It is suggested that sex steroids (i.e. estradiol and progesterone) have a central role in migraine etiology (Gupta et al., 2007; V.T. Martin & Behbehani, 2006b) especially in menstrual migraine. 35-51% of female migraineurs have menstrually related migraine, even though 7-19% has pure menstrual migraine. Interestingly only attacks of migraine without aura occur during the perimenstrual time period and attacks of migraine with aura happen equally during the menstrual cycle. The main trigger of menstrual migraine seems to be withdrawal of estrogen rather than the maintenance of continuous high or low estrogen levels. On the other hand, sustained changes in estrogen levels related to pregnancy (augmented levels) and menopause (declined levels) likewise affect headaches (V.T. Martin & Behbehani, 2006b).

2.3.2.1 Possible mechanisms

The neurosteroids and ovarian steroids may exert their effects on vascular and nervous system via cytosolic and nuclear receptors (genomic pathway) and membrane receptors (non-genomic pathway) and initiate a migraine attack (V.T. Martin & Behbehani, 2006a). These steroids can lead to neuronal excitation via increase in calcium and decrease in magnesium concentration, vasodilatation and activation of trigeminal nerve through synthesis and release of nitric oxide, neuropeptides (i.e. calcitonin gene related peptide), increase or decrease in inhibitory or excitatory neurotransmitters synthesis and opioids and their impacts on receptors. However there are some contradictory results of negative or positive effects of steroids on onset of migraine attack (Gupta et al., 2007; V.T. Martin & Behbehani, 2006a).

2.3.3 Genetic background

Any change in activity of involved gene in hormonal and vascular function causes increase in susceptibility to migraine. Recently, it has been suggested that the association between migraine and dysfunction of genes involved in progesterone and/or estrogen receptor 1, might play a role in increased susceptibility to migraine (Colson et al., 2006). Moreover, diamine oxidase activity in histamine breakdown in the intestine might be important in those who are sensitive to food containing histamine. It seems that vitamin B6 supplementation enhances diamineoxidase activity, and in that way decreases histamine-induced migraine attacks (Ross, 2011).

3. Treatment

Introducing the concept of brain disorder in migraine etiology led to a new approach in treatment options in migraine disorder (Monteith & Goadsby, 2011). Migraine treatment can be classified into medical and non-medical treatment. Non-medical treatments include patient education and behavioral therapy for the prevention of trigger factors involved in migraine. The pharmacotherapy for migraine can be categorized into preventive drugs, which are administrated daily regardless of the presence of headache and acute drugs, which are taken by patients immediately after symptoms appearing (Goadsby et al, 2002).

3.1 Drugs

Acute treatment is classified into nonspecific treatments, including non-steroidal anti-inflammatory drugs (NSAIDs), and migraine-specific treatments, including ergot derivatives and the triptans (Table 2) (Goadsby et al, 2002). However, only one third of patients in clinical trials feel pain-free 2 hours after taking a triptan orally, so novel treatment options are still required. Recently, new drugs have been developed by targeting neural sites. Interestingly, safety and efficiency of some of these drugs have been confirmed in phase II and some other in phase III clinical trials (Monteith & Goadsby, 2011).

Preventive therapy (prophylaxis) including beta-blockers, anticonvulsants like valproate and topiramate, and calcium channel blockers are preferred choice for treatment of patients unresponsive to acute-attack medications (Table 2). In the U.S, therapeutic guidelines regular migraine prophylaxis for patients with more than two acute attacks per week are recommended, but in the Europe the regular preventive treatment therapeutic guidelines are recommended on the basis of two or more acute attacks per month (Goadsby & Sprenger, 2010).

3.2 Complementary alternative medicine

Despite some controversy regarding formal definition for Complementary Alternative Medicine, the National Center for Complementary and Alternative Medicine, defines it as "a group of diverse products, medical and health care systems, practices that are not presently considered to be part of conventional medicine." Using complementary alternative medicine along with conventional medical treatments as part of a multidisciplinary treatment strategy has higher probability to result in appropriate responses. Although, some evidences are available in favor of these treatments, more extensive studies are required to fully elucidate their efficacies (Sun-Edelstein & Mauskop, 2011). Here nutritional supplements and medicinal herbs will be explained further.

Acute attack drugs in migraine[a]
Specific drugs
• Ergot derivatives
• (ergotamine and dihydroergotamine)
• Serotonin 5-HT receptor agonists
• 5-$HT_{1B/1D}$ receptor agonists
• Triptans: almotriptan, eletriptan, frovatriptan, naratriptan, rizatriptan, Sumatriptan, and zolmitriptan.
• Serotonin 5-HT_{1F} receptor agonists*
• Other receptors antagonists*
• Calcitonin gene-related peptide (Olcegepant and telcagepant)
• Glutamate AMPA/kainate
• Transient receptor potential vanilloid-1
• Prostanoid EP4
• Inducible and neuronal nitric oxide synthase inhibitors*
Nonspecific drugs
• Non-steroidal anti-inflammatory drugs (Aspirin, acetaminophen),
• Opiates, and combination analgesics
Preventive drugs in migraine[b]
• Beta-blockers (Propranolol, Metoprolol)
• Anticonvulsants (Valproate, Topiramate)
• Calcium channel blockers (Flunarizine)
• Antidepressants (dosulepin (dothiepin), Venlafaxine)
• Serotonin antagonists (Pizotifen, Methysergide)
• ACE inhibitors (Lisinopril, Candesartan)
• Cortical spreading depression inhibitors (tonabersat) *
• Neuromodulators (the stimulation of the greater occipital nerve) *
• Botulinum toxin type-A*
• Patent foramen ovale closure*

* These drugs are under investigation in phase II or III clinical trial. [a](Goadsby et al., 2002; Goadsby & Sprenger, 2010; Monteith & Goadsby, 2011); [b](Goadsby & Sprenger, 2010).

Table 2. Acute and preventive drugs for migraine treatment.

3.2.1 Riboflavin

Riboflavin (vitamin B_2) is critical for membrane stability, cellular energy production and the maintenance of cellular functions (Rios & Passe, 2004; Sun-Edelstein & Mauskop, 2009). It is thought a deficit in brain mitochondrial energy reserve, causes biochemical changes that trigger the trigeminovascular system, and therefore play an important role in migraine attacks (Rios & Passe, 2004). Riboflavin can increase the mitochondrial energy efficiency. It is reported an attenuation of the frequency of migraine attack after supplementation with high dose riboflavin (400 mg/day) for three months (Sun-Edelstein & Mauskop, 2009) (Rios & Passe, 2004). Despite minor side effects of high-dose of riboflavin (including diarrhea and polyuria), no identified complication is reported for riboflavin in pregnancy (Rios & Passe, 2004). However, there is no consensus that riboflavin is to significantly operative in migraine preventive.

3.2.2 Coenzyme Q10

Due to its function on mitochondrial respiratory chain and antioxidant activity, it seems to be helpful to prevent migraine (Sun-Edelstein & Mauskop, 2009; 2011). Moreover, efficacy of coenzyme Q10 supplementation in migraine pediatric prophylaxis has been reported (Ross, 2011; Sun-Edelstein & Mauskop, 2009; 2011) and approximately 300 mg of coenzyme Q10 is thought to be effective in migraine prevention (Sun-Edelstein & Mauskop, 2009). However, these results require further approval before to be suggested as an effective treatment.

3.2.3 Alpha-lipoic acid

Similar to riboflavin and coenzyme Q10, alpha-lipoic acid improves oxygen metabolism in mitochondria and adenosine triphosphate production (Sun-Edelstein & Mauskop, 2011). Although no defined supplementation dose for alpha-lipoic acid have been approved by the U.S Food and Drug Administration, it is reported that supplementation with 600 mg of alpha-lipoic acid once a day for three months attenuated the frequency of migraine attacks (Sun-Edelstein & Mauskop, 2009).

3.2.4 Magnesium

Based on results of several investigations, failure in calcium-magnesium balance in patients with migraine plays a key role in pathogenesis of this disease. In addition to possible role of magnesium as a biomarker for migraine (described previously), regarding its physiological functions in energy production, maintaining blood vessel tone and stability of neurons, it may be beneficial in patients with migraine (Ross, 2011; Sun-Edelstein & Mauskop, 2009; 2011). Although oral magnesium can prevent migraine attacks and intravenous magnesium can reduce acute headache, the use of magnesium has shown controversial results (Sun-Edelstein & Mauskop, 2009; 2011). The daily supplementation with 400 mg of chelated magnesium (Sun-Edelstein & Mauskop, 2009), magnesium oxide or 600 mg of trimagnesium dicitrate (Rios & Passe, 2004) is thought to be effective in treatment of migraine. These remarks have not been confirmed yet. The high dose of magnesium can cause diarrhea, loss of appetite, nausea, vomiting and gastric irritation. Also, owing due to involvement of high dose of magnesium in decreasing fluoroquinolones absorption, it is not recommended for patients with ulcerative colitis, diverticulitis, or renal failure and in pregnant or nursing women (Rios & Passe, 2004).

3.2.5 Dietary avoidance

Elimination of food allergens (including cow's milk; wheat; eggs) (Ross, 2011) or dietary triggers (described in external triggers previously) (V.T Martin & Behbehani, 2001; Millichap & Yee, 2003), which initiate a migraine attack, can lead to elimination or reduction of frequency and severity of migraine attacks. Thus, they can be considered as candidate for treatment of migraine. Though, due to daily need to some of the mentioned foods for cellular function, it is impossible to eliminate them from dietary completely, so they are replaced with either (Millichap & Yee, 2003).

4. Herbal medicine

4.1 History

Before the advent of modern synthetic drugs, herbs were considered as first choice for treatment of human diseases. In spite of the fact that using herbs has been diminished in modern medicine, fortunately, there is a growing trend, particularly in migraine disorder. There have been few studies examining herbal remedy effectiveness and most of our information is based on traditional experiences. However, mechanism of action of many of them have not been fully understood.

In traditional medicine in Iran, China and India and some older societies, factors such as geographic location and experience in the proven effectiveness of herbs, affect their acceptance as medicine. The famous scientists gathered their ancestor's experiences and their own researches which remained as useful references for the future. *Qanoon fel teb* (*The Canon of Medicine*) by Ebn-e-Sina *(Avicenna,* 980–1037), *al-hawi* (*Continens*) by Zakariya Râzi (Rhazes, 860–940) and *Kitab-al-Maliki* (*Liber Regius*) by Ali Ebn Al-Abbas-al-Majusi (Haly Abbas, 949–982) are good examples in this regard (Gorji, 2003; Gorji & Khaleghi Ghadiri, 2002). On the other hand, using new techniques to analyze the active ingredients of plants and methods for the study of underlying mechanism, can confirm their effectiveness and safety. Due to the easier and faster access to medical information resources of traditional medicine for treatment, as well as new technology in various countries to identify the mechanism of action of herbal ingredients, it is possible to clarify more aspects of mechanism underlying treatment of several diseases, such as migraine.

4.2 Herbs application for migraine treatment

4.2.1 Analgesic effects

Analgesics are widely used for pain relief worldwide. Many herbal remedies have been proved to be effective in painful situations like migraine headache empirically and/or in clinical trials. Some of these botanical analgesics which have shown pain killing effects are listed in Table 3 (Yarnell, 2002; Zareba, 2009; Zengion & Yarnell, 2011). Although some aspects of herbs mechanism of action have been understood, more studies are required to elucidate anodyne herb's function.

Herbs containing salicylates and those with anti-inflammatory effects are usually safe and beneficial for pains caused by inflammation (Yarnell, 2002; Zareba, 2009; Zengion & Yarnell, 2011). *Salix alba* is a good example which decreases pain due to its salicin content and is reported for migraine treatment (Gorji, 2003; Gorji & Khaleghi Ghadiri, 2002). Feverfew and ginger (Mustafa & Srivastava, 1990) are two important anti-inflammatory herbs with proved anti-migraine activity. Hypnotic anodynes have more general analgesic properties and are ideal when pain contributes to insomnia. Some studies recommended Valerian to be used in migraine treatment. Numerous centrally-acting herbs have stronger analgesic effect and they should be used with lower doses to avoid adverse effects. Topically used herbs like *Capsicum frutescens* could propose a useful way to relieve neuropathic pain, and other pain syndromes due to capsaicin as an effective component. Intranasal application of capsaicin for relief of migraine is reported (Yarnell, 2002).

Anti-inflammatory herbs
- *Curcuma Longa* (Turmeric)
- *Angelica sinensis* (Dang Gui, Tang Kui, Dong Kuai),
- *Harpagophytum procumbens* (Devil's Claw)*
- *Boswellia serrata* (Frankincense)*
- *Zingiber officinalis* (Ginger)*
- *Tanacetum parthenium* (Feverfew)*

Centrally-acting herbs
- *Cannabis sativa* (Cannabis)*
- *Hypericum perforatum* (St. John's Wort)*
- *Corydalis yanhusuo*
- *Bryonia alba* (White Bryony)

Hypnotic herbs
- *Valeriana officianalis* (Valerian)*
- *Piscidia piscipula, P. erythrina* (Jamaican Dogwood)
- *Eschscholtzia californica* (California Poppy)

Salicylate-containing herbs
- *Salix alba* (White Willow)*
- *Populus tremuloides* (Quaking Aspen)

Topical herbs
- *Capsicum frutescens* (Cayenne)*
- *Urtica dioica* (Stinging Nettle)
- *Symphytum officinale* (Comfrey)

Miscellaneous
- *Ginkgo biloba* (Ginkgo)*
- *Centella asiatica* (Gotu Kola)
- *Viburnum opulus* (Cramp Bark)
- *Viburnum prunifolium* (Black Haw)
- *Scutellaria laterifolia* (Skullcap)
- *Scutellaria baicalensis* (Huang qin)
- *Rosa canina**
- *Solidago chilensis* (Brazilian Arnica)

* analgesic herbs which are traditionally used for relief of migraine headache (Gorji, 2003; Gorji & Khaleghi Ghadiri, 2002; Yarnell, 2002; Zareba, 2009)..

Table 3. Analgesic herbs used for pain relief (Yarnell, 2002; Zareba, 2009; Zengion & Yarnell, 2011).

4.2.2 Prophylactic effects

Efficacy for prophylactic drugs is defined as a reduction in migraine frequency of more than 50%. Also it could refer to reduction in attack severity, or significant reductions in nausea, vomiting, photophobia and phonophobia. Feverfew and butterbur were the first herbs that have been utilized for migraine preventive therapy.

4.2.2.1 Feverfew

Although, feverfew (*Tanacetum parthenium*) is a perennial herb native to Balkan Mountains in Eastern Europe, in more recent times it has become naturalized widely in Europe, North America, and South America (Sun-Edelstein & Mauskop, 2011). Several studies have been reported that feverfew has anti-inflammatory and anti-platelet aggregation properties, thereby having promising results in the treatment of migraine (Rios & Passe, 2004; Ross, 2011). Its anti-migraine action is probably related to its active compound i.e. parthenolide (Sun-Edelstein & Mauskop, 2011). Although optimal supplementation dose have not been established, daily supplementation with 100 mg (Sun-Edelstein & Mauskop, 2009) or 50-145 mg of feverfew supplements, containing at least 0.2% parthenolide (Rios & Passe, 2004; Ross, 2011) is thought to be effective in migraine treatment. The usage of these doses is associated with side effects like nausea, and diarrhea, mouth ulcerations (only when chewing leaves), and withdrawal symptoms including muscle stiffness, anxiety, and rebound migraine headache. It is noted that the use of feverfew supplements is not recommended in pregnancy (due to uterus contraction), nursing women, children below 2 years, patients with high sensitivity to plants of *Asteraceae* family (Rios & Passe, 2004; Ross, 2011), and patients undergoing surgery, due to its function as an inhibitor of platelet aggregation (Ross, 2011).Using feverfew as an approved medication require further investigations.

4.2.2.2 Butterbur

Butterbur (*Petasites hybridus*) also known as pestwurz, blatterdock, bog rhubarb, and butter-dock (Rios & Passe, 2004), is an herb, found throughout Europe and parts of Asia (Sun-Edelstein & Mauskop, 2011). It seems to be a promising drug for reduction of frequency and severity of migraine attacks (Rios & Passe, 2004; Ross, 2011), especially in children (Oelkers-Ax, et al., 2008). Butterbur is rich in pharmacologically active compounds called sesquiterpenes; such as petasin and isopetasin (Sun-Edelstein & Mauskop, 2011). Despite uncertainty about its optimal dose, similar to feverfew, by Food and Drug Administration (Rios & Passe, 2004), 75 mg of butterbar twice daily for a month, following 50 mg twice a day (Sun-Edelstein & Mauskop, 2009) or 50-100 mg twice a day, containing at least 7 mg of petasin and isopetasin (Rios & Passe, 2004*)* is believed to be beneficial for migraine headaches. So, until performing further studies, it cannot be supported as an effective treatment for migraine. Pyrrolizidine alkaloids found in butterbur are recognized as toxins with carcinogenic and hepatotoxic effects. For this reason, it is necessary to eliminate these alkaloids from commercial butterbur extracts (Sun-Edelstein & Mauskop, 2011). It is not recommended for the pregnant or nursing mothers (Rios & Passe, 2004).

4.2.2.3 MigriHeal®

Recently a novel herbal remedy was introduced with prophylactic effect against migraine attacks which lasts even after the discontinuation of therapy (Fallah et al., 2005). This herbal drug which is used as inhalation up to 4 months can decrease headache frequency and severity (www.araamesh.com). No adverse effects were reported by patients and animal study proved its safety even in higher doses. Investigating the effect of M*igriHeal®* extracts on nitric oxide production in mouse endothelial cell-line showed reduced production in a dose-dependent manner (Ansari et al., 2005; 2007).

4.3 Possible mechanisms of medicinal herbs used in migraine

On the contrary to primary products, such as carbohydrates, lipids, proteins, heme, chlorophyll, and nucleic acids, which participate in modulation of cellular metabolism and maintenance of plant cells, the benefits of phytomedicine typically may be caused by the combined action of secondary plant compounds. Although, up to now, there are some *in vivo* and *in vitro* studies about role of phytomedicine in migraine treatment as well as its possible mechanism, further investigation is required. Therefore, studies exploring the effect of phytomedicine on frequency and severity of migraine attacks can help us to understand the etiology of migraine. Besides, investigation of plant derivatives can lead to new drugs for migraine treatment.

Here, we discuss possible mechanisms of several medicinal plants, used in migraine headache treatment.

4.3.1 Compensatory components

Due to high level of some molecules in medicinal plants, which are reduced in patients with migraine, it seems that they can be used as compensatory mechanism for migraine treatment. It has been shown that some medicinal plants including *Tripleurospermum disciforme, Viola odorata* and *Tanacetum parthenium* used in treatment of migraine headache, contain high concentration of melatonin (Ansari et al., 2010). Notably, these results are in line with other studies about other medicinal plants used in treatment of neurologic disorders, *Tanacetum parthenium, Hypericum perforatum,* and *Scutellaria biacalensis* (Murch et al., 1997) and Chinese medicinal plants are used in treatment oxidative abnormality-related diseases (Chen et al., 2003). Plasma level of melatonin is decreased in migraine and its therapeutic use in this disorder has been reported (Peres et al., 2006). In the other hand, owing to increase in plasma concentration of melatonin in human (Oba et al., 2008) and rat (Reiter et al., 2005) following phytomelatonin administration, the high content of melatonin (from picograms to micrograms per gram of plant material) in these medicinal plants is thought to be responsible of reduction of migraine attack and can be considered as potential candidate for migraine prevention.

Interestingly, *In vivo* studies have been shown that extract of some medicinal plants can enhance gene expression and activity of enzyme involved in melatonin synthesis, N-acetyltransferase, thereby increasing melatonin level (Qu et al., 2008). In addition, it seems that the extract of some plants has large affinity for the serotonin (5-HT_{4e}, 5-HT_6, and 5-HT_7) and melatonin (ML1 and ML2) receptors (Abourashed et al., 2004). In spite of some discrepancies between the studies on role of enzymes involved in melatonin synthesis and melatonin receptors in migraine etiology, the involvement of melatonin in migraine pathogenesis is notable. Accordingly, further studies are required to elucidate possible impact of medicinal plants on reduction or treatment of migraine attacks as well as underlying mechanism.

In addition of melatonin, high level of several metabolites of tryptophan metabolism including 5-Hydroxytryptophan, as a direct precursor of the neurotransmitter serotonin, (used to boost levels of this compound in the human brain thereby treating cases of serotonin deficiency syndrome) (Lemaire & Adosraku., 2002), tryptamine and serotonin (Badria, 2002) have been considered in some medicinal plants. It seems that the metabolites will be a potent term in phytomedicine research reports, particularly in migraine treatment.

4.3.2 Effects on signaling and expression regulation

4.3.2.1 Effects on nitric oxide formation and calcitonin gene related peptide

These effects can result from elimination of nitric oxide, inhibition of gene expression of enzymes and removal of calcium ion from environment and its influence on calcium channels and calcitonin gene related peptide. For example, some medicinal plants such as Lavender, Coriander, Chamomile and Viola can decrease nitric oxide as stated in Ansari et al. report. There have been noted that different forms (e.g. aqueous extract, essential oil) of these herbs significantly suppress nitric oxide production in a dose-dependent manner (Ansari et al., 2005; 2007) and possibly thereby reducing migraine attacks. These herbs with analgesic and/or prophylactic effects are also summarized in Gorji et al. reviews (Gorji, 2003; Gorji & Khaleghi Ghadiri, 2002).

It is believed that the parthenolide as a sesquiterpene lactone in feverfew prevents migraine. The parthenolide has been found to inhibit, lipopolysaccharide-induced nitric oxide formation and lipopolysaccharide-induced activation of the inducible isoform of nitric oxide synthase. It should be noted that several flavonoid glycosides in feverfew have shown vasodilation and anti-inflammatory properties, but parthenolide in other plants have not shown anti-migraine effects. Interestingly, extract with high parthenolide showed a low tolerability, in comparison with purified parthenolide.

Treatment of rat trigeminal ganglia cultures with *Theobroma cacao* extract, following exposure to depolarizing stimuli was shown to block calcium channel activity and to inhibit the HCl and capsain-stimulated enhancement in calcitonin gene related peptide secretion. According to in vivo study, this extract was demonstrated to decrease nitric oxide release and inflammatory cytokines from macrophages significantly (Abbey et al., 2008). Nutritional coca in a similar manner, can suppress calcitonin gene related peptide expression in neurons and inducible nitric oxide synthase activity, thereby it is involved in migraine pathophysiology, pain feeling and inflammation-related responses. Interestingly, cocoa can suppress neuronal increased expression of the mitogen-activated protein kinase p38 and extracellular signal-regulated kinases after stimulation with acute or chronic peripheral inflammation (Cady & Durham, 2010). It is noted that mitogen-activated protein kinase signal transduction participated in initiation and stimulation of inflammatory responses and pain feeling. It has been suggested that high level of borocyanides in *Arace catechu* as well as inhibitory influence on inducible nitric oxide synthase activity can be involved in its underlying mechanism in anti-migraine properties (Bhandare et al., 2011).

4.3.2.2 Effects on Arachidonic pathway

The feverfew (parthenolide) is known to inhibit prostaglandin, thromboxane B4 and leukotriene B_4 release by phospholipase A_2 inhibition (Summer et al., 1992). Main active ingredients of butterbur are petasin and isopetasin, inhibiting both lipoxygenase pathway and leukotriene synthesis –related anti-inflammatory effects (Rios & Passe, 2004; Ross, 2011). On the other hand, the inhibitory properties of ginger in prostaglandins, thromboxanes and leukotriene have been linked to its anti-migraine effects (Mustafa & Srivastava, 1990).

4.3.2.3 Effects on platelet activity

Regarding to decrease in platelet 5-hydroxytryptamine content, change in 5-hydroxytryptamine transport as well as platelet cytosolic free-calcium concentration, in patients with migraine, it is evident that abnormalities in platelet function may participate in migraine pathogenesis (Rogers et al., 2001). According to results of a study, for quantification of the antiplatelet effect of Australian plants extracts via testing adenosine di phosphate induced platelet aggregation and the release of 5-hydroxytryptamine, it has been demonstrated that these extracts through regulation of cyclooxygenase pathway may contribute to inhibition of platelet 5-hydroxytryptamine release (Rogers et al., 2000). Previously, Rogers et al reported that *E. vespertilio* and *C. ambiguous* can be served as traditional treatments for headache due to inhibitory effect of their extracts on platelet activation (Rogers et al., 2001).

In view of the several studies about function of gingkolide B (an herbal constituent extract from *Ginko biloba* leaves) as a natural antiplatelet activating factor, recently it has been shown that its administration can be effective in patients with primary headache (Usai et al., 2011). Based on investigation of ginsenosides (active constituent of *Genus Panax*, ginseng) effects on rats, it has been shown that they inhibit thrombin or collagen-induced platelet aggregation. In addition, it has been reported that enough concentrations of allicin, a primary constituent of garlic (*Allium sativum*) can result into platelet aggregation and degranulation blockage. Despite of in vitro studies, it is noted that after administration of these plants in healthy individuals, the platelet function does not change (Beckert et al., 2007).

On the other hand, goshoyoto as an herbal drug seems to be effective in treatment of migraine headaches by suppression of platelet aggregation. Its two herbal components, zingiberis and evodiae, have been shown to inhibit collagen-induced platelet aggregation. Interestingly, 6-gingerol and 6-shogaol as two constituents of zingiberis can inhibit platelet aggregation by inhibition of cyclooxygenase-1 activity (Hibino et al., 2008). In another study, anti-migraine properties of *Sapindustrifoliatus* water extract has been linked to both inhibition of 5-HT_{2B} receptor and release of platelet serotonin (Arulmozhi et al., 2004).

4.3.2.4 Effects on ion channels

Evidences link the ion channel gene mutations, particularly those encoding voltage-gated calcium channels, to rare and severe hemiplegic migraine. Accordingly, use of L-type voltage-gated calcium channels blockers for the prophylactic relief of migraine seems occasionally reasonable. Studies show that extracts of *E. bignoniiflora*, *A. symphyocarpa* and *E. vespertilio* have potential antagonists of neuronal voltage- gated calcium channels (Rogers et al., 2002). In addition, due to combined effects of $Ca_v2.1$-inhibitory properties of petasins (as the main constituents of the anti-migraine herb *P. hybridus*) and sulfur containing petasins in these herbs, it can be considered as appropriate approach to migraine prophylaxis (Horak et al., 2009). These findings prompt further electrophysiological studies to investigate the modulatory capacity of these compounds on other ion channels implicated in hemiplegic migraine pathophysiology.

4.3.2.5 Others

In addition to mentioned mechanism underlying the effect of herbal medicine in migraine treatments, several pathways is thought to be involved in this regard. For example, based on results of one study (Arulmozhi et al., 2005), it has been suggested that the high level of saponin in *Sapindus trifoliatus* can have a regulatory role in dopaminergic and adrenergic receptors. Also, anti-inflammatory, analgesic and narcotic properties of this herb can be responsible for its effects in migraine treatment. It is worth mentioning that these receptors can associate with migraine pathogenesis.

5. Conclusion

It seems that future researches should be emphasized to unravel the hidden area of migraine pathophysiology using metabolomics and proteomics study which could also lead to find some biomarkers to discriminate patient and healthy people. The latter could be used in new classification of the disease, and also as a strong diagnostic tool.

6. References

Abbey, M.J., Patil, V.V., Vause, C.V. & Durham, P.L. (2008). Repression of calcitonin gene-related peptide expression in trigeminal neurons by a Theobroma cacao extract. *Journal of Ethnopharmacology,* Vol.115, No.2, pp.238-248, ISSN 0378-8741

Abokrysha, N. (2009). Ibn Sina (Avicenna) on Pathogenesis of Migraine Compared With the Recent Theories. *Headache,* Vol.49, No.6, pp.923-937, ISSN 0017-8748

Abourashed, E.A., Koetter, U. & Brattström, A. (2004). In vitro binding experiments with a Valerian, Hops and their fixed combination extract (Ze91019) to selected central nervous system receptors. *Phytomedicine,* Vol.11, No.7-8, pp.633-638, ISSN 0944-7113

Acuña-Castroviejo, D., Escames, G., López, L.C., Hitos, A.B. & León, J. (2005). Melatonin and Nitric Oxide: Two Required Antagonists for Mitochondrial Homeostasis. *Endocrine,* Vol.27, No.2, pp.159-168, ISSN 1355-008X

Ambriz-Tututi, M., Rocha-González, H.I., Cruz, S.L., Granados-Soto, V. (2009). Melatonin: A hormone that modulates pain. *Life Sciences,* Vol.84, No.15-16, pp.489-498, ISSN 0024-3205

Ansari, M., Mahrooz, A., Sharif Tabrizi, A., Vardasbi, S. & Naimi, S.M. (2005). The effect of antimigraine herbal extract on nitric oxide level in cultured vascular endothelial cells. *Proceedings of Cephalalgia 2005 12th Congress of the International Headache Society,* pp.918, Kyoto, Japan, October 9-12, 2005

Ansari, M., Naeemi, S.M., Paknejad, M., Soukhtalou, M & Ansari A. (2007). Effect of Althaea officinalis and citrus Bigaradia water Extracts on Nitric Oxide Production in cultured vascular Endotelioma cells. *The 9th Iranian Congress of Biochemistry and the 2nd International congress of Biochemistry and Molecular Biology,* Shiraz, Iran, Oct.29-Nov.1, 2007

Ansari, M., Paknejad, M., Ansari, A. (2007). Effects of three Medicinal Herbs Essontial oil on Nittric Oxide Production in Cultured vascular endothelioma cell line. *11th Asian Pacific Congress of Clinical Biochemistry,* Beijing, China, October 14-19, 2007

Ansari, M., Rafiee, Kh., Yasa, N., Vardasbi, S., Naimi, S.M & Nowrouzi, A. (2010). Measurement of melatonin in alcoholic and hot water extracts of *Tanacetum parthenium, Tripleurospermum disciforme* and *Viola odorata. DARU,* Vol.18, No.3, pp. 173-178, ISSN 1560-8115

Anttila, V., Stefansson, H., Kallela, M., Todt, U., Terwindt, G M., Calafato, M S., Nyholt, D.R., Dimas, A.S., Freilinger, T., Müller-Myhsok, B., Artto, V., Inouye, M., Alakurtti, K., Kaunisto, M.A., Hämäläinen, E., de Vries, B., Stam, A.H., Weller, C.M., Heinze, A., Heinze-Kuhn, K., Goebel, I., Borck, G., Göbel, H., Steinberg, S., Wolf, C., Björnsson, A., Gudmundsson, G., Kirchmann, M., Hauge, A., Werge, T., Schoenen, J., Eriksson, J G., Hagen, K., Stovner, L., Wichmann, H-E., Meitinger, T., Alexander, M., Moebus, S., Schreiber, S., Aulchenko, Y.S., Breteler, M.M.B., Uitterlinden, A.G., Hofman, A., van Duijn, C.M., Tikka-Kleemola, P., Vepsäläinen, S., Lucae, S., Tozzi, F., Muglia, P., Barrett, J., Kaprio, J., Färkkilä, M., Peltonen, L., Stefansson, K., Zwart, J-A., Ferrari, M.D., Olesen, J., Daly, M., Wessman, M., van den Maagdenberg, A.M., Dichgans, M., Kubisch, C., Dermitzakis, E.T., Frants, R.R. & Palotie, A. (2010). Genome-wide association study of migraine implicates a common susceptibility variant on 8q22.1. *Nature Genetic,* Vol.42, No.10, pp.869-873, ISSN 1061- 4036

Arulmani, U., Van Den Brink, A.M., Villalón, C.M. & Saxenaa, P.R. (2004). Calcitonin gene-related peptide and its role in migraine pathophysiology. *European journal of pharmacology,* Vol.500, No.1-3, pp.315-330, ISSN 0014-2999

Arulmozhi, D.K., Sridhar, N., Bodhankar, S.L., Veeranjaneyulua, A. & Arora, S.K. (2004). In vitro pharmacological investigations of Sapindus trifoliatus in various migraine targets. *Journal of Ethnopharmacology,* Vol.95, No.2-3, pp.239-245, ISSN 0378-8741

Arulmozhi, D.K., Veeranjaneyulu, A., Bodhankar, S.L. & Arora, S.K. (2005). Pharmacological studies of the aqueous extract of Sapindus trifoliatus on central nervous system: possible antimigraine mechanisms. *Journal of Ethnopharmacology,* Vol.97, No.3, pp.491-496, ISSN 0378-8741

Badria, F.A. (2002). Serotonin, tryptamine and melatonin in some Egyptian food and medicinal plants. *J. Med. Food,* Vol.5, No.3, pp.53-57, ISSN 1557-7600

Bartleson J.D. & Cutrer M. (2010). Migraine Update: Diagnosis and Treatment . Clinical and Health Affairs. Minnesota Medicine, Vol.93, No.5, pp.36-41, ISSN 0026-556X

Beckert, B.W., Concannon, M.J., Henry, S.L., Smith, D.S. & Puckett, C.L. (2007). The Effect of Herbal Medicines on Platelet Function: An In Vivo Experiment and Review of the Literature. *Plastic and Reconstructive Surgery,* Vol.120, No.7, pp.2044-2050, ISSN 0032-1052

Bhandare A., Kshirsagar A., VyawahareN., Sharma P., Mohitea R. (2011). Evaluation of anti-migraine potential of Areca catechu to prevent nitroglycerin-induced delayed inflammation in rat meninges: Possible involvement of NOS inhibition. *Journal of Ethnopharmacology,* Vol.136, pp.267–270, ISSN 0378-8741

Brainard, J.B. (1976). Salt load as a trigger formigraine. *Minnesota Medicine,* Vol.59, No.4, pp.232-233, ISSN 0026-556X

Cady, R.J. & Durham, P.L. (2010). Cocoa-enriched diets enhance expression of phosphatases and decrease expression of inflammatory molecules in trigeminal ganglion neurons. *Brain Research,* Vol.1323, pp.18-32, ISSN 0006-8993

Casado-Vela, J., Cebrián, A., Gómez Del Pulgar, M.T. & Lacal, J.C. (2011). Approaches for the study of cancer: towards the integration of genomics, proteomics and metabolomics. *Clin Transl Oncol,*Vol.13, No.9, pp.617-628, ISSN 1699-048X

Charbit, A.R., Akerman, S. & Goadsby, P.J. (2010). Dopamine: what's new in migraine? *Current Opinion in Neurology,* Vol.23, No.3, pp.275-281, ISSN 0006-8993

Charles, A. (2009). Advances in the basic and clinical science of migraine. *Ann Neurol,* Vol.65, No.5, pp.491-498, ISSN 1531-8249

Chen, G., Huo, Y., Tan, D-X. & Liang, Z. (2003). Melatonin in Chinese medicinal herbs. *Life Sciences,* Vol.73, No.1, pp.19-26, ISSN 0024-3205

Colson, N.J., Lea, R.A. & Quinlan, S. (2006). The role of vascular and hormonal genes in migraine susceptibility. *Molecular Genetics and Metabolism,* Vol.88, No.2, pp.107-113, ISSN 1096-7192

de Vries, B., Haan, J., Frants, R.R., Van den Maagdenberg, A.M. & Ferrari, M.D. (2006). Genetic Biomarkers for Migraine. *Headache,* Vol.46, No.7, pp.1059-1068, ISSN 0017-8748

de Vries, B., Frants, R.R., Ferrari, M.D. & van den Maagdenberg, A.M. (2009). Molecular genetics of migraine. *Human Genetic,* Vol.126, No.1, pp.115-132, ISSN 0340-6717

Donma, O. & Donma, M.M. (2002). Association of Headaches and the Metals. *Biological Trace Element Research,* Vol.90, No.1-3, pp.1-14, ISSN 0163-4984

Durham, P.L. (2006). Emerging Neural Theories of Migraine Pathogenesis Calcitonin Gene-Related Peptide (CGRP) and Migraine. *Headache,* Vol.46, No.,Sup.1, pp.S3-S8, ISSN 0017-8748

Edvinsson, L. (2006). Neuronal Signal Substances as Biomarkers of Migraine. *Headache,* Vol.46, No.7, pp.1088-1094, ISSN 0017-8748

Fallah, M.S., Ansari, M., Roudbari, S.A., & Rezaei, F. (2005). Prophylactic treatment of migraine with a novel herbal remedy. *Proceedings of Cephalalgia 2005 12th Congress of the International Headache Society,* pp.945, Kyoto, Japan, October 9-12, 205

Fischer, M.J.M. (2010). Calcitonin gene-related peptide receptor antagonists for migraine. *Expert Opin. Investig. Drugs,* Vol.19, No.7, pp.815-823, ISSN 1354-3784

Fooladsaz, K., Ansari, M., Rasaie, M.J. (2004). Evaluation and Comparison of Serum Melatonin Determination in Normal Individuals and Migraine Patients. *Tehran University Medical Journal,* Vol.62, No.1, pp.43-48, ISSN 16831764

Gallai, V., Floridi, A., Mazzotta, G., Codini, M., Tognoloni, M., Vulcano, M.R., Sartori, M., Russo, S., Alberti, A., Michele, F. & Sarchielli, P. (1996). L-arginine/nitric oxide pathway activation in platelets of migraine patients with and without aura. *Acta Neurol Scand,* Vol.94, No.2, pp.151-160, ISSN 0001-6314

Goadsby, P.J. (2006). Biomarkers in Migraine — Glimpses into the Future. *Journal Watch Neurology,* ISSN 1524-0207

Goadsby, P.J., Lipton, R.B. & Ferrari, M.D. (2002). Migraine - Current understanding and treatment. *The New England Journal of Medicine,* Vol.346, No.4, pp.257-270, ISSN 1533-4406

Goadsby, P.J. & Sprenger, T. (2010). Current practice and future directions in the prevention and acute management of migraine. *Lancet Neurology,* Vol.9, No.3, pp.285-298, ISSN 1474-4422

Gonçalves, F.M., Martins-Oliveira, A., Speciali, J.G., Izidoro-Toledo, T.C., Luizon, M.R., Dach, F. & Tanus-Santos, J.E. (2010). Vascular Endothelial Growth Factor Genetic Polymorphisms and Haplotypes in Women with Migraine. *DNA and Cell Biology,* Vol.29, No.7, pp.357-362, ISSN 1044-5498

Gonçalves, F.M., Martins-Oliveira, A., Speciali, J.G., Luizon, M.R., Izidoro-Toledo, T.C., Silva, P.S., Dach, F. & Tanus-Santos, J.E. (2011). Endothelial Nitric Oxide Synthase Haplotypes Associated with Aura in Patients with Migraine. *DNA and Cell Biology,* Vol.30, No.6, pp.363-369, ISSN 1044-5498

Gorji A. (2003). Pharmacological treatment of headache using traditional Persian medicine. TRENDS in Pharmacological Sciences, Vol.24, No.7, pp.331-334, ISSN 0165-6147

Gorji A & Khaleghi Ghadiri M. (2002). History of headache in medieval Persian medicine. THE LANCET Neurology, Vol.1, No.8, pp.510-515, ISSN 1474-4422

Gupta, S., Mehrotra, S., Villalón, CM., Perusquía, M., Saxena, P.R. & MaassenVanDenBrink, A. (2007). Potential role of female sex hormones in the pathophysiology of migraine. *Pharmacology & Therapeutics,* Vol.113, No., pp.321-340, ISSN 0163 -7258

Hamel, E. (2007). Serotonin and migraine: biology and clinical implications. *Cephalalgia,* Vol.27, No., pp.1295-1300, ISSN 0333-1024

Hardeland, R., Cardinali, D.P., Srinivasan, V., Spence, W., Brown, G.M. & Pandi-Perumal, S.R. (2011). Melatonin—A pleiotropic, orchestrating regulator molecule. Progress in *Neurobiology,* Vol.93, No., pp.350-384, ISSN 0301-0082

Harrington, M.G. (2006). Cerebrospinal Fluid Biomarkers in Primary Headache Disorders. *Headache,* Vol.46, No., pp.1057-1087, ISSN 0017-8748

Harrington, M.G., Fonteh, A.N., Cowan, R.P., Perrine, K., Pogoda, J.M., Biringer, R.G. & Hühmer, A.F. (2006). Cerebrospinal Fluid Sodium Increases in Migraine. *Headache,* Vol.46, No., pp.1128-1135, ISSN 0017-8748

Hauge, A.W., Kirchmann, M. & Olesen, J. (2010). Trigger factors in migraine with aura. *Cephalalgia,* Vol.30, No.3, pp.346-353, ISSN 0333-1024

Hibino, T., Yuzurihara, M., Terawaki, K., Kanno, H., Kase, Y. & Takeda, A. (2008). Goshuyuto, a Traditional Japanese Medicine for Migraine, Inhibits Platelet Aggregation in Guinea-Pig Whole Blood. *Journal of Pharmacological Sciences,* Vol.108, No., pp.89-94, ISSN 1347-8613

Horak, S., Koschak, A., Stuppner, H. & Striessnig, J. (2009). Use-Dependent Block of Voltage-Gated $Ca_v2.1$ Ca^{2+} Channels by Petasins and Eudesmol Isomers. *The Journal of Pharmacology and experimental Therapeutics,* Vol.330, No.1, pp.220-226, ISSN 0022-3565

International Classification of Headache Disorders II. (2004). *Cephalalgia,* Vol.24, Sup.1, pp.1-160, ISSN 0333-1024

Jensen, R. & Stovner, L.J. Epidemiology and comorbidity of headache. (2008). *Lancet Neurology,* Vol.7, No., pp.354-361, ISSN 1474-4422

Jia, S., Ni, J., Chen, S., Jiang, Y., Dong, W. & Gao, Y. (2011). Association of the Pentanucleotide Repeat Polymorphism in NOS2 Promoter Region with Susceptibility to Migraine in a Chinese Population. *DNA and Cell Biology,* Vol.30, No.2, pp.117-122, ISSN 1044-5498

Kallela, M., Farkkila, M., Saijonmaa, O. & Fyhrquist, F. (1998). Endothelin in migraine patients. *Cephalalgia,* Vol.18, No., pp.329-332, ISSN 0333-1024

Lafrenière, R.G., Cader, M.Z., Poulin, J-F., Andres-Enguix, I., Simoneau, M., Gupta, N., Boisvert, K., Lafrenière, F., McLaughlan, S., Dubé, M-P., Marcinkiewicz, M.M., Ramagopalan, S., Ansorge, O., Brais, B., Sequeiros, J., Pereira-Monteiro, J., Griffiths, L.R., Tucker, S.J., Ebers, G. & Rouleau, G.A. (2010). A dominant-negative mutation in the TRESK potassium channel is linked to familial migraine with aura. *Nature Medicine,* Vol.16, No.10, pp.1157-11605, ISSN 1078-8956

Lauritzen, M. (1994). "Pathophysiology of the migraine aura. The spreading depression theory". *Brain,* Vol.117, No.1, pp.199-210, ISSN 1078-8956

Lemaire, P.A. & Adosraku, R.K. (2002). An HPLC method for the direct assay of the serotonin precursor, 5-hydroxytrophan, in seeds of Griffonia simplicifolia. *Phytochem. Anal,* Vol.13, No., pp.333-337, ISSN 09580344

Liu, H., Liu, M., Wang, Y., Wang, X-M., Qiu, Y., Long, J-F. & Zhang, S-P. (2011). Association of 5-HTT gene polymorphisms with migraine: A systematic review and meta-analysis. *Journal of the Neurological Sciences,* Vol.305, No., pp.57-66, ISSN 0022-510X

Loder, E. (2006). Biomarkers in Migraine: Their Promise, Problems, and Practical Applications. *Headache,* Vol.46, No., pp.1046-1058, ISSN 0017-8748.

Martin, P.R. (2010). Behavioral Management of Migraine Headache Triggers: Learning to Cope with Triggers. *Curr Pain Headache Rep,* Vol.14, No., pp.221-227, ISSN 1531-3433

Martin, V.T. & Behbehani, M.M. (2006a). Ovarian Hormones and Migraine Headache: Understanding Mechanisms and Pathogenesis—Part I. *Headache,* Vol.46, No., pp.3-23, ISSN 0017-8748

Martin, V.T. & Behbehani, M.M. (2006b). Ovarian Hormones and Migraine Headache: Understanding Mechanisms and Pathogenesis—Part 2. *Headache,* Vol.46, No., pp.365-386, ISSN 0017-8748

Martin, V.T. & Behbehani, M.M. (2001). Toward a rational understanding of migraine trigger factors. *Medical Clinics of North America,* Vol.85, No.4, pp.911-941, ISSN 0025-7125

Masruha, M.R., de Souza Vieira, D.S., Minett, T.S.C., Cipolla-Neto, J., Zukerman, E., Vilanova, L.C.P. & Peres, M.F.P. (2008). Low urinary 6-sulphatoxymelatonin concentrations in acute migraine. *J Headache Pain,* Vol.9, No., pp.221-224, ISSN 1129-2369

Mauskop, A. & Altura, B.M. (1998). Role of magnesium in the pathogenesis and treatment of migraines. *Clinical Neuroscience,* Vol.5, No., pp.24-27, ISSN 0967-5868

Mayeux, R. (2004). Biomarkers: Potential Uses and Limitations. *The Journal of the American Society for Experimental Neuro Therapeutics,* Vol.1, No., pp.182-188, ISSN 1545-5343

Menon, S., Cox, H.C., Kuwahata, M., Quinlan, S., MacMillan, J.C., Haupt, L.M., Lea, R.A. & Griffiths, L.R. (2011). Association of a Notch 3 gene polymorphism with migraine susceptibility. *Cephalalgia,* Vol.31, No.3, pp.264-270, ISSN 0333-1024

Messlinger, K. (2009). Migraine: where and how does the pain originate?. *Exp Brain Res,* Vol.196, No., pp.179-193, ISSN 0014-4819

Miano, S., Parisi, P., Pelliccia, A., Luchetti, A., Paolino, M.C. & Villa, M.P. (2008). Melatonin to prevent migraine or tension-type headache in children. Neurol Sci, Vol.29, No., pp.285-287, ISSN 0022-510X

Millichap, J.G. & Yee, M.M. (2003). The Diet Factor in Pediatric and Adolescent Migraine. *Pediatr Neurol,* Vol.28, No., pp.9-15, ISSN 0887-8994

Monteith, T. S. & Goadsby, P. J. (2011). Acute Migraine Therapy: New Drugs and New Approaches. *Current Treatment Options in Neurology,* Vol.13, No., pp.1-14, ISSN 1092-8480

Murch, S.J., Simmons, C.B. & Saxena, P.X. (1997). Melatonin in feverfew and other medicinal plants. *Lancet,* Vol.350, No., pp.1598-1599, ISSN 0140-6736

Mustafa, T. & Srivastava, K.C. (1990). Ginger (*ZINGIBER OFFICINALE*) in migraine headache. *Journal of Ethnopharmacology,* Vol.29, No., pp.267-273, ISSN 0378-8741

Nagata, E., Hamada, J., Shimizu, T., Shibata, M., Suzuki, S., Osada, T., Takaoka, R., Kuwana, M. & Suzuki, N. (2007). Altered levels of serotonin in lymphoblasts derived from migraine patients. *Neuroscience Research,* Vol.57, No., pp.179-183, ISSN 0168-01

Nyholt, D.R., LaForge, K.S., Kallela, M., Alakurtti, K., Anttila, Verneri., Färkkilä, M., Hämäläinen, E., Kaprio, J., Kaunisto, M.A., Heath, A.C., Montgomery, G.W., Hartmut, G., Todt, U., Ferrari, M.D., Launer, L.J., Frants, R.R., Terwindt, G.M., de Vries, B., Verschuren, W.M.M., Brand, J., Freilinger, T., Pfaffenrath, V., Straube, A., Ballinger, D.G., Zhan, Y., Daly, M.J., Cox, D.R., Dichgans, M., van den Maagdenberg, A.M., Kubisch, C., Martin, N.G., Wessman, M., Peltonen, L. & Palotie, A. (2008). A high-density association screen of 155 ion transport genes for involvement with common migraine. *Human Molecular Genetics,* Vol.17, No.21, pp.3318-3331, ISSN 0964-6906

Oba, S., Nakamura, K., Sahashi, Y., Hattori, A. & Nagata, C. (2008). Consumption of vegetables alters morning urinary 6-sulfatoxymelatonin concentration. *Journal of Pineal Research,* Vol.45, No., pp.17-23, ISSN 0742-3098

Oelkers-Ax, R., Leins, A., Parzer, P., Hillecke, T., Bolay, H.V., Fischer, J., Bender, S., Hermanns, U. & Resch, F. (2008). Butterbur root extract and music therapy in the prevention of childhood migraine: An explorative study. *European Journal of Pain,* Vol.12, No., pp.301-313, ISSN 10903801

Olesen, J. (2008). The role of nitric oxide (NO) in migraine, tension-type headache and cluster headache. *Pharmacology & Therapeutics,* Vol.120, No., pp.157-171, ISSN

Panconesi, A. (2008). Serotonin and migraine: a reconsideration of the central theory. *J Headache Pain,* Vol.9, No., pp.267-276, ISSN 1129-2369

Pandi-Perumal, S.R, Srinivasan, V., Maestroni, G.J., Cardinali, M., Poeggeler, B. & Hardeland R. (2006). Melatonin Nature's most versatile biological signal? *FEBS Journal,* Vol.273, No., pp.2813-2838, ISSN 1742464X

Papandreou, O., Soldatou, A., Tsitsika, A., Kariyannis C., Papandreou, T., Zachariadi, A., Papassotiriou, I., Chrousos, G.P. (2005). Serum S100β protein in children with acute recurrent headache: a potentially useful marker for migraine. Headache, Vol.45, No., pp.1313-1316, ISSN 0017-8748

Peres, M.F.P. (2005). Melatonin, the pineal gland and their implications for headache disorders. *Cephalalgia,* Vol.25, No., pp.403-411, ISSN 0333-1024

Peres, M.F.P., Masruha, M.R. & Rapoport, A.M. (2007). Melatonin Therapy for Headache Disorders. *Drug Development Research,* Vol.68, No., pp329.334-, ISSN 0272-4391

Peres, M.F.P., Masruha, M.R., Zukerman, E. , Alberto, C., Moreira-Filho, & Cavalheiro, E.A. (2006). Potential therapeutic use of melatonin in migraine and other headache disorders. *Expert Opin Investig Drugs,* Vol.15, No.4, pp.367-375, ISSN 1354-3784

Peres, M.F.P., Zukerman, E., Da Cunha, T.F., Moreira, F.R. & Cipolla-Neto, J. (2004). Melatonin, 3 mg, is effective for migraine prevention. *Neurology,* Vol.63, No., pp.757, ISSN 0028-3878

Pietrobon, D. & Striessnig, J. (2003). Neurobiology of migraine. *Nature review,* Vol.4, No., pp.386-398, ISSN 1471-00

Qu, H-G., Cheng, S-W., Tian, R-B., Li, Z-L., Lei, W-L., Wang, H-Q., Yao, Z-B. & He, H-W. (2008). Effects of the Aqueous Extract of the Chinese Medicine Danggui-Shaoyao-San on Rat Pineal Melatonin Synthesis. *Neuroendocrinol Lett,* Vol.29, No.3, pp.366-372, ISSN 0172–780X

Rainero, I., Rubino, E., Gallone, S., Fenoglio, P., Picci, L.R., Giobbe, L., Ostacoli, L. & Pinessi, L. (2011). Evidence for an association between migraine and the hypocretin receptor 1 gene. *J Headache Pain,* Vol.12, No., pp.193-199, ISSN 1129-2369

Ravishankar K. (2006) 'Hair wash' or 'head bath' triggering migraine – observations in 94 Indian patients. *Cephalalgia,* Vol.26, No., pp.1330-1334, ISSN 0333-1024

Reiter, R.J., Manchester, L.C. & Tan, D.X. (2005). Melatonin in walnuts: Influence on levels of melatonin and total antioxidant capacity of blood. *Nutrition,* Vol.21, No., pp.920-924, ISSN 0899-9007

Rios, J. & Passe, M.M. (2004). Evidenced-Based Use of Botanicals, Minerals, and Vitamins in the Prophylactic Treatment of Migraines. *Journal of the American academy of nurse practitioners,* Vol.16, No.6, pp.251-256, ISSN 1041-2972

Roda, A. (2005). Genetic variants of angiotensin converting enzyme and methylenetetrahydrofolate reductase may act in combination to increase migraine susceptibility. *Brain research,* Vol.136, No.1-2, pp.112-117, ISSN 0006-8993

Rogers, K.L., Fong, W.F., Redburn, J. & Griffiths, L.R. (2002). Fluorescence detection of plant extracts that affect neuronal voltage-gated Ca^{2+} channels. *European Journal of Pharmaceutical Sciences,* Vol.15, No., pp.321-330, ISSN 0928-0987

Rogers, K.L., Grice, I.D. & Griffiths, L.R. (2000). Inhibition of platelet aggregation and 5-HT release by extracts of Australian plants used traditionally as headache treatments. *European Journal of Pharmaceutical Sciences,* Vol.9, No., pp.355-363, ISSN 0928-0987

Rogers, K.L., Grice, I.D. & Griffiths, L.R. (2001). Modulation of in vitro platelet 5-HT release by species of Erythrina and Cymbopogon. *Life Sciences,* Vol.69, No., pp.1817-1829, ISSN 0024-3205

Ross, S.M. (2011). Clinical Applications of Integrative Therapies for Prevention and Treatment of Migraine Headaches. *Holistic Nursing Practice,* Vol.25, No.1, pp.49-52, ISSN 0887-9311

Roudbari SA, Ansari M, Fallah MS, Abbasi F, Abrishamizadeh AA. (2005). Serum ionized magnesium and calcium level in adult migraineurs during interictal period in comparison with control group. *Proceedings of Cephalalgia 2005 12th Congress of the International Headache Society,* pp.889, Kyoto, Japan, October 9-12, 2005

Russell, M.B. & Ducros, A. (2011). Sporadic and familial hemiplegic migraine: pathophysiological mechanisms, clinical characteristics, diagnosis, and management. *Lancet Neurol,* Vol.10, No., pp.457-470, ISSN 1474-4422

Scher, A.I., Bigal, M.E. & Lipton, R.B. (2005). Comorbidity of migraine. *Current Opinion in Neurology,* Vol.18, No., pp.305-310, ISSN 1350-7540

Schürks, M., Rist, P.M. & Kurth, T. (2010). *MTHFR* 677C>T and *ACE* D/I Polymorphisms in Migraine: A Systematic Review and Meta-Analysis. Published in final edited form as: *Headache,* Vol.50, No.4, pp.588-599, ISSN 0017-8748

Silberstein, S.D. (2004). Migraine. *Lancet,* Vol.363, No., pp.381-391, ISSN 0140-6736

Summer, H., Salan U.,Knight D.W., Hoult, J.R.S. (1992). Inhibition of 5-lipoxygenase and cyclo-oxygenase in leukocytes by feverfew. Involvement of sesquiterpene lactones and other components. *Biochemical Phamacology,* Vol.43, No.11, pp.2313-2320, ISSN 0006-2952

Sun-Edelstein, C. & Mauskop, A. (2009). Role of magnesium in the pathogenesis and treatment of migraine. *Expert Rev Neurother,* Vol.9, No.3, pp.369-379, ISSN 1473-7175

Sun-Edelstein, C. & Mauskop, A. (2011). Alternative Headache Treatments: Nutraceuticals, Behavioral and Physical Treatments. *Headache,* Vol., No., pp.469-483, ISSN 0017-8748

Tan, D-X., Manchester, L.C., Terron, M.P., Flores, L.J. & Reiter, R.J. (2007). One molecule, many derivatives: A never-ending interaction of melatonin with reactive oxygen and nitrogen species? *J. Pineal Res,* Vol.42, pp.28-42, ISSN 0742-3098

Usai, S., Grazzi, L. & Bussone, G. (2011). Gingkolide B as migraine preventive treatment in young age: results at 1-year follow-up Neurol Sci, Vol.32, No.1, pp.s197-s199, ISSN 0022-510X

Wood, H. (2010). Familial migraine with aura is associated with a mutation in the TRESK potassium channel. *Nature reviews neurology,* Vol.6, No., pp.643, ISSN 1759-4758

Yarnell, E. (2002). Phytotherapy for the treatment of pain. *Modern Phytotherapist,* Vol.7, No.1, pp.3-12, ISSN 1322-2775

Zareba, G. (2009). Phytotherapy for pain relief. *Drugs of To*day, Vol.45, No.6, pp.445-467, ISSN 00257656

Zengion A. & Yarnell E. (2011). Chapter 20 - Herbal and Nutritional Supplements for Painful Conditions, In: *Pain Procedures in Clinical Practice,* 3rd Edition, pp.187-204, Saunders, ISBN: 978-1-4160-3779-8, USA

Part 4

Neuropsychiatry of Drug and Alcohol Dependence

9

Substance Dependence as a Neurological Disorder

William Meil, David LaPorte and Peter Stewart
Indiana University of Pennsylvania
USA

1. Introduction

Traditionally, explanations of drug addiction adhered to a moralistic perspective. This perception, still held by many individuals and policy makers, suggests addiction is a problem to be addressed through the criminal justice system (Brown, 2011; Leshner, 1997). However, this approach has yielded little success in addressing the problem (Lee et al., 2010) and may serve to stigmatize addicts and act as a barrier to initiating treatment (Brown, 2011). Moreover, early theories of addiction grounded in learning theory have proven insufficient in explaining several key aspects of addictive behaviour (Robinson & Berridge, 1993). More recently, addiction has been viewed as disease which is characterized as a chronic relapsing disorder in which behavior is marked by a compulsion to seek and take drugs, a loss of control in limiting intake, and the emergence of a negative emotional state upon withdrawal (Koob & Le Moal, 1997). With recent advances in neuroscience and more widespread adoption of the disease model of addiction, current theories have shifted their emphasis to explaining addiction as a brain disease, subserved by varying degrees of cellular, molecular and neurocircuitry dysfunction (Koob & Le Moal, 1997; Volkow et al., 2011).

The defining features of what constitutes a "disease" varies (White et al., 2002). Most current theories focus squarely on the issue of voluntary control (Hyman, 2007; Lyvers, 2000). More specifically, they view addiction as a disease involving the erosion of voluntary control (Hyman, 2007; London et al., 2000; Lubman et al., 2004). It is noteworthy that addicts themselves most often attribute relapse to impulsive action with no known cause (Miller & Gold, 1994). While a comprehensive review of the neural underpinnings of addiction and how it informs the disease model is beyond the scope of this chapter, this review will emphasize how changes in neurological function related to the loss of voluntary control serve as a thread that runs through the addiction literature. The neural circuitry most often linked to the voluntary control of behaviour are the various regions of the prefrontal cortex and their interconnections with limbic and striatal regions (Feil et al., 2010; Goldstein & Volkow, 2002; Lubman et al., 2004; Volkow & Fowler, 2000). The role of dysfunction within this circuitry is bolstered by the observation that addicts show, hypofunction in various regions of the prefrontal cortex (Li et al., 2009; Volkow et al., 1991), perform poorly on measures related to behavioural control (Fishbein et al., 2007; Ornstein et al., 2000; Rubio et al., 2008), and often perform similarly on neuropsychological tests as those who have suffered damage to the prefrontal cortex (Rogers et al., 1999).

The prefrontal cortex represents a complex and heterogeneous structure with multiple subregions interacting with various subcortical circuits (Feil et al., 2010; Tekin & Cummings, 2002). The functions of the prefrontal cortex have been broadly characterized as executive functions. The construct of voluntary control of behavior overlaps considerably with that of executive function, the latter of which is more commonly used in the literature and will be used for the remainder of this chapter. Executive function includes a set of higher order regulatory and supervisory functions including: planning, cognitive flexibility, abstract thinking, rule acquisition, initiating appropriate actions and inhibiting inappropriate actions, and selecting relevant sensory information (Stuss, 2007). The initial part of this chapter describes the various subdivisions of the prefrontal cortex and links between these areas and executive function domains.

While the dependence profile of the classes of addictive drugs varies somewhat (Fernandez-Serrano et al., 2011), research in recent decades suggests that the neurochemical adaptations and neural circuitry underlying the addictive process is remarkably similar across abused substances (Feil et al., 2010; Robinson & Berridge, 2003; Volkow et al., 2011). This chapter will review research implicating the prefrontal cortex and executive abilities for each major class of addictive drugs (Psychostimulants, Opioids, Alcohol, and Nicotine). Many drug addicts use and/or are dependent on multiple substances (Degenhardt & Hall, 2003) and therefore research investigating executive dysfunction among polysubstance users will be addressed in an additional subsection.

Currently much of the focus in addiction research is to understand how various neural states are related to different aspects of addiction (Crews & Bottiger, 2009; Goldstein & Volkow, 2002; Volkow et al., 2011). Within each drug class discussed in this chapter three major areas will be addressed 1) the degree to which executive abilities are able to predict vulnerability to develop compulsive drug use; 2) impairment of executive abilities and cortical neurocircuitry among drug addicts related to the maintenance of addictive behaviour and continued risk of relapse; 3) the relationship between neurological functioning and recovery from addiction and how treatment interacts with this process.

Substance dependent individuals represent a highly heterogeneous group, and the variables related to the development of this disorder are many (e.g., temperament, social and environmental factors, genetics, etc.)(Conner et al., 2010). Drug addicts show impaired executive function and decreased activity in the prefrontal cortex (Dom et al., 2005; Feil et al., 2010). Several prospective studies suggest lower scores on measures of executive abilities among adolescents is predictive of future vulnerability to drug dependence suggesting executive dysfunction is among the variables conferring vulnerability for drug addiction (Mezzich et al., 2007; Najam et al., 1997). Moreover, the delayed maturation of the prefrontal cortex may be related to vulnerability of developing drug problems during adolescence (Bickel et al., 2007).

In addition to predating the development of addiction other studies, suggest chronic drug exposure may impair executive abilities and associated cortical function. The severity of drug use has been linked to the degree of executive impairment (Bolla et al., 1999; Verdejo-Garcia et al., 2006). Today, several theories of addiction are based on specific executive dysfunctions including: inhibitory response control and impulsivity (Crews & Boettiger, 2009; Feil et al., 2010; Jentsch & Taylor, 1999; Lubman et al., 2004; McNamee et al., 2008;

Volkow et al., 2003), decision making (Dom et al., 2005; London et al., 2000; Schoenbaum et al., 2006), affect dysregulation (Cheetham et al., 2011; Tekin & Cummings, 2002) cognitive performance (Pfefferbaum et al., 1997), and temporal discounting (Mackillop et al., 2011). A variety of hypotheses exist to explain how individuals with compromised executive abilities might be more predisposed to cyclical patterns of drug dependence. For example, impaired outcome expectancies may decrease the ability to make adaptive decisions and recognize the negative consequences of decisions (Schoenbaum et al., 2006). Attenuated inhibitory control may impair functional goal directed behaviours and promote participation in poorly conceived, prematurely expressed risky behaviour (Crews & Boettiger, 2009). Moreover, executive impairments in temporal discounting may render addicted individuals less likely to choose the delayed rewards of sobriety by minimizing the perceived benefits of future rewards (Bickel et al., 2007). Alternately, failure of inhibitory control mechanisms may result in maladaptive and uncontrolled drug use even when faced with disastrous consequences (Lubman et at., 2004).

Given that impairment of executive abilities and their neural substrates appear central to the development and maintenance of addictive behaviour, presumably, the recovery process should involve improvement of executive functions. This literature is in its infancy and this chapter will review research examining the relationship between improvement in executive function and recovery from substance dependence. It has been suggested that treatments that focus on improving executive abilities (such as cognitive behavioural therapy and motivational interviewing) may be effective in promoting recovery (Bickel et al., 2007; Lubman et al., 2004) and that recognition of this relationship may generate novel treatment approaches centered on augmenting activation of the prefrontal cortex and executive abilities, such as biofeedback, electrical or magnetic stimulation, and cognitive enhancing drugs (Bickel et al., 2007, Crews & Boettiger, 2009; Ersche & Sahakian, 2007). Longitudinal studies investigating treatment efficacy and related neural and behavioural changes are methodologically challenging and difficult to interpret, but may promote advances regarding the timing of treatment and matching clients to effective interventions (Bickel et al., 2007).

2. The prefrontal cortex and executive function

The frontal lobes represent arguably the most advanced structure of evolution and reach their zenith in humans, comprising almost one third of the total cortex. The prefrontal cortex, the most anterior portion of the frontal lobes, is a heterogeneous area that has been further subdivided based on their neuroanatomical connectivity and functionality, the latter of which is often revealed through deficits on neuropsychological tests or impairments resulting from lesions to the frontal regions. Multiple classification schemes based on neuropsychological and anatomical features have also been articulated (Stuss, 2007; Tekin & Cummings, 2002). One useful nomenclature for the regions of the frontal lobes has been described by Tekin & Cummings (2002) characterizes five frontal subcortical circuits. The circuits originate in the supplementary motor area, frontal eye field, dorsolateral prefrontal region, lateral orbitofrontal region, and anterior cingulate region. In some cases lesions within this circuitry have been linked to behavioral deregulation. Dorsolateral prefrontal circuit lesions are associated with executive dysfunction, orbitofrontal circuit lesions have been linked to disinhibition of behavior and anterior cingulate circuit lesions are associated with apathy (Tekin & Cummings, 2002).

Stuss (2007) has proposed dividing the prefrontal cortex into lateral and ventromedial regions. According to this nomenclature, these regions subserve four somewhat overlapping functions. The first, *executive cognitive,* involves the control and direction of more basic automatic functions. The functions of this unit include the ability to plan behavior, monitor the outcome of behaviors, and switch behaviors when necessary. Impairments in these behaviors are typically seen following lesions to the lateral prefrontal cortex. The second functional unit, *behavioral-emotional self-regulatory,* which is subserved largely by the ventromedial prefrontal cortex, are behaviors invoked when an adaptive response is required in a novel situation but when habitual ways of responding are not appropriate or environmental cues and cognitive processing of the situation are inadequate in arriving at the most adaptive response. This region processes emotional information as they are related to rewards, which aids in higher level decision making. *Energization regulating,* the third function, involves the ability to generate and maintain both cognitive and behavioral actions. Deficits in this ability result in the syndromes of abulia and apathy in which the individual is unable to sustain behaviors. Moreover, this function is seen as providing energy for the other frontal functions to operate. Lastly, *metacognitive* processes involve self-awareness, aspects of personality, and social cognition.

The use of neuropsychological tests to measure frontal lobe functions is notoriously difficult due, in part, to the fact that these abilities are typically invoked in novel problem-solving situations (Kramer & Quitania, 2007). Moreover, most neuropsychological tasks are multifaceted in terms of the component skills necessary to successfully complete the task. As a result, lesions of a diffuse nature can result in impairments on "frontal lobe" tasks. Additionally, given the abundant connections of prefrontal cortex to various neural circuits a lesion to any non-frontal area can also result in deficits on executive measures (Tekin & Cummings, 2002). There are many tasks utilized in research on the prefrontal cortex and many of these clinical measures began their life in laboratory settings only to find their way into clinical situations. While most of these measures likely tap more than one aspect of executive functioning, it is believed that certain measures may be more selective for specific executive domains. Fernandez-Serrano et al., (2011) provides a summary of the various measures used to assess each executive domain.

3. Alcohol

3.1 Executive dysfunction and vulnerability to alcohol dependence

Genetics have clearly emerged as a risk factor for developing alcoholism and some research suggests genetic polymorphism related to impulsivity may play a role in this vulnerability, yet research in this area remains equivocal (Verdejo-Garcia et al., 2008). Moreover, the genetic vulnerability for alcoholism does not appear to be alcohol-specific, but represents a general vulnerability toward sociopathy, impulsivity, and substance abuse and dependence, complicating causal attributions (Kendler et al., 2003). It remains difficult to delineate whether impairment in executive abilities among alcoholics results from a genetic vulnerability, alcohol use itself, or a combination of these factors. Some studies report the offspring of alcoholics who do not themselves abuse alcohol at the time of testing show evidence of executive dysfunction, suggesting vulnerability may pre-date use induced impairment (Lovallo et al., 2006; Sher et al., 1991). Other research suggests that a family history of alcoholism and adolescent substance use represent unique risk factors for poor neuropsychological functioning during adolescence (Tapert & Brown, 2000).

Longitudinal studies are emphasized in the section below because they consider the variability in maturation of executive abilities across time. The relationship between cortical development during adolescence and alcohol dependence have been reviewed extensively elsewhere (Brown et al., 2008, Crews et al., 2007) and underscore the importance of neural development of executive functions and alcohol exposure during adolescence as a risk factor for alcoholism. Corral et al. (2003) compared neuropsychological test results between young children with a high-density of alcoholism within their families to those with no family history. Testing was conducted when participants averaged 11 years of age and then again 3.5 years later. Performance across time on a digit span procedure was shown to increase in those with a high-density of familial alcoholism until it was comparable to those in the control group. Performance on the Wisconsin Card Sorting Test among high-density children did not show the same degree of improvement over time compared to controls.

Other studies have examined executive abilities, family history, and antisocial behaviour as predictive factors in the development of alcohol dependence. Nigg et al., (2004) employed the longitudinal approach to examine the executive functioning of boys who varied in familial risk for alcoholism and antisocial behaviour. Participants were followed between 3 and 14 years of age. Executive dysfunction (response inhibition, response speed, and symbol-digit modalities) was greatest among those with a family history of alcoholism who did not possess antisocial comorbidity. However, the relationship between executive dysfunction, antisocial behaviour, and substance abuse remains to be clarified. Nigg et al., (2006) study of individuals tested repeatedly across early and late adolescence (15-17 years of age) found that poor response inhibition predicted combined alcohol related problems, number of illicit drugs used, and comorbid alcohol and drug use. In contrast to their previous results, these findings were independent of both familial alcohol history and antisocial personality disorder, leading them to stress that alterations in response inhibition across time may be an important variable in the development of drug and alcohol related problems.

Brain imaging studies have also implicated executive dysfunction in the development of alcoholism. Functional Magnetic Resonance Imaging applied during performance of a visual oddball task to reveal bilateral attenuated activity among male sons of male alcoholics in the inferior parietal lobule and inferior frontal gyrus, suggesting dysfunction within the frontoparietal circuitry is linked to working memory (Rangaswamy et al., 2004). Deckel et al., (1995) examined young adult males and found that neuropsychological measures of executive function predicted the age of first drink, and scores on the Michigan Alcoholism Screening Test. Moreover, the age subjects reported their first drink and frequency of drinking to "get high" were associated with left-frontal slow alpha electroencephalograph activity. Similarly, Chanraud et al., (2007) reported the age of first drinking was linked with decreased gray matter volume in frontal cortex, cerebellum, and pons using Magnetic Resonance Imaging suggesting that these regions may be more vulnerable to the neurotoxic effects of alcohol during adolescence.

Two recent imaging studies further suggest that disruption of various regions of the prefrontal cortex and related executive abilities is antecedent to significant drug and alcohol exposure. Hill et al., (2009) used Magnetic Resonance Imaging to investigate orbitofrontal cortex anatomy among a sample of high-risk offspring from multiplex alcohol dependent families (defined by the presence of a pair of adult alcoholic brothers) compared to controls lacking a family history of alcohol dependence. High-risk participants with decreased right/left orbitofrontal volumes and attenuated white matter ratios, which were associated with elevated scores on the Multidimensional Personality Questionnaire control scales, suggesting reduced white matter in the orbitofrontal cortex is related to increased impulsivity. In addition, Andrews et al., (2011) examined neural activation via Functional Magnetic Resonance Imaging during a monetary reward task sensitive to multiple components of addictive behaviour in individuals without past or present alcohol or substance abuse histories, but who differed in family history of alcoholism. Overall, the results suggest impulsivity and differential reward sensitivity are associated with a positive family history of alcoholism.

3.2 Impairment of executive function in alcohol dependence

Anatomical deficits and functional impairment in various regions of the prefrontal cortex and across multiple executive domains has been well documented in alcohol dependent individuals and has been extensively reviewed elsewhere (Lyvers, 2000; Sullivan & Pfefferbaum, 2005; Verdejo-Garcia et al., 2008). This section will highlight research that integrates neuroimaging and neuropsychological testing in the study of executive function and alcoholism. Chanraud et al., (2007) using Magnetic Resonance Imaging and voxel-based Morphometry found bilateral attenuation of gray matter was most pronounced within the dorsolateral prefrontal cortex among alcohol dependent individuals. Gray matter deficits correlated with decreased executive performance on the Trail Making Test-B, letter number sequencing subtest, and Wisconsin Card Sorting Test performance, but not scores on the Stroop Interference Test. Similarly, Akine et al., (2007) reported young alcohol dependent individuals showed reduced activation in the right dorsolateral prefrontal cortex, anterior cingulate, left pulvinar of the thalamus, and right striatum using Functional Magnetic Resonance Imaging during a modified False Recognition Task designed to engage frontal lobe activity, though performance on this task did not differ from controls. These results are consistent with several other reports linking reduced activity within the prefrontal cortex and performance on specific executive measures (Dao Castella et al., 1998; Noel et al., 2001).

3.3 Executive function, treatment, recovery and alcohol dependence

Several studies have investigated the role of executive function during short-term abstinence from alcohol. Noel et al., (2002) reported subjects who relapsed two months after completing an inpatient treatment program showed lower bilateral activity in the medial frontal gyrus and poorer performance on frontal lobe tasks compared to abstainers. Similarly, Bowden-Jones et al., (2005) observed recently detoxified alcoholics who were more impulsive according to the Barratt Impulsiveness Scale, sampled significantly more cards from bad decks on a gambling task, and consistently risked more points across all odds on a decision making task were more likely to relapse within 3 months compared to abstainers. These findings are bolstered by recent research using a combined cross sectional and longitudinal approach examining abstainers, resumers, (based on 12 month abstinence), and controls using an arterial spin labelling perfusion Magnetic Resonance Imaging. After 7 days of abstinence, resumers showed reduced frontal and parietal gray matter perfusion compared to controls and abstainers. When assessed at 35 days, resumers had significantly lower frontal perfusion than the other groups (Durazzo et al., 2010). Overall, research suggests greater executive function and related activity in the prefrontal cortex may be central to maintaining short-term abstinence from alcohol.

Research examining the effects of chronic alcohol use on executive abilities and cortical function remains equivocal. Some studies suggest these deficits are deeply ingrained, long-lasting, and predispose individuals to continued problems (Mann et al., 1995; Fein et al., 1990). Other studies suggest there is significant potential for recovery of executive abilities during prolonged abstinence from alcohol dependence. Fein et al., (2006) reported a sample middle-aged, long-term alcoholics averaging 6.7 years of abstinence performed similarly to a sample of non-alcohol users on eight domains of neuropsychological abilities including frontal lobe tasks. In another longitudinal study, alcoholic men who had achieved abstinence for a month were repeatedly assessed using a battery of tests of executive function, motor function, and Magnetic Resonance Imaging. Abstainers showed increased improvement than relapsers on measures of delayed recall of drawings, visuospatial function, attention, gait, and balance. Shrinkage in 3rd ventricle was significantly correlated with improvement in nonverbal short-term memory in all participants (Sullivan et al., 2000).

A limitation of the literature described above is that these studies fail to identify and/or provide significant depth regarding the treatments that study participants received in order to achieve abstinence and therefore, little is known regarding whether specific therapeutic approaches may be more amenable than others to promoting executive abilities and abstinence. The results of research examining the effectiveness of treatment for alcohol addiction as a function of the degree of cognitive impairment are also mixed (Leber et al., 1985; Teichner et al. 2002). However, recent research suggests activating cortical circuitry related to executive functions or strengthening executive abilities themselves may be advantageous in treatment. Boggio et al., (2008) reported transcranial direct current stimulation of the dorsolateral prefrontal cortex was able to reduce cue-induced craving for alcohol compared to sham stimulation in a sample of recently abstinent alcoholics. Problem drinkers who received working memory training over 25 days were found to both improve working memory and reduce alcohol consumption for more than a month post-training (Houben et al., 2011).

4. Psychostimulants

4.1 Executive dysfunction and vulnerability to psychostimulant dependence

Numerous genetic targets have been implicated in the vulnerability to develop psychostimulant addiction (Kreek et al., 2005). Among these targets, recent research suggests that gene/environment interactions may influence gray matter volumes within the prefrontal cortex. Alia-Klein et al., (2011) compared cocaine dependent men to controls using Magnetic Resonance Imaging and genotyping for Monoamine Oxidase A (MAOA) polymorphism. Cocaine addicted individuals possessed attenuation of gray matter volume in the orbitofrontal, dorsolateral, temporal cortex, and hippocampus. Reductions in the orbitofrontal cortex were solely related to genotyping and lifetime cocaine use. Decreases in the prefrontal cortex and hippocampus were associated with lifetime alcohol use beyond genotyping. Similarly, methamphetamine addicts may show a genetic vulnerability related to executive impairment, as prevalence of the dopamine receptor type 2 (DRD2)- Taq A1 allele and the number of perseverative errors on the Wisconsin Card Sorting Test was found to be increased in methamphetamine addicts compared to controls (Han et al., 2008).

High impulsivity has also been suggested as a predisposing factor for psychostimulant use. Elevated scores on self-report measures of impulsivity have been reported in young stimulant users (Leland & Paulus, 2005) and reports of impulsivity among cocaine dependent subjects were related to age of initial cocaine use (Moeller et al., 2002.) Psychological variables may also interact with impulsivity and other executive functions to increase vulnerability to psychostimulant dependence. It has been recently reported that childhood trauma was linked to executive dysfunction on the Wisconsin Card Sort test and impulsivity using the Barratt Impulsivity Scale in a sample seeking treatment for crack cocaine use (Narvaez et al., 2011).

Other research supports the role of cocaine exposure itself in executive impairment and cortical dysfunction. For example, Ersche et al., (2011), has shown anatomical changes in the orbitofrontal cortex, insular and striatal regions are related to the duration of cocaine dependence, inattention, and compulsivity of cocaine consumption. Makris et al., (2008) has reported thinner gray matter in the prefrontal cortex was linked to reduced judgement and decision making in a cocaine dependent sample, though some thickness differences were associated with cocaine use independent of nicotine and alcohol consumption leading these authors to suggest brain structure abnormalities in addicts trace their origin to drug use as well as toward a predisposition to drug addiction.

4.2 Impairment of executive function in psychostimulant dependence

Deficits across multiple domains of executive dysfunction have been reported among psychostimulant dependent populations (Camchong et al., 2011; Ersche et al., 2011; Henry et al., 2010; King et al., 2010; Kubler et al. 2005; Leland & Paulus, 2005; Verdejo-Garcia et al., 2008). Recent research suggests executive deficits in psychostimulant addicts revealed through the use of neuropsychological measures translate into deficits in everyday functional impairment, as methamphetamine dependent subjects reported greater impairment in measures of daily functioning and performed poorly on a measure of performance-based skills compared to controls (Henry et al., 2010).

These executive impairments among psychostimulant addicts are likely the result of anatomical and functional deficits within regions of the prefrontal cortex. Magnetic Resonance Imaging has revealed cocaine and methamphetamine dependent individuals possess reduced grey matter densities across multiple regions of the frontal cortex including the ventromedial orbitofrontal cortex, lateral orbitofrontal cortex, and cingulate cortex (Ersche, et al., 2011; Franklin et al., 2002). Functional imaging has also revealed reduced activity within the orbitofrontal regions of the prefrontal cortex among psychostimulant dependent populations (Volkow et al., 2001).

Studies assessing executive function concomitantly with functional imaging methods have revealed varing degrees of cortical and subcortical activation are linked to executive changes. Goldstein et al., (2002) reported metabolism in the orbitofrontal gyrus is correlated with aspects of behavioural control via a self-report measure in abstinent methamphetamine addicts. Kubler et al., (2005) demonstrated significant deficits on working memory and visuospatial performance in a cocaine dependent sample compared to controls. However, on a verbal task in which cocaine users and controls performed similarly, reduced activation within the prefrontal, cingulate corticies and striatal regions was observed among cocaine dependent subjects. Recently, Camchong et al., (2011) showed cocaine addicts possess increased functional connectivity within the perigenual anterior cingulate network in the left medial frontal gyrus and middle temporal gyrus compared to control subjects. Abnormalities in functional connectivity were positively associated with task performance in delayed discounting and reversal learning in cocaine dependent subjects.

4.3 Executive function, treatment, recovery and psychostimulant dependence

Significant variability exists within the literature regarding the persistence of executive deficits (Chang et al., 2002; Hoffman et al., 2006) and structural and functional differences (Chang et al., 2002; Kim et al., 2005) during abstinence from psychostimulant dependence. While this literature generally supports the persistence of executive deficits within these samples, some research suggests gross deficits in executive function may be less durable (Fernadez-Serrano et al., 2011).

The majority of the research cited above involves cross sectional comparisons between abstinent psychostimulant addicts and non-using control subjects. Longitudinal studies of executive abilities are generally lacking and show disparate results. Di Sclafani et al., (2002) reported greater executive impairment in a sample of crack-cocaine dependent subjects compared to controls at 5-6 weeks of abstinence. After 6 months of abstinence these deficits were still present. In contrast, adolescents with a diagnosis of methamphetamine abuse or dependence who showed poor neuropsychological performance compared to controls demonstrated improvements on the PEG Board Test and forward digit span task that were related to the length of abstinence (King et al., 2010).

Few studies have examined executive abilities as a function of abstinence greater than a year. Selby & Azrin, (1998) found no significant improvement in neuropsychological function following 36 months of cocaine abstinence among incarcerated adult male felons with a history of cocaine dependence, however this was not surprising as these participants' neuropsychological performance was similar to matched control subjects. However, limited research suggests some improvement in executive abilities with prolonged abstinence. Toomey et al., (2003) examined neuropsychological function between 50 pairs of twins in which only one twin had a history of heavy stimulant abuse ending at least a year prior to assessment. Twins with a history of psychostimulant abuse performed poorly compared to those without a history of abuse on measures of attention and motor function, but better on a measure of visual vigilance. In addition, Salo et al., (2009) has demonstrated recently abstinent methamphamine addicts show augmented stroop reaction time interference compared to control participants and compared to methamphetamine addicts who initiated abstinence more than a year prior to being assessed. Stroop reaction time interference was also positively correlated with the length of participants' abstinence suggesting that protracted psychostimulant abstinence may yield improvement in executive function.

Studies examining executive abilities among abstinent stimulant users often fail to report details of treatment that participants received in order achieve abstinence and therefore, little is known regarding the interaction between treatment modality, executive function and recovery from psychostimulant addiction. However, research employing Transcranial Magnetic Stimulation has linked decreased cocaine craving to activation of the dorsolateral prefrontal cortex (Camprodon et al., 2007).

5. Opiates

5.1 Executive dysfunction and vulnerability to opiate dependence

Several studies linking executive abilities and vulnerability to substance dependence have included opiate users (Najam et al., 1997; Tarter et al., 2003; Mezzich et al., 2007), however there are few studies specifically examining neurological functioning as a predictor of opiate dependence. Bauer et al., (1999) found that a family history of paternal opiate dependence was not related to P300 event related potentials during performance of the Stroop Task.

5.2 Impairment of executive function in opiate dependence

There is a relative lack of empirical studies examining deficits in executive function specific to opiate addicts (Feil et al., 2010, Gruber et al., 2007). However, a growing body of evidence has demonstrated impaired performance among opiate dependent subjects on executive measures including; the Stroop Task, Ruff Figural Fluency Test, Go/No go task, measures of impulsivity, gambling tasks, delay discounting tasks, attention, and working memory (Brand et al., 2008; Fishbein et al., 2007; Forman et al. 2004; Lee & Pau, 2002; Kirby & Petry, 2004; Mintzer & Stitzer, 2002; Ornstein et al., 2000; Rapeli et al., 2006; Pirastu et al., 2006). However, reports of executive deficits among opiate addicts are not universal (Ersche & Shakian, 2007; Pau et al., 2002), may be less significant than observed in psychostimulant addicts (Ersche & Shakian, 2007), and research suggests that some of defícts may be highly transient and reflect changes related to recent abstinence (Rapeli et al., 2006).

Studies have investigated structural deficits associated with chronic opiate use. Pezawas et al., (1998) using Computerized Tomography found that compared to controls opiate dependent individuals showed significant cortical volume loss and that this loss in the frontal cortex was associated with a shorter period of abstinence before relapse. Lyoo et al., (2006) using Magnetic Resonance Imaging and voxel-based morphometry found reduced gray matter density in the bilateral prefrontal cortex and several other regions in opiate dependent subjects compared to controls. Using similar imaging methods, Liu et al., (2009) reported gray matter reductions in the right prefrontal cortex, left supplementary motor cortex, and bilateral cingulate cortex among opiate addicts.

Functional imaging research also implicates hypofrontality and executive impairment as a consequence of chronic opiate use. Forman et al., (2004) using event-related Functional Magnetic Resonance Imaging in individuals performing the Go/No go task found that relative to controls, opiate dependent subjects had reduced anterior cingulate error signal activation and poorer task performance. Using Functional Magnetic Resonance Imaging while heroin dependent subjects and controls performed the Arrow Task (which assesses cognitive regulation and impulsivity) it was found that heroin addicts had greater impulsivity and performed more errors. Neural activation of heroin dependent subjects was attenuated in the anterior cingulate cortex and augmented in the left dorsolateral prefrontal cortex, bilateral inferior parietal, and left medial temporal regions relative to controls (Lee et al., 2005). Another study combining Positron Emission Tomography with performance on the Cambridge Risk Task revealed heroin dependent subjects had significant under-activation in the lateral orbitofrontal region compared to controls and that abnormal task related activation was correlated with duration of intravenous heroin use. Being conservative following loss of points on the task was negatively associated with activation of the pregenual anterior cingulate and insula cortex in controls, but not opiate users (Ersche et al., 2006).

5.3 Executive function, treatment, recovery and opiate dependence

Abstinence from opiate dependence has been linked to persisting executive and cortical deficits. Fu et al., (2008) used functional Magnetic Resonance Imaging to examine the neural mechanisms of response inhibition while abstinent heroin addicts performed the Go/no go Task. Neural response inhibition in the anterior cingulate cortex, medial prefrontal, and inferior frontal lobe activity was linked to response inhibition and competition on the behavioural measure. Moreover, heroin dependent subjects showed impaired response inhibition that persisted several months into abstinence. These results are further supported by studies reporting heroin addicts who had been abstinent for between 3 and 18 months performed more poorly than controls on the Porteus Maze Test of impulse control (Lee & Pau., 2002) and significant deficits in episodic memory and impulsivity following three months of abstinence (Prosser et al., 2006). Other studies support executive impairment lasting as long as a year into abstinence in verbal fluency (Davis et al., 2001) and impulsivity but not attention, mental flexibility and abstract reasoning (Pau et al., 2002).

Research has also investigated the extent to which executive function changes in response to treatment and is predictive of clinical outcome. Passetti et al., (2008) found that performance on two measures of decision making (Cambridge Gambling Task and Iowa Gambling Task), but not on measures of planning, motor inhibition, reflection impulsivity or delay discounting were predictive of abstinence from illicit drug use at 3 months in opiate dependent subjects following 6 weeks of community drug treatment. Similarly, Gruber at al., (2006) examined subjects upon entering methadone maintenance therapy and again following two months of treatment. Improvements in verbal learning and memory, visuospatial memory, psychomotor performance, and decreased frequency of drug use were observed compared to baseline.

In an unpublished study from our lab changes in executive function on a battery of neuropsychological tests administered an average of 47 days post-admission and then again 90 days later among 16 heroin dependent individuals undergoing Methadone Maintenance Therapy were investigated. At the time of initial testing, participants showed significant deficits in the: Stroop Color Word Test, Porteus Mazes Test, and a trend toward poorer performance on the Wisconsin Card Sorting Test compared to the normative population. Methadone maintained clients showed significant improvement in Figural Fluency Test and the Stroop Interference Score between the two test times. Six family members of the Methadone maintained participants completed the Frontal Systems Behavioral Scale and reported significantly greater levels of disinhibition and a trend towards increased apathy among study participants. Family members also reported a trend towards improvement in apathy and executive function across the three months of Methadone Maintenance Therapy. In addition, Stroop Interference Scores at both time points were predictive of opiate abstinence. Stroop Interference Scores after 4 months of treatment were also predictive of cocaine and opiate abstinence. Participants who were opiate negative after 4 months showed improved performance on the Stroop Interference Test while those testing positive for opiates did not show improvement across time. While caution in warranted when interpreting these results due to the small sample size, these results are consistent with a growing literature that suggests recovery from opiate addiction is accompanied by improved executive abilities and may be predictive of clinical outcomes. (Meil et al., 2008).

6. Nicotine

6.1 Executive dysfunction and vulnerability in nicotine dependence

There is a lack of research directly examining executive dysfunction as a predictive factor in the development of nicotine dependence. However, childhood attention problems were shown to be a significant predictor of adult smoking (Kahalley et al., 2010). In addition, impairment in working memory has been shown to be related to an earlier age of onset of smoking. Further, male smokers initiated smoking at an earlier age and were more impaired during tests of attention than female smokers and non-smokers, leading these authors to suggest that neurotoxic effects of nicotine are more severe when use occurs earlier (Jacobsen et al., 2005). Research has also began to link impulsivity to the development of nicotine dependence in adolescent smokers (Chase & Hogarth, 2011).

6.2 Impairment of executive function in nicotine dependence

Until recently, executive dysfunction associated with nicotine dependence has recieved relatively little attention. Impairment in nicotine dependent populations has been documented in specific aspects of executive functionins such as working memory, cognitive flexibility, emotion regulation, and inhibitory control (Billieux et al., 2010; Jacobsen et al., 2005; Kahalley et al., 2010; Razani et al., 2004). In addition, Spinella (2003) found self-reported scores on the apathy, disinhibition, and executive dysfunction subscales of the Frontal Systems Behavioral Scale were related to nicotine dependence.

Limited imaging studies have also examined deficits in prefrontal cortical function in nicotine dependent individuals. Cigarette smokers showed smaller gray matter volumes and lower gray matter densities than nonsmokers in the prefrontal cortex, along with smaller volumes in the left dorsal anterior cingulate cortex and lower gray matter densities in the right cerebellum (Brody et al., 2004). Gallin et al., (2006) reported decreases in grey matter volume and lower grey matter density were observed in smokers in the frontal regions which were inversely associated with the magnitide of lifetime exposure to tobacco smoke. Research also finds increased activation of frontal regions associated with inhibitory control (such as the left orbitofrontal cortex and dorsolateral prefrontal cortex) in response to smoking related cues, suggesting the importance of these regions in resisting the urge to smoke (Brody et al., 2002).

6.3 Executive function, treatment, recovery in nicotine dependence

Studies also found evidence of persistent deficits amongst former smokers over varying periods of abstinence. Neuhaus et al., (2006) revealed persistent fronto-striatal dysfunction in former smokers despite a mean of 11 years of abstinence from cigarette smoking. In addition to other functional differences, they reported decreased cortical activation in orbitofrontal and left dorsolateral prefrontal regions amongst previous smokers when completing an auditory oddball task. These results are grossly consistent with Dawkins et al., (2009) who found no evidence of improvement on a measure of attentional bias in a small group of successful quitters over a period of three months. The successful quitters also showed no improvement on two different indices of response inhibition.

Limited reserach has also investigated executive function and treatment outcomes for nicotine dependence. Brega et al., (2008) reported participants' scores on the Behavioral Dyscontrol Scale was a significant predictor of whether they had achieved abstinence. Moreover, research employing brain stimulation of the dorsolateral prefrontal cortex in nicotine dependent subjects suggests this procedure may be effective in combatting nicotine dependence and further implicates executive abilities in the recovery process (Eichhammer et al., 2003).

7. Polysubstance dependence

7.1 Executive dysfunction and vulnerability in polysubsubstance dependence

The genetic predisposition for drug addiction may involve impulsivity (Kreek et al., 2005). Self-reported impulsivity has been recently shown to be a predictor of current and future substance use in a 3 year longitudinal study of adolescents (Krank et al., 2011). Broader aspects of executive function have also been linked to the familial factors in the development of drug addiction. Najam et al., (1997) administered children with a high and low risk for drug abuse, based on a history of paternal diagnosis, a battery of neuropsychological tests at 10-12 years of age and a drug use measure two years later. Poorer executive function performance on the Stroop task, Memory Scan, Motor restraint, and the Wechsler Intelligence Scale for Children III, was significantly associated with subsequent substance abuse. Executive cognitive functioning discriminated between children who were at high and low risk of abuse based on familial history.

A series of longitudinal studies by Tarter and colleagues have suggested that Neurobehavioral disinhibition, a construct combining affective, behavioural, and cognitive indicators of self-regulation, is a significant predictor of substance dependence between childhood and young adulthood (Kirisci et al., 2006; Mezzich et al., 2007; Tarter et al., 2003). For example, Mezzich et al., (2007) reported that neurobehavioral disinhibition in boys, measured at age 10-12 and again at age 16 significantly predicted substance use disorders by age 19. Included in their measure of neurobehavioral disinhibition are several common test of executive function including Stroop test, Porteus Maze Test, Vigilance Test, Forbidden Toys Test, Block Design Test, and Motor Restraint Test. The executive functioning component of this composite accounted for 30% of the variance at each time point, implicating it as a major component of this trait, though it should be noted that many consider other aspects of neurobehavioral disinhibition (e.g., aspects of self-regulation) as falling under the executive function umbrella. In addition, Functional Magnetic Resonance Imaging has revealed that scores on the neurobehavioral disinhibition trait are negatively correlated with frontal cortical activation (McNamee et al., 2008). It has also been suggested that drug use itself may be related to the development of executive impairment among drug addicts as Verdejo-Garcia et al., (2006) reported that the severity of use was predictive of executive deficits in a sample of poly-substance abusers. Specifically, the severity of cannabis use predicted apathy and executive dysfunction and the severity of cocaine use was predictive of greater behavioural disinhibition.

7.2 Impairment of executive function in polysubstance dependence

A recent review comparing the specific and generalized effects of abused substances on neuropsychological performance by Fenandez- Serrano et al., (2011) concluded that drugs of abuse are commonly associated with significant impairment in multiple neuropsychological domains including episodic memory, emotional processing, including updating and decision making. However, some drugs were linked to greater impairment of certain neuropsychological abilities such as enhanced effects of alcohol and psychostimulants on impulsivity and cognitive flexibility compared to other drugs. Individual studies in which polysubstance dependent subjects are compared to controls support the idea that polysubstance dependence produces significant executive impairment (Cunha et al., 2010). Studies directly comparing neuropsychological profiles between individuals dependent on different drugs suggest widespread executive deficits, but that distinct patterns of deficits may be observed between drugs (Ershe & Sahakian, 2007; Ornstein et al., 2000). Neural imaging studies also support the idea that polysubstance use yields deficits in prefrontal cortical gray matter volume (Liu et al., 1998).

7.3 Executive function, treatment, recovery and in polysubstance dependence

Research regarding the longevity of executive deficits among polysubstance user suggests impairment may persist at least up to a year (Grant et al., 1978). Fernandez-Serrano et al., (2010) recently reported that polysubstance dependent individuals enrolled in therapeutic communities averaging 24 weeks of abstinence showed substantial deficits on multiple measures of executive function including measures of working memory, fluency, shifting, planning, multi-tasking, and interference. A second study by this author also found widespread executive impairment in a population of abstinent polysubstance abusers following an average of 32 weeks of abstinence (Fernandez-Serrano et al., 2010). A recent long-term longitudinal study by Hanson et al., (2011) examined adolescents with and without alcohol and substance dependence, who were tested repeatedly for neuropsychological performance for 10 years. Ninety-four percent of substance dependent participants met criteria for alcohol dependence and dependence on at least one other drug. At baseline and subsequently, controls performed better on neuropsychological measures than substance dependent participants. Heavy use patterns over time were associated with impaired neuropsychological functioning on measures of verbal learning and memory, visuospatial memory and verbal/attention/working memory. In addition, participants who discontinued alcohol and drug use during this period showed improvement in cognitive function.

Studies investigating the effectiveness of treatment among abstinent polysubstance dependent subjects suggest the degree of neuropsychological deficits may be important in determining clinical outcomes. Fals-Stewart and Schafer, (1992) reported that in substance abusers admitted to a therapeutic community, performance on the Digit Symbol and Block Design Subtests of the Wechsler Adult Intelligence Scale were predictive of time in treatment. In another study, the decision to stop drug use following a prevention intervention during adolescence was predicted by the severity of childhood neurobehavioral disinhibition (Kirisci et al., 2006).

8. Conclusion

This chapter is unique compared to other papers reviewing the relationship between anatomical and functional changes in the prefrontal cortex, executive abilities, and substance dependence (Feil et al., 2010; Goldstein & Volkow, 2002; Fernandez-Serrano et al., 2011; Schoenbaum et al., 2006). This chapter emphasizes the breadth of this topic by describing this relationship across multiple classes of drugs and polysubstance dependence. In addition, it examines this relationship across the vulnerability to develop substance dependence, the impairment observed among addicts, and the persistence and recovery of executive functions during abstinence and as a function of treatment.

Several conclusions can be drawn from this literature review. Pre-existing variability in executive function and the effects of drug use itself are among the variables which influence an individuals' risk of developing substance dependence. A significant body of literature shows that substance dependent individuals are impaired across multiple domains of executive functioning, and possess decreased grey matter and impaired activity within the prefrontal cortex. Moreover, multiple studies combining brain imaging and neuropsychological measures link impairment of performance on tests of executive function with anatomical and functional impairments of the prefrontal cortex. The persistence of executive deficits across time is highly variable, however research suggests that following short-term and long-term abstinence many individuals show recovery of executive functions which appears to be related to their ability to maintain abstinence across time. A growing body of research suggests specific treatments focused on augmenting activity within the prefrontal cortex or strengthening executive abilities may represent viable treatment approaches. While some differences in impairment of executive abilities have been observed across drugs, there are remarkable similarities in the executive deficits observed among drug addicts.

There are several limitations of this review. The purpose of this chapter is to illustrate the role of executive dysfunction in substance dependence, however it does not represent an exhaustive review of this topic. The research described here illustrates the major findings of studies in this area but does not emphasize results that were not consistent with the premise of this review. Based on this review it is evident that specific areas of the prefrontal cortex appear to show a greater degree of impairment than others (orbitofrontal, anterior cingulate, and dorsolateral regions) and that substance dependent populations appear to show greater deficits on certain executive domains (response inhibition, impulsivity, working memory); this chapter did not systematically evaluate these differences. This review focussed on the role of prefrontal cortical regions and executive dysfunction in addiction. Regions of the prefrontal cortex have also been implicated in other addiction related processes including craving, reward, and withdrawal (Goldstein & Volkow, 2002), however, a broader neural circuitry and associated behavioral dysregulation is likely involved in drug dependence.

The typical definition of a "disease" emphasizes that it involves abnormal structure and function of the body (Leshner, 1997). This chapter argues that according to this broad conceptualization, substance dependence should be considered a disease given its association with deficits in cortical function and related executive abilities. Addiction also shows several similarities with other chronic conditions considered diseases, such as a similar vulnerability toward relapse (Leshner, 1997). While these deficits are not unique to drug addiction (Rogers et al., 1999), in combination with compulsive drug use and other neurobiological markers this body of research strengthens the argument for defining addiction as a disease.

9. References

Akine, Y.; Kato, M., Muramatsu, T., Umeda, S., Mimura, M., Asai, Y., Tanada, S., Obata, T., Ikehira, H., Kashima, H. & Suhara, T. (2007). Altered Brain Activation by a False Recognition Task in Young Abstinent Patients with Alcohol Dependence. *Alcoholism: Clinical and Experimental Reserach,* Vol. 31, No. 9, (September 2007), pp. 1589-1597, ISSN 1530-0277

Alia-Klein, N.; Parvaz, M., Woicik, P., Konova, A., Maloney, T., Shumay, E., Wang, R., Telang, F., Biegon, A., Wang, G., Fowler, J., Tomasi, D., Volkow, N. & Goldstein, R. (2011). Gene x Disease Interaction on Orbitofrontal Gray Matter in Cocaine Addiction. *Archives of General Psychiatry*, Vol. 68, No. 3, (March 2011), pp. 283-294, ISSN 0003-990x

Andrews, M.; Meda, S, Thomas, A., Potenza, M., Krystal, J., Worhunsky, P., Stevens, M., O'Malley, S., Book, G., Reynolds, B. & Pearlson, G. (2011). Individuals Family History Positive for Alcoholism Show Functional Magnetic Resonance Imaging Differences in Reward Sensitivity that are Related to Impulsivity Factors. *Biological Psychiatry*, Vol. 69, No. 7, (April 2011), pp. 675-683, ISSN 0006-3223

Bauer, L., & Hesselbrock, V. (1999). Subtypes of family history and conduct disorder: effects on P300 during the stroop test. *Neuropsychopharmacology*, Vol. 21, No. 1, (July 1999), pp. 51-62, ISSN 0893-133X

Bickel, W.; Miller, M., Yi, R., Kowal, B., Lindquist, D. &, Pitcock, J. (2007). Behavioral and Neuroeconomics of Drug Addiction: Competing Neural Systems and Temporal Discounting Processes, *Drug and Alcohol Dependence*, Vol. 90, No. 1, (September 2007), pp. 85-91, ISSN 0376-8716

Billieux, J.; Gay, P., Rochat, L., Khazaal, Y., Zullino, D. & Van der Linden, M. (2010). Lack of Inhibitory Control Predicts Cigarette Smoking Dependence: Evidence From a Non-Deprived Sample of Light to Moderate Smokers. *Drug and Alcohol Dependence*, Vol. 112, No. 1-2 (November 2010), pp. 164-167, ISSN 0376-8716

Boggio, P.; Sultani, N., Fecteau, S., Merabet, L., Mecca, T., Pascual-Leone, A., Basaglia, A. & Fregni, F. (2008). Prefrontal Cortex Modulation Using Transcranial DC Stimulation Reduces Alcohol Craving: A Double-blind, Sham-controlled Study. *Drug and Alcohol Dependence*, Vol. 92, No. 1-3, (January 2008), pp. 55-60, ISSN 0376-8716

Bowden-Jones, H.; McPhillips, M., Rogers, R., Hutton, S. & Joyce, E. (2005). Risk-taking on Tests Sensitive to Ventromedial Prefrontal Cortex Dysfunction Predicts Early Relapse in Alcohol Dependency: A Pilot Study. *Journal of Neuropsychiatry and Clinical Neuroscience,* Vol. 17, No. 3, (Summer 2005), pp. 417-420, ISSN 0895-0172

Brand, M., Roth-Bauer, M., Driessen, M., & Markowitsch, H. (2008). Executive Functions and Risky Decision-making in Patients with Opiate Dependence. *Drug and Alcohol Dependence*, Vol. 97, No. 1-2, (September 2008), pp. 64-72, ISSN 0376-8716

Brega, A.; Grigsby, J., Kooken, R., Hamman, F. & Baxter, J. (2008). The Impact of Executive Cognitive Functioning on Rates of Smoking Cessation in the San Luis Valley Health and Aging Study. *Age and Ageing*, Vol. 37, No. 5, pp. 521 -525 ISSN 0002-0729

Brody, A.; Mandelkern, M., Jarvik, M., Lee, G., Smith, E., Huang, J., Bota, R., Bartzokis, G. & London, E. (2004). Differences Between Smokers and Nonsmokers in Regional Gray Matter Volumes and Densities. *Biological Psychiatry*, Vol. 55, No. 1, (January 2004), pp. 77-84, ISSN 0006-3223

Brody, A.; Mandelkern, M., London, E., Childress, A., Lee, G., Bota, R., Ho, M., Saxena, S., Baxter, L., Madsen, D. & Jarvik, M. (2002). Brain Metabolic Changes During Cigarette Craving. *Archives of General Psychiatry*, Vol. 59, No. 12, (December 2002), pp. 1162-1172 ISSN 0003-990x

Brown, P. (2011). Standardized Measures for Substance Use Stigma. *Drug and Alcohol Dependence*, Vol. 116, No. 1, (July 2011), pp. 137-141, ISSN 0376-8716

Brown, S.; McGue, M., Maggs, J., Schulenberg, J., Hingson, R., Swartzwelder, S., Martin, C., Chung, T., Tapert, S., Sher, K., Winters, K., Lowman, C. & Murphy, S. (2008). A Developmental Perspective on Alcohol and Youths 16 to 20 Years of Age. *Pediatrics*, Vol. 121, No. 4, (April 2008), pp. 290-310, ISSN 0031-4005

Camchong, J.; MacDonald, A. 3rd, Nelson, B., Bell, C., Mueller, B., Specker, S. & Lim, K. (2011). Frontal Hyperconnectivity Related to Discounting and Reversal Learning in Cocaine Subjects. *Biological Psychiatry*, Vol. 69, No. 11, (June 2011). pp. 1117-1123, ISSN 0006-3223

Camprodon, J.; Martínez-Raga, J., Alonso-Alonso, M., Shih, M. & Pascual-Leone, A. (2007). One Session of High Frequency Repetitive Transcranial Magnetic Stimulation (rTMS) to the Right Prefrontal Cortex Transiently Reduces Cocaine Craving. *Drug and Alcohol Dependence*, Vol. 86, No. 1, (January 2007), pp. 91-94, ISSN 0376-8716

Chang, L.; Ernst, T., Speck, O., Patel, H., DeSilva, M., Leonido-Yee, M. & Miller, E. (2002). Perfusion MRI and Computerized Cognitive Test Abnormalities in Abstinent Methamphetamine Users. *Psychiatry Research*, Vol. 114, No. 2, (June 2002), pp. 65-79, ISSN 0165-1781

Chanraud, S.; Martelli, C., Delain, F., Kostogianni, N., Douaud, G., Aubin, H., Reynaud, M. & Martinot, J. (2007). Brain Morphometry and Cognitive Performance in Detoxified Alcohol-dependents with Preserved Psychosocial Functioning. *Neuropsychopharacology*, Vol. 32, No. 2, (February 2007), pp. 429-438, ISSN 0893-133X

Chase, H. & Hogarth, L. (2011). Impulsivity and Symptoms of Nicotine Dependence in a Young Adult Population, *Nicotine and Tobacco Research*, ISSN 1462-2203

Cheetham, A.; Allen, N., Yücel, M. &, Lubman, D. (2010). The Role of Affective Dysregulation in Drug Addiction. *Clinical Psychology Review*, Vol. 30, No. 6, (August 2010), pp. 621-634, ISSN 0272-7358

Conner, B.; Hellemann, G., Ritchie, T. & Nobel, E. (2010). Genetic, Personality, and Environmental Predictors of Drug Use in Adolescents. *Journal of Substance Abuse Treatment*, Vol. 38, No. 2, (March 2010), pp. 178-190, ISSN 0740-5472

Corral, M.; Holguín, S. & Cadaveira, F. (2003). Neuropsychological Characteristics of Young Children from High-density Alcoholism Families: A Three-year Follow-up. *Journal of Alcohol Studies*, Vol. 64, No. 2, (March 2003), pp. 195-199, ISSN 1937-1888

Crews, F. & Boettiger, C. (2009). Impulsivity, Frontal Lobes and Risk for Addiction. *Pharmacology, Biochemistry and Behavior*, Vol. 93, No. 3, (September 2009), pp. 237-247, ISSN 0091-3057

Crews, F.; He, J. & Hodge, C. (2007). Adolescent Cortical Development: A Critical Period of Vulnerability for Addiction. *Pharmacology, Biochemistry and Behavior*, Vol. 86, No. 2, (February 2007), pp. 189-199, ISSN 0091-3057

Cunha, P.; Nicastri, S., de Andrade, A. & Bolla, K. (2010). The Frontal Assessment Battery (FAB) Reveals Neurocognitive Dysfunction in Substance-dependent Individuals in

Distinct Executive Domains: Abstract Reasoning, Motor Programming, and Cognitive Flexibility, *Addictive Behavior*, Vol. 35, No. 10, (October 2010), pp. 875-881, ISSN 0306-4603

Davis, P.; Liddiard, H. & McMillan, T. (2002). Neuropsychological Deficits and Opiate Abuse. *Drug and Alcohol Dependence,* Vol. 67, No. 1, (June 2002), pp. 105-108, ISSN 0376-8716

Dawkins, L.; Powell, J., Pickering, A., Powell, J. & West, R. (2009). Patterns of Change in Withdrawal Symptoms, Desire to Smoke, Reward Motivation and Response Inhibition Across 3 Months of Smoking Abstinence. *Addiction*, Vol. 104, No. 5, (May 2009), pp. 850-858, ISSN 1360-0443

Deckel, A.; Bauer, L., & Hesselbrock, V. (1995). Anterior Brain Dysfunctioning as a Risk Factor in Alcoholic Behaviors. *Addiction*, Vol. 90, No. 10, (October, 1995), pp. 1323-1334, ISSN 1360-0443

Degenhardt, L. & Hall, W. (2003). Patterns of Co-morbidity Between Alcohol Use and other Substance Use in the Australian Population. *Drug and Alcohol Review,* Vol. 22, No. 1, (March 2003), pp. 7 - 13, ISSN 1465-3362

Di Sclafani, V.; Tolou-Shams, M., Price, L. & Fein, G. (2002). Neuropsychological Performance of Individuals Dependent on Crack-cocaine, or Crack-cocaine and Alcohol, at 6 Weeks and 6 Months of Abstinence. *Drug and Alcohol Dependence*, Vol. 66, No. 2, (April 2002), pp. 161-171, ISSN 0376-8716

Dao-Castellana, M.; Samson, Y., Legault, F., Martinot, J., Aubin, H., Crouzel, C., Feldman, L., Barrucand, D., Rancurel, G., Féline, A. & Syrota, A. (1998). Frontal Dysfunction in Neurologically Normal Chronic Alcoholic Subjects: Metabolic and Neuropsychological Findings. *Psychological Medicine*, Vol. 28, No. 5, (September 1998), pp. 1039-1048, ISSN 0033-2917

Dom, G.; Sabbe, B., Hulstijn, W. & van den Brink, W. (2005). Substance Use Disorders and the Orbitofrontal Cortex: Systematic Review of Behavioural Decision-making and Neuroimaging Studies, *British Journal of Psychiatry*, Vol. 187, (September 2005), pp. 209-220, ISSN 0007-1250

Durazzo, T.; Gazdzinski, S., Mon, A. & Meyerhoff, D. (2010). Cortical Perfusion in Alcohol-Dependent Individuals During Short-term Abstinence: Relationships to Resumption of Hazardous Drinking After Treatment. *Alcohol*, Vol. 44, No. 3, (May 2010), pp. 201-210, ISSN 0741-8329

Eichhammer. P.; Johann, M., Kharraz, A., Binder, H., Pittrow, D., Wodarz, N. & Hajak, G. (2003). High-frequency Repetitive Transcranial Magnetic Stimulation Decreases Cigarette Smoking. Journal of Clinical Psychiatry, Vol. 64, No. 8, (August 2003), pp. 951-953, ISSN 0160-6689

Ershe, K.; Barnes, A., Jones, P., Morein-Zamir, S., Robbins, T. & Bullmore, E. (2011). Abnormal Structure of Frontostriatal Brain Systems is Associated with Aspects of Impulsivity and Compulsivity in Cocaine Dependence, *Brain*, ISSN 0006-8950

Ersche, K., Fletcher, P., Roiser, J., Fryer, T., London, M., Robbins, T., & Sahakian, B. (2006). Differences in Orbitofrontal Activation During Decision-making Between Methadone-maintained Opiate Users, Heroin Users and Healthy Volunteers. *Psychopharmacology*, Vol. 188, No. 3, (September 2006), pp. 364-373, ISSN 0033-3158

Ersche, K. & Sahakian, B. (2007) The Neuropsychology of Amphetamine and Opiate Dependence: Implications for Treatment. *Neuropsychology Review*, Vol. 17, No. 3, (September, 2007), pp. 317-336, ISSN 1040-7308

Fals-Stewart, W. & Schafer, J. (1992). The Relationship Between Length of Stay in Drug-free Therapeutic Communities and Neurocognitive Functioning. *Journal of Clinical Psychology*, Vol. 48, No. 4, (July, 1992), pp. 539-543, ISSN 0021-9762

Feil, J.; Sheppard, D., Fitzgerald, P., Yucel, M., Lubman, D. & Bradshaw, J. (2010). Addiction, Compulsive Drug Seeking, and the Role of Frontostriatal Mechanisms in Regulating Inhibitory Control. *Neuroscience and Biobehavioral Reviews*, Vol. 35, No. 2, (November 2010), pp. 248-275, ISSN 0149-7634

Fein, G.; Bachman, L., Fisher, S. & Davenport, L. (1990). Cognitive Impairments in Abstinent Alcoholics. *The Western Journal of Medicine*, Vol. 152, No. 5, (May 1990), pp. 531-537, ISSN 0093-0415

Fein, G.; Torres, J., Price. L. &Di Sclafani, V. (2006). Cognitive Performance in Long-term Abstinent Alcoholic Individuals. *Alcoholism: Clinical and Experimental Research*, Vol. 30, No. 9, (September 2006), pp. 1538-1544, ISSN 1530-0277

Fernández-Serrano, M., Pérez-García, M., Perales, J. & Verdejo-García, A. (2010). Prevalence of Executive Dysfunction in Cocaine, Heroin and Alcohol Users Enrolled in Therapeutic Communities. *European Journal of Pharmacology*, Vol. 626, No. 1, (January 2010), pp. 104-112, ISSN 0014-2999

Fernandez-Serrano, M.; Perez-Garcia, M. & Verdejo-Garcia, A. (2011). What Are the Specific vs. Generalized Effects of Drugs of Abuse on Neuropsychological Performance. *Neuroscience and Biobehavioral Reviews*, Vol. 35, No. 3, (January 2011), pp. 377-406. ISSN 0149-7634

Fishbein, D.; Krupitsky, E., Flannery, B., Langevin, D., Bobashev, G., Verbitskaya, E., Augustine, C., Bolla, K., Zvartau, E., Schech, B., Egorova, V., Bushara, N. & Tsoy, M. (2007). Neurocognitive Characterizations of Russian Heroin Addicts Without a Significant History of Other drug Use. *Drug and Alcohol Dependence*, Vol. 90, No 1, (September 2007), pp. 25-38, ISSN 0376-8716

Forman, S., Dougherty, G., Casey, B., Siegle, G., Braver, T., Barch, D., Stenger, V., Wick-Hull, C., Pisarov, L., & Lorensen, E. (2004). Opiate Addicts Lack Error-dependent Activation of Rostral Anterior Cingulate. *Biological Psychiatry*, Vol. 55, No. 5, (March 2004), pp. 531-537, ISSN 0006-3223

Franklin, T.; Acton, P., Maldjian, J., Gray, J., Croft, J., Dackis, C., O'Brien, C. & Childress, A. (2002). Decreased Gray Matter Concentration in the Insular, Orbitofrontal, Cingulate, and Temporal Cortices of Cocaine Patients. *Biological Psychiatry*, Vol. 51, No. 2, (January 2002), pp. 134-142, ISSN 0006-3223

Fu, L., Bi, G., Zou, Z., Wang, Y., Ye, E., Ma, L., Ming-Fan, & Zheng, Y. (2008). Impaired Response Inhibition Function in Abstinent Heroin Dependents: An fMRI study. *Neuroscience Letters*, Vol. 438, No. 3, (June 2008), pp. 322-326, ISSN 0304-3940

Gallinat, J.; Meisenzahl, E., Jacobsen, L., Kalus, P., Bierbrauer, J., Kienast, T., Witthaus, H., Leopold, K., Seifert, F., Schubert, F. & Staedtgen, M. (2006). Smoking and Structural Brain Deficits: A Volumetric MR Investigation. *European Journal of Neuroscience*, Vol. 24, No. 6, (September 2006), pp. 1744-1750, ISSN 1460-9568

Goldstein, R. & Volkow, N. (2002). Drug Addiction and its Underlying Neurobiological Basis: Neuroimaging Evidence for Involvement of the Frontal Cortex. *American Journal of Psychiatry*, Vol. 159, No. 10, (October 2002), pp. 1642-1652, ISSN 0002-953X

Grant, I.; Adams, K., Carlin, A., Rennick, P. Judd, L. & Schooff, K. (1978). The Collaborative Neuropsychological Study of Polydrug Users. *Archives of General Psychiatry*, Vol. 35, No. 9, (September 1978), pp. 1063-1074, ISSN 0003-990x

Gruber, S., Silveri, M., & Yurgelun-Todd, D. (2007). Neuropsychological Consequences of Opiate Use. *Neuropsychology Review*, Vol. 17, No. 3, (September 2007), pp. 299-315, ISSN 1040-7308

Gruber, S.; Tzilos, G., Silveri, M., Pollack, M., Renshaw, P., Kaufman, M. & Yurgelun-Todd, D. (2006). Methadone Maintenance Improves Cognitive Performance After Two Months of Treatment. *Experimental and Clinical Psychopharmacology*, Vol. 14, No. 2, (May 2006), pp. 157-164, ISSN 1064-1297

Han, D.; Yoon, S., Sung, Y., Lee, Y., Kee, B., Lyoo, I., Renshaw, P. & Cho, S. (2008). A Preliminary Study: Novelty Seeking, Frontal Executive Function, and Dopamine Receptor (D2) TaqI A Gene Polymorphism in Patients with Methamphetamine Dependence. *Comprehensive Psychiatry*, Vol. 49, No. 4, (July-August 2008), pp. 387-392, ISSN 0010-440X

Hanson, K.; Cummins, K., Tapert, S. & Brown, S. (2011). Changes in Neuropsychological Functioning Over 10 Years Following Adolescent Substance Abuse Treatment. *Psychology of Addictive Behavior*, Vol. 25, No. 1, (March 2011), pp. 127-142, ISSN 0893-164X

Henry, B.; Minassian, A. & Perry, W. (2010). Effect of Methamphetamine Dependence on Every Day Functional Ability. *Addictive, Behaviors*, Vol. 35, No. 6, (June 2010), pp. 593-598, ISSN 0306-4603

Hill, S.; Wang, S., Kostelnik, B., Carter, H., Holmes, B., McDermott, M,, Zezza, N., Stiffler, S. & Keshavan, M. (2009). Disruption of Orbitofrontal Cortex Laterality in Offspring from Multiplex Alcohol Dependence Families. *Biological Psychiatry*, Vol. 65, No. 2, (January 2009), pp. 129-136, ISSN 0006-3223

Hoffman, W.; Moore, M., Templin, R., McFarland, B., Hitzemann, R.& Mitchell, S. (2006). Neuropsychological Function and Delay Discounting in Methamphetamine-Dependent Individuals. *Psychopharmacology*, Vol. 188, No. 2, (October 2006), pp. 162-170, ISSN 0033-3158

Houben, K.; Wiers, R. & Jansen, A. (2011). Getting a Grip on Drinking Behavior: training Working Memory to Reduce Alcohol Abuse, *Psychological Science*, Vol. 22, No. 7, (July 2011), pp. 968-975, ISSN 0956-7976

Hyman, S. (2007). The Neurobiology of Addiction: Implications for Voluntary Control of Behavior. *The American Journal of Bioethics*, Vol. 7, No. 1, (January 2007), pp.8-11, ISSN 1526-5161

Jacobsen, L.; Krystal, J. Mencl, W., Westerveld, M., Fros,t S. & Pugh, K. (2005). Effects of Smoking and Smoking Abstinence on Cognition in Adolescent Tobacco Smokers. *Biological Psychiatry*, Vol. 57, No. 1, (January 2005), pp. 56-66, ISSN 0006-3223

Jentsch, J. & Taylor, J. (1999). Impulsivity Resulting from Frontostriatal Dysfunction in Drug Abuse: Implications for the Control of Behavior by Reward-related Stimuli. *Psychopharmacology*, Vol. 146, No. 4, (October 1999), pp. 373–390, ISSN 0033-3158

Kahalley, L.; Robinson, L., Tyc, V., Hudson, M., Leisenring, W., Stratton, K., Zeltzer, L., Mertens, A., Robison, L. & Hinds, P. (2010). Attentional and Executive Dysfunction as Predictors of Smoking Within the Childhood Cancer Survivor Study Cohort. *Nicotine and Tobacco Research*, Vol. 12, No. 4, (April 2010), pp. 344-354, ISSN 1462-2203

Kendler, K.; Prescott, C., Myers, J. & Neale, M. (2003). The structure of genetic and environmental risk factors for common psychiatric and substance use disorders in men and women. *Archives of General Psychiatry*, Vol. 60, No. 9, (September 2003), pp. 929-937, ISSN 0003-990x

Kim, S.; Lyoo, I., Hwang, J., Sung, Y., Lee, H., Lee, D., Jeong, D. & Renshaw, P. (2005). Frontal Glucose Hypometabolism in Abstinent Methamphetamine Users. *Neuropsychopharmacology*, Vol. 30, No. 7, (July 2005), pp. 1383-1391, ISSN 0893-133X

King, G.; Alicata, D., Cloak, C. & Chang, L. (2010). Neuropsychological Deficits in Adolescent Methamphetamine Abusers. *Psychopharmacology,* Vol. 212, No. 2, (October 2010), pp. 243-249, ISSN 0033-3158

Kirby, K., & Petry, N. (2004). Heroin and Cocaine Abusers Have Higher Discount Rates for Delayed Rewards Than Alcoholics or Non-drug-using Controls. *Addiction*, Vol. 99, No. 4, (April 2004), pp. 461-471, ISSN 1360-0443

Kirisci, L.; Tarter, R., Reynolds, M. & Vanyukov, M. (2006). Individual Differences in Childhood Neurobehavior Disinhibition Predict Decision to desist Substance Use During Adolescence and Substance Use Disorder in Young Adulthood: A Prospective Study. *Addictive Behavior*, Vol. 31, No. 4, (April 2006), pp. 686-696, ISSN 0306-4603

Koob, G. & Le Moal, M. (1997). Drug Abuse: Hedonic Homeostatic Dysregulation. *Science*, Vol. 278, No. 5335, (October 1997), pp. 52-58, ISSN 0036-8075

Kramer, J. & Quitania, L. (2007). *Bedside frontal lobe testing*. In: *The Human Frontal Lobes, (2nd Edition)*. B.L. Miller & J.L. Cummings (Eds.). 279-291. Guilford Press, New York, United States

Krank, M.; Stewart, S., O'Connor, R., Woicik, P., Wall, A. & Conrod, P. (2011). Structural, Concurrent, and Predictive Validity of the Substance Use Risk Profile Scale in Early Adolescence. *Addictive Behavior*, Vol. 36, No. 1-2 (January-February 2011), pp. 37-46, ISSN 0306-4603

Kübler, A.; Murphy, K. & Garavan, H. (2005). Cocaine Dependence and Attention Switching Within and Between Verbal and Visuospatial Working Memory. *European journal of Neuroscience*, Vol. 21, No. 7, (April 2005), pp. 1984-1992, ISSN 1460-9568

Kreek, M.; Nielsen, D., Butelman, E. & LaForge, K. (2005). Genetic Influences on Impulsivity, Risk Taking, Stress Responsivity and Vulnerability to Drug Abuse and Addiction. *Nature Neuroscience*, Vol. 8, No. 11, (November 2005), pp. 1450-1457, ISSN 1097-6256

Leber, W.; Parsons, O. & Nichols, N. (1985). Neuropsychological Test Results are Related to Ratings of Men Alcoholics' Therapeutic Progress: a Replicated Study. *Journal of Studies on Alcohol*, Vol. 42, No. 2, (March 1985), pp. 116-121, ISSN 1937-1888

Lee, P.; Lee, D. & Arch, P. (2010). 2010: U.S. Drug and Alcohol Policy, Looking Back and Moving Forward. *Journal of Psychoactive Drugs*, Vol. 42, No.2, (June 2010), pp. 99-111, ISSN 0279-1072

Lee, T., & Pau, C. (2002). Impulse Control Differences Between Abstinent Heroin Users and Matched Controls. *Brain Injury,* Vol. 16, No. 10, (October 2002), pp. 885-889, ISSN 0269-9052

Lee, T., Zhou, W., Luo, X., Yuen, K., Ruan, X., & Weng, X. (2005). Neural Activity Associated with Cognitive Regulation in Heroin Users: A fMRI study. *Neuroscience Letters*, Vol. 382, No. 3, (July 2005), pp. 211-216. ISSN 0304-3940

Leland, D. & Paulus, M. (2005). Increased Risk-aking Decision-making But Not Altered Response to Punishment in Stimulant-using Young Adults. *Drug and Alcohol Dependence*, Vol. 78, No. 1, (April 2005), pp. 83-90, ISSN 0376-8716

Leshner, A. (1997). Addiction is a Brain disease, and it Matters. *Science,* Vol. 278, No. 5335, (October 1997), pp. 45-47, ISSN 0036-8075

Li, C.; Luo, X., Yan, P., Bergquist, K. & Sinha, R. (2009).Altered Impulse Control in Alcohol Dependence: Neural Measures of Stop Signal Performance. *Alcohol: Clinical Experimental Research,* Vol. 33, No. 4 (January 2009), pp. 740-750, ISSN 1530-0277

Liu, H., Hao, Y., Kaneko, Y., Ouyang, X., Zhang, Y., Xu, L., Xue, Z., & Liu, Z. (2009). Frontal and Cingulate Gray Matter Volume Reduction in Heroin Dependence: Optimized Voxel-based Morphometry. *Psychiatry and Clinical Neurosciences,* Vol. 63, No. 4, (August 2009), pp. 563-568, ISSN 1440-1819

Liu, X.; Matochik, J., Cadet, J. & London, E. (1998). Smaller Volume of Prefrontal Lobe in Polysubstance Abusers: A Magnetic Resonance Imaging Study. *Neuropsychopharmacology,* Vol 18, No. 4, (April 1998), pp. 243-252, ISSN 0893-133X

London, E.; Ernst, M, Grant, S., Bonson, K. & Weinstein, A. (2000). Orbitofrontal Cortex and Human Drug Abuse: Functional Imaging. *Cerebral Cortex,* Vol. 10, No. 3, (March 2000), pp. 334-342, ISSN 1047-3211

Lovallo, W.; Yechiam, E., Sorocco, K., Vincent, A. & Collins, F. (2006). Working Memory and Decision-making Biases in Young Adults with a Family History of Alcoholism: Studies From the Oklahoma Family Health Patterns Project. *Alcohol Clinical and Experimental Research,* Vol. 30, No. 5, (May 2006), pp. 763 - 773 ISSN 1530-0277

Lubman, D.; Yucel, M. & Pantelis, C. (2004). Addiction, a Condition of Compulsive Behavior? Neuroimaging and Neuropsychological Evidence of Inhibitory Dysregulation. *Addiction,* Vol. 99, No. 12, (August 2004), pp. 1491-1502, ISSN 1360-0443

Lyoo, I., Pollack, M., Silveri, M., Ahn, K., Diaz, C., Hwang, J., Kim, S., Yurgelun-Todd, D., Kaufman, M, & Renshaw, P. (2005). Prefrontal and Temporal Gray Matter Density Decreases in Opiate Dependence. *Psychopharmacology,* Vol. 184, No. 2, (December 2005), pp. 139-144, ISSN 0033-3158

Lyvers, M. (2000). Loss of Control in Alcoholism and Drug Addiction: A Neuroscientific Interpretation. *Experimental and Clinical Psychopharmacology,* Vol. 8, No. 2, (May 2000), pp.225-249, ISSN 1064-1297

MacKillop, J.; Amlung, M., Few, L., Ray, L., Sweet, L. & Munafò, M. (2011). Delayed Reward Discounting and Addictive Behavior: A Meta-analysis. *Psychopharmacology,* Vol. 216, No. 3, (August 2011), pp. 305-321, ISSN 0033-3158

Makris, N.; Gasic, G., Kennedy, D., Hodge, S., Kaiser, J., Lee, M., Kim, B., Blood, A., Evins, A., Seidman, L., Iosifescu, D., Lee, S., Baxter, C., Perlis, R., Smoller, J., Fava, M. & Breiter H. (2008). Cortical Thickness Abnormalities in Cocaine Addiction--a

Reflection of Both Drug Use and a Pre-existing Disposition to Drug Abuse? *Neuron,* Vol. 60, No. 1, (October 2009), pp. 174-188, ISSN 0896-6273

Mann, K.; Mundle, G., Strayle, M. & Wakat, P. (1995). Neuroimaging in Alcoholism: CT and MRI Results and Clinical Correlates. *Journal of Neural Transmission, General section,* Vol. 99, No. 1-3, pp. 145–155, ISSN 0300-9564

McNamee, R.; Dunfee, K., Luna, B., Clark, D., Eddy, W. & Tarter, R. (2008). Brain activation, response inhibition, and increased risk for substance use disorder. *Alcohol: Clinical Experimental Research,* Vol. 32, No. 3, (March 2008), pp. 405-413, ISSN 1530-0277

Meil, W.; Kugler, L. & Verbiest, R. (2008). Improvement in Executive Function and Prediction of Abstinence During Early Methadone Maintenance Therapy. *Society for Neuroscience Annual Meeting,* Washington D.C., United States

Mezzichk, A.; Tarter, R., Feske, U., Kirisci, L., McNamee, R. & Day, B. (2007). Assessment of Risk for Substance Use Disorder Consequent to Consumption of Illegal Drugs: Psychometric Validation of the Neurobehavior Disinhibition Trait. *Psychology of Addictive Behavior,* Vol. 21, No. 3, (December 2007), pp. 508-515, ISSN 0893-164X

Miller, N. & Gold, M. (1994). Dissociation of 'Conscious Desire'(craving) from and Relapse in Alcohol and Cocaine Dependence. *Annals of Clinical Psychiatry,* Vol. 6, pp. 99-106, ISSN 1040-1237

Mintzer, M., & Stitzer, M. (2002). Cognitive Impairment in Methadone Maintenance Patients. *Drug and Alcohol Dependence,* Vol. 67, No. 1, (June 2002), pp. 41-51, ISSN 0376-8716

Moeller, F.; Dougherty, D., Barratt, E., Oderinde, V., Mathias, C., Harper, R. & Swann, A. (2002). Increased Impulsivity in Cocaine Dependent Subjects Independent of Antisocial Personality Disorder and Aggression. *Drug and Alcohol Dependence,* Vol. 68, No. 1, (Septemeber 2002), pp. 105-111, ISSN 0376-8716

Najam, N.; Moss, H., Kirisci, L. & Tarter, R. (1997). Executive Cognitive Functioning Predicts Drug Use in Youth, *Journal of Indian Academy of Applied Psychology,* Vol. 23, No. 1-2, (January-July 1997), pp 3-12, ISSN 0019-4247

Narvaez, J.; Magalhães, P., Trindade, E., Vieira, D., Kauer-Sant'anna, M., Gama, C., von Diemen, L., Kapczinski, N. & Kapczinski, F. (2011). Childhood Trauma, Impulsivity, and Executive Functioning in Crack Cocaine Users. *Comprehensive Psychiatry,* (June 2011), ISSN 0010-440X

Neuhaus A., Bajbouj, M., Kienast, T., Kalus, P., von Haebeler, D., Winterer, G. & Gallinat, J. (2006). Persistent Dysfunctional Frontal Lobe Activation in Former Smokers. *Psychopharmacology,* Vol. 186, No. 2, pp. 191-200, ISSN 0033-3158

Nigg, J.; Glass, J., Wong, M., Poon, E., Jester, J., Fitzgerald, H., Puttler, L., Adams, K. & Zucker, R. (2004). Neuropsychological Executive Functioning in Children at Elevated Risk for Alcoholism: Findings in Early Adolescence. *Journal of Abnormal Psychology,* Vol. 113, No. 2, (May 2004), pp. 302-314, ISSN 0021-843X

Nigg, J.; Wong, M., Martel, M., Jester, J., Puttler, L., Glass, J., Adams, K., Fitzgerald, H. & Zucker, R. (2006). Poor Response Inhibition as a Predictor of Problem Drinking and Illicit Drug Use in Adolescents at Risk for Alcoholism and Other Substance Use Disorders. *Journal of the American Academy of Child and Adolescent Psychiatry,* Vol. 45, No. 4, (April 2006), pp. 468-475, ISSN 0890-8567

Noël, X.; Paternot, J., Van der Linden, M., Sferrazza, R., Verhas, M., Hanak, C., Kornreich, C., Martin, P., De Mol, J., Pelc, I. & Verbanck, P. (2001). Correlation Between

Inhibition, Working Memory and Delimited Frontal Area Blood Flow Measure by 99mTc-Bicisate SPECT in Alcohol-dependent Patients. *Alcohol and Alcoholism,* Vol. 36, No. 6, (November-December 2001), pp. 556-563, ISSN 0735-0414

Noël, X.; Sferrazza, R., Van Der Linden, M., Paternot, J., Verhas, M., Hanak, C., Pelc, I. & Verbanck, P. (2002). Contribution of Frontal Cerebral Blood Flow Measured by (99m)Tc-Bicisate Spect and Executive Function Deficits to Predicting Treatment Outcome in Alcohol-dependent Patients. *Alcohol and Alcoholism,* Vol. 37, No. 4, (July-August 2002), pp. 347-354, ISSN 0735-0414

Ornstein, T.; Iddon, J., Baldacchino, A., Sahakian, B., London, M., Everitt, B. & Robbins, T. (2000). Profiles of Cognitive Dysfunction in Chronic Amphetamine and Heroin Abusers. *Neuropsychopharmacology,* Vol. 23, No. 2, (August 2000), pp. 113-126, ISSN 0893-133X

Passetti, F.; Clark, L., Mehta, M., Joyce, E. & King, M. (2008). Neuropsychological predictors of Clinical Outcome in Opiate Addiction. *Drug and Alcohol Dependence,* Vol. 94, No. 1-3, (April 2008), pp. 82-91, ISSN 0376-8716

Pau, C., Lee, T., & Chan, S. (2002). The Impact of Heroin on Frontal Executive Functions. *Archives of Clinical Neuropsychology,* Vol. 17, No. 7, (October 2002), pp. 663-670. ISSN 0887-6177

Pezawas, L., Fischer, G., Diamant, K., Schneider, C., Schindler, S., Thurnher, M., Ploechl, W., Eder, H., & Kasper, S. (1998). Cerebral CT Findings in Male Opioid-dependent Patients: Stereological, Planimetric and Linear Measurements. *Psychiatry Research: Neuroimaging,* Vol. 83, No. 3, (September 1998), pp. 139-147, ISSN 0925-4927.

Pfefferbaum, A.; Sullivan, E., Mathalon, D. & Lim, K. (1997). Frontal Lobe Volume Loss Observed with Magnetic Resonance Imaging in Older Chronic Alcoholics. *Alcoholism: Clinical and Experimental Research,* Vol. 21, No. 3, (May 1997), pp. 521–529, ISSN 1530-0277

Prosser, J., Cohen, L., Steinfeld, M., Eisenberg, D., London, E., & Galynker, I. (2006). Neuropsychological Functioning in Opiate-dependent Subjects Receiving and Following Methadone Maintenance Treatment. *Drug and Alcohol Dependence,* Vol. 84, No. 3, (October 2006), pp. 240-247, ISSN 0376-8716

Rangaswamy, M.; Porjesz, B., Ardekani, B., Choi, S., Tanabe, J., Lim, K. & Begleiter, H. (2004). A Functional MRI Study of Visual Oddball: Evidence for Frontoparietal Dysfunction in Subjects at Risk for Alcoholism. *Neuroimage,* Vol. 21, No. 1,(January 2004), pp. 329-339, ISSN 1053-8119

Rapeli, P., Kivisaari, R., Autti, T., Kähkönen, S., Puuskari, V., Jokela, O., & Kalska, H. (2006). Cognitive Function During Early Abstinence from Opioid Dependence: A Comparison to Age, Gender, and Verbal Intelligence Matched Controls. *BMC Psychiatry,* Vol. 6, (February 2006), pp. 9, ISSN 1471-244X

Razani, J.; Boone, K., Lesser, I. & Weiss, D. (2004). Effects of Cigarette Smoking History on Cognitive Functioning in Healthy Older Adults. *The American Journal of Geriatric Psychiatry,* Vol. 12. No. 4, (July-August 2004), pp. 404-411, ISSN 1064-7481

Robinson, T. & Berridge, K. (1993). The Neural Basis of Drug Craving: An Incentive-Senstization Theory of Addiction. *Brain Research Reviews,* Vol. 18, No. 3, (September/December 1993), pp. 247-291, ISSN 0165-0173

Robinson, T. & Berridge, K. (2003). Addiction. *Annual Review of Psychology,* Vol. 54, pp. 25-53, ISSN 0066-4308

Rogers, R.; Everitt, B., Baldacchino, A., Blackshaw, A., Swainson, R., Wynne, K., Baker, N., Hunter, J., Carthy, T., Booker, E., London, M., Deakin, J., Sahakian, B. & Robbins, T. (1999). Dissociable Deficits in the Decision-making Cognition of Chronic Amphetamine Abusers, Opiate Abusers, Patients with Focal Damage to Prefrontal Cortex, and Tryptophan-Depleted Normal Volunteers: Evidence for Monoaminergic Mechanisms. *Neuropsychopharmacology,* Vol. 20, No. 4, (April 1999), pp. 322-339, ISSN 0893-133X

Rubio, G.; Jimenez, M., Rodriguez-Jimenez, R., Martinez, I., Avila, C., Ferre, F., Jimenez-Arriero, M., Ponce, G. & Palomo, T. (2008). The Role of Behavioral Impulsivity in the Development of Alcohol Dependence: A 4-year Follow-up Study. *Alcohol: Clinical Experimental Research*, Vol. 32, No. 9, (September 2008), pp. 1681-1687, ISSN 1530-0277

Salo, R.; Nordahl, T., Galloway, M., Moore, C., Water, C. & Leamon, M. (2009). Drug Abstinence and Cognitive Control in Methamphetamine Dependent Individuals, *Journal of Substance Abuse Treatment,* Vol. 37, No. 3, (October 2009), pp. ISSN 0740-5472

Schoenbaum, G.; Roesch, M. & Stalnaker, T. (2006). Orbitofrontal Cortex, Decision-making and Drug Addiction. *Trends in Neuroscience,* Vol. 29, No. 2, (February 2006), pp 116-124, ISSN 0166-2236

Selby, M. & Azrin, R. (1998). Neuropsychological Functioning in Drug Abusers. *Drug and Alcohol Dependence,* Vol. 50, No. 1, (March 1998), pp. 39-45, ISSN 0376-8716

Sher, K.; Walitzer, K., Wood, P. & Brent, E. (1991). Characteristics of Children of Alcoholics: Putative Risk Factors, Substance Use and Abuse Psychopathology. *Journal of Abnormal Psychology,* Vol. 100, No. 4, (November 1991), pp. 427-448, ISSN 0021-843X

Spinella, M. (2003). Relationship Between Drug Use and Prefrontal-associated Traits. *Addiction Biology,* Vol. 8, No. 1, (March 2003), pp 67-74, ISSN 1369-1600

Stuss, D. (2007). New Approaches to Frontal Lobe Testing. In *The Human Frontal Lobes* (2nd *Edition.),* B.L. Miller & J.L. Cummings (Eds.). 292-305. Guildford Press, New York, United States

Sullivan, E. & Pfefferbaum, A. (2005). Neurocircuitry in Alcoholism: A Substrate of Disruption and Repair. *Psychopharmacology,* Vol. 180, No. 4, (August 2005), pp. 583-594, ISSN 0033-3158

Sullivan, E.; Rosenbloom, Margaret, J., Lim, K. & Pfefferbaum, A. (2000). Longitudinal Changes in Cognition, Gait, and Balance in Abstinent and Relapsed Alcoholic Men: Relationships to Changes in Brain Structure. *Neuropsychology,* Vol. 14, No. 2, (April 2000), pp. 178-188, ISSN 1385-4046

Tapert, S. & Brown, S. (2000). Substance Dependence, Family History of Alcohol Dependence, and Neuropsychological Functioning in Adolescence. *Addiction,* Vol. 95, No. 7, (July 2000), pp. 1043–1053, ISSN 1360-0443

Tarter, R.; Kirisci, L., Mezzich, A., Cornelius, J., Pajer, K., Vanyukov, M., Gardner, W., Blackson, T., & Clark, D. (2003). Neurobehavioral Disinhibition in Childhood Predicts Early Age at Onset of Substance Use Disorder. *American Journal of Psychiatry,* Vol. 160, No. 6, (June 2003), pp. 1078-1085, ISSN 0002-953X

Teichner, G.; Horner, M., Roitzsch, J., Herron, J. & Thevos, A. (2002). Substance Abuse Treatment Outcomes for Cognitively Impaired and Intact Outpatients, *Addictive Behavior*, Vol. 27, No. 5, (September-October 2002), pp. 751-763, ISSN 0306-4603

Tekin, S. & Cummings, J. (2002). Frontal-subcortical Neuronal Circuits and Clinical Neuropsychiatry An Update. *Journal of Psychosomatic Research*, Vol. 53, No. 2, (August 2002), pp. 647-654, ISSN 0022-3999

Toomey, R.;, Lyons, M., Eisen, S., Xian, H., Chantarujikapong, S., Seidman, L., Faraone, S. & Tsuang, M. (2003). A Twin Study of the Neuropsychological Consequences of Stimulant Abuse. *Archives of General Psychiatry*, Vol. 60, No. 3, (March 2003), pp. 303-310, ISSN 0003-990x

Verdejo-García, A.; Lawrence, A. & Clark, L. (2008). Impulsivity as a Vulnerability Marker for Substance-use Disorders: Review of Findings from High-risk Research, Problem Gamblers and Genetic Association Studies. *Neuroscience Biobehavioral Reviews*, Vol. 32, No. 4, (January 2008), pp. 777-810, ISSN 0149-7634

Verdejo-García, A.; Rivas-Pérez, C., López-Torrecillas, F. & Pérez-García, M. (2006). Differential Impact of Severity of Drug Use on Frontal Behavioral Symptoms. *Addictive Behavior*, Vol. 31, No.8, (August 2006), pp. 1373-1382, ISSN 0306-4603

Volkow, N. & Fowler, J. (2000). Addiction a Disease of Compulsion and Drive: Involvement of the Orbitofrontal Cortex, *Cerebral Cortex*, Vol. 10, No. 3, (March 2000), pp. 318-325, ISSN 1047-3211

Volkov, N.; Fowler, J., Wang, G., Hitzemann, R., Logan. J., Schyler, D., Dewey, S. & Wolf, A. (1993). Decreased Dopamine D2 Receptor Availability is Associated with Reduced Frontal Metabolism in Cocaine Abusers. *Synapse*, Vol. 14, No. 2, (June 1993), pp. 169-177, ISSN 1098-2396

Volkow, N.; Wang, G., Fowler, J., Tomasi, D. & Telang, F. (2011). Addiction: Beyond Dopamine Reward Circuitry, *Proceedings of the National Academy of Sciences United States of America,* (March 2011), ISSN 1091-6490

White, W.; Boyle, M. & Loveland, D. (2002). Alcoholism/Addiction as a Chronic Disease: From Rhetoric to Clinical Reality. *Alcoholism Treatment Quarterly*, Vol. 20, No. 3-4, (July 2002), pp. 107-130, ISSN 0734-7324